# TOPICS IN ANTIBIOTIC CHEMISTRY
## Volume 2

**Antibiotics from Marine Organisms, Oligosaccharides, Anthracyclines and their Biological Receptors**

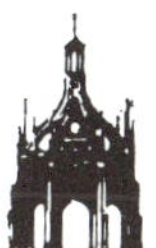

## TOPICS IN ANTIBIOTIC CHEMISTRY

*Series Editor:*

P. G. SAMMES, Professor of Chemistry, The City University, London

The object of this continuation series is to keep all interested workers informed on the advances of our knowledge concerning the role of antibiotics in nature, and on the mechanisms by which they act against pathogenic organisms. Future volumes have been planned and will appear regularly.

**Volume 1 AMINOGLYCOSIDES AND ANSAMYCINS**

**The Aminoglycosides** – D. A. Cox, K. Richardson and B. C. Ross, Pfizer Central Research, Sandwich, Kent.

**The Ansamycins** – M. Brufani, University of Siena, Italy.

**Volume 2 ANTIBIOTICS FROM MARINE ORGANISMS, OLIGOSACCHARIDES, ANTHRACYCLINES AND THEIR BIOLOGICAL RECEPTORS.**

**Antibiotics from Marine Organisms** – D. J. Faulkner, Scripps Institution of Oceanography, University of California, San Diego.

**Oligosaccharide Antibiotics** – A. K. Ganguly, Schering Corporation, Bloomfield, New Jersey.

**Daunomycin and Related Antibiotics** – F. Arcamone, Farmitalia – Ricerca Chimica, Milan.

**Interactions of Daunomycin and Related Antibiotics with Biological Receptors** – S. Neidle, Department of Biophysics, King's College, University of London.

**Volume 3 In preparation.**

**The topics planned will include:**

**New β-Lactam Antibiotics**
**Modes of Action of Nalidixit Acid and its Congeners**
**Peptide Antibiotics of High Oxidation State**

# Topics in Antibiotic Chemistry

# Volume 2

**Antibiotics from Marine Organisms, Oligosaccharides Anthracyclines and their Biological Receptors**

*Editor:*
P. G. SAMMES
Professor of Chemistry, The City University, London

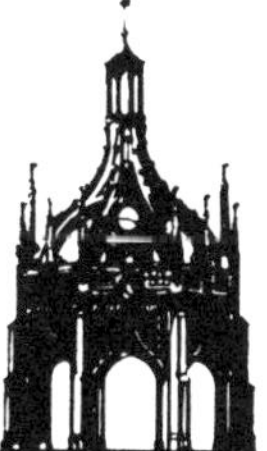

ELLIS HORWOOD LIMITED
Publishers Chichester

Halsted Press: a division of
JOHN WILEY & SONS
Chichester, New York, Brisbane, Toronto

*The publisher's colophon is reproduced from James Gillison's drawing of the ancient Market Cross, Chichester.*

First published in 1978 by

**ELLIS HORWOOD LIMITED**
Market Cross House, Cooper Street, Chichester, Sussex, England

**Distributors:**

*Australia, New Zealand, South-east Asia:*
Jacaranda-Wiley Ltd., Jacaranda Press,
JOHN WILEY & SONS INC.,
G.P.O. Box 859, Brisbane, Queensland 4001, Australia.

*Canada:*
JOHN WILEY & SONS CANADA LIMITED
22 Worcester Road, Rexdale, Ontario, Canada.

*Europe, Africa:*
JOHN WILEY & SONS LIMITED
Baffins Lane, Chichester, Sussex, England.

*North and South America and the rest of the world:*
HALSTED PRESS, a division of
JOHN WILEY & SONS
605 Third Avenue, New York, N.Y. 10016, U.S.A.



**British Library Cataloguing in Publication Data**

Topics in antibiotic chemistry.
Vol. 2: Antibiotics from marine organisms,
oligosaccharides, anthracyclines and their
biological receptors.
1. Antibiotics
I. Title II. Sammes, Peter George
615'.329 RS431.A6 78-40228

ISBN 0-85312-121-4 (Ellis Horwood Ltd., Publishers)
ISBN 0-470-26365-2 (Halsted Press)



Typeset in Press Roman by Coll House Press, Chichester, Sussex.

Printed in Great Britain by Biddles of Guildford

# Editor's Preface

As defined in Volume 1 the object of this continuing series is to keep all interested workers informed on the advances being made in our knowledge on the role antibiotics play in nature and on the mechanisms by which they act against pathogenic organisms. The emphasis is on the chemical nature of such interactions, although due account will be taken of related factors, such as the function of pharmaco-kinetics and on inbuilt resistance mechanisms.

Contributions to *Topics in Antiobiotic Chemistry* are sought from experts who are actively engaged in research in the fields covered by their articles. This precedent was set in Volume 1 and has been rigorously followed in this second volume of the series which contains four topical articles, each reflecting different aspects of the subject.

In Part A, Dr. John Faulkner, from the Scripps Institution of Oceanography, La Jolla, California, has written a timely survey of antibiotics isolated from marine organisms. The sea has long been recognised as a rich source of natural products and the variety of chemical structures found is only limited by the ability of chemists to unravel them. Despite a number of screening programmes, up to this point in time few viable antibiotics have so far been isolated from marine organisms and Dr. Faulkner critically reviews the reasons for this.

In Part B, Dr. Ashit Ganguly details the current state of the art in work on the oligosaccharide group of antibiotics. In a chemical sense these structures are very complex, many having molecular weights well in excess of 1000. Manipulation of such structures needs new techniques and methodology and Dr. Ganguly emphasises the approaches used by his group in dealing with compounds such as the everninomycins.

The final Parts of this volume, Parts C and D, are complementary articles describing the anthracycline group of antibiotics. These compounds, such as daunomycin and adriamycin, have extremely important anti-tumour properties. Chemical aspects of these compounds are highlighted in Dr. Federico Arcamone's article in Part C. As one of the world's leading experts in this area Dr. Arcamone has presented a comprehensive survey of work carried out, including synthetic work, metabolic studies and structure-activity relationships. In Part D Dr. Stephen Neidle, an X-ray crystallographer specialising in drug-substrate interactions, has collated all the important information concerning the mode of action of the anthracyclines at the molecular level, and details models used to explain the intercalating properties of these agents.

As editor of this series I have been greatly encouraged by the interest generated in Volume 1. I wish to thank all those who have made constructive comments about the previous volume and to extend an invitation for constructive and critical comments on this volume of *Topics in Antibiotic Chemistry*. Any suggestions for future articles will be very welcome and will all receive serious consideration. As before, it is not our intention to restrict the scope of articles to purely chemical aspects of the subject but to also include associated areas of interest, such as modern methods for screening, isolation, and production of this very important group of drugs.

The production of these volumes depends a great deal on a large number of people, especially the cooperation of the staff at Ellis Horwood Ltd., our publishers. May I acknowledge all their help and encouragement.

February 1978

P. G. Sammes,
Department of Chemistry,
The City University,
London.

# CONTENTS

# PART A

# ANTIBIOTICS FROM MARINE ORGANISMS

by

**D. JOHN FAULKNER**

SCRIPPS INSTITUTION OF OCEANOGRAPHY
UNIVERSITY OF CALIFORNIA, SAN DIEGO, LA JOLLA, CALIFORNIA

## PART A

## CONTENTS

# 1 INTRODUCTION

Marine biologists have long been aware that many marine organisms produce antimicrobial substances. Early studies of antibiosis within the marine environment were principally ecological studies which focussed on the antimicrobial properties of whole organisms or simple extracts of organisms. The legacy of this research can be found in large compilations of data recording *in vitro* antimicrobial activity of marine organisms often collected at random. Identification of the metabolites responsible for antimicrobial activity is a relatively recent field of study which has rewarded the chemist with a variety of interesting marine natural products.

Chemical studies of antibiotics from marine organisms have evolved from both ecological and pharmaceutical research. This dual genesis is reflected in two very different definitions of the terms antibiosis and antibiotic. The marine biologists have tended to adopt a broader view of antibiosis which includes almost every example of the production of chemicals by one organism in order to affect a second organism in some detrimental manner. The pharmaceutical industry has adopted a stricter definition of antibiotic which includes only those substances which can destroy or inhibit the growth of a microorganism at low concentrations. Marine natural products chemists have tended to adopt a rather pragmatic definition of an antibiotic as a substance which inhibits the growth of a microorganism in an *in vitro* assay. The fault in such a practical definition is that there is an element of uncertainty associated with subjective interpretation of *in vitro* assays. Unfortunately, relatively few antimicrobial compounds have been subjected to quantitative *in vitro* assays to obtain minimum inhibitory concentrations (M.I.C.'s) against a broad spectrum of test organisms or to *in vivo* testing.

The ecology of marine antibiotics and coral reefs was reviewed in detail by Burkholder [1]. He presented a survey of marine antibiotics from a viewpoint of a marine microbiologist, concentrating on their ecological importance. At the time that Burkholder was writing, there had been many studies which demonstrated the existence of marine antibiotics, but few of the antibiotic substances had been identified. This review concentrates on the chemical studies of marine antibiotics; readers should consult Burkholder's review for a more complete account of the ecological role of marine bacteria and marine antibiotics.

Seawater itself is a poor medium for bacterial growth. Organic substrates are essential for the growth of marine bacteria, so that high concentrations of marine bacteria are generally associated with organic detritus. However, marine bacteria may be required to survive for weeks in a resting state until contact is made with a suitable substrate. Thus one may take the view that marine organisms exist in a hostile medium, one containing bacterial predators. Since many marine organisms produce antimicrobial substances, one may ask whether antibacterial production is a defense against or a response to bacterial predation. In the case of antimicrobial substances produced by marine bacteria, it seems unlikely that the marine bacteria which produce antibacterial substances ever reach the density required to produce sufficient concentrations of antibiotic compounds to inhibit the growth of other marine bacteria in the vicinity. Photoplankton blooms, which must be regarded as abnormal events, may produce sufficiently high concentrations of extracellular metabolites to inhibit the growth of marine bacteria. Multicellular organisms do not appear to excrete antibiotics; the antibiotics are released only when the organism is injured and could help to ward off bacterial attack while the injury heals. For chemists, it is best to leave such speculation, into the evolution and ecological function of antibiotics, to the marine biologists and concentrate on the progress which has been made toward the chemical identification of marine antibiotics.

Studies [2] recording the results of large-scale screening of marine organisms for antibiotic activity have been of limited use to the marine products chemist. Those surveys which have presented results in terms of the percentage of organisms of a particular phylum which inhibited a test microorganism are of minimal value. Surveys which have recorded the antimicrobial activity of individual species, or, better still, of different solvent extracts of individual species, have proved to be quite useful guides for the organic chemist. There is, however, no real substitute for a research program in which marine organisms are collected by the chemist and the subsequent natural product study is guided by an antibiotic assay, which is among the simplest assays to perform. If the antibiotic assay is also used to guide the collection of organisms, the chemist can study antibiotics from marine organisms while doing the minimum of ecological damage.

The compounds which are reviewed are those which have been isolated and identified and which have been shown to inhibit the growth of microorganisms. The majority of these compounds have been subjected to limited *in vitro* antimicrobial screening, although a few compounds have been tested *in vivo* without success. The general picture which has evolved is a rather dismal one. Those compounds with high *in vitro* antimicrobial activity are often highly toxic and are best termed antiseptic agents. At present there does not appear to be an antibiotic from a marine organism to rival the fungal metabolites. However, the marine antibiotics are often compounds which contain features not previously found in terrestrial organisms and, as such, are worthy of the chemist's attention.

## 2 ANTIBIOTICS FROM MICROORGANISMS

The production of antibiotics by marine microorganisms has been assumed to be a relatively common phenomenon. However, few chemical constituents of marine microorganisms have been described, probably because this research requires close collaboration between the marine microbiologist and the natural products chemist. The culture of marine microorganisms is a rather specialized task which requires the attention or, at the very least, the advice of a specialist. Some of the marine bacteria which produce antibiotics are very difficult to culture due to autotoxicity. It is not unknown for microorganisms to mutate in culture so that an organism which showed some antibiotic activity when freshly isolated may lose some or all of its potency. For these and other reasons, it is best to study freshly isolated microorganisms. Having isolated an antibiotic-producing microorganism, several weeks may be required to find the best culture medium, but the effort will be rewarded by increased yields of the antibiotic. This is particularly important because the extraction of very large volumes of culture medium may be a limiting factor in the isolation procedure. In this laboratory, the major problem experienced while working on antibiotics from marine bacteria is the isolation of sufficient quantities of the antibiotics to permit chemical identification.

The first antibiotic substance from marine bacteria to be isolated and identified was 2-(3′,5′-dibromo-2′-hydroxyphenyl)-3,4,5-tribromopyrrole (**1**). The

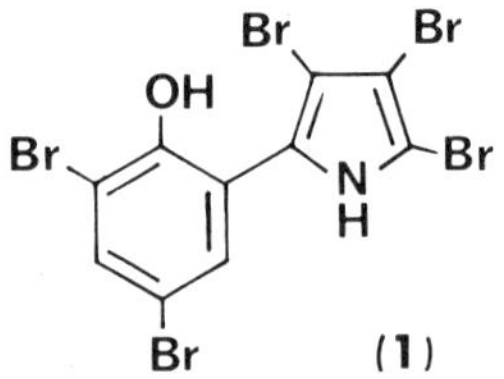

(**1**)

marine bacterium *Pseudomonas bromoutilis* was isolated by Burkholder *et al.* [3] from *Thalassia* (turtle grass) in Puerto Rico. The chemical structure was elucidated by Lovell [4] using X-ray crystallography, and the compound was synthesized by Hanessian and Kaltenbronn [5], using the route outlined in Scheme 2.1. This highly brominated antibiotic was shown to be highly active against gram positive bacteria. Strains of *Staphylococcus aureus, Diplococcus pneumoniae* and *Streptococcus pyogenes* were inhibited at antibiotic concentrations of 0.0063 μg/ml in broth culture. However, the antibiotic (**1**) failed to show a therapeutic value against *S. aureus* when administered subcutaneously to mice. In addition, the antibiotic was fairly toxic to mice (25–50 mg/kg i.v.). The antibiotic inhibited many marine bacteria but did not inhibit *P. bromoutilis.*

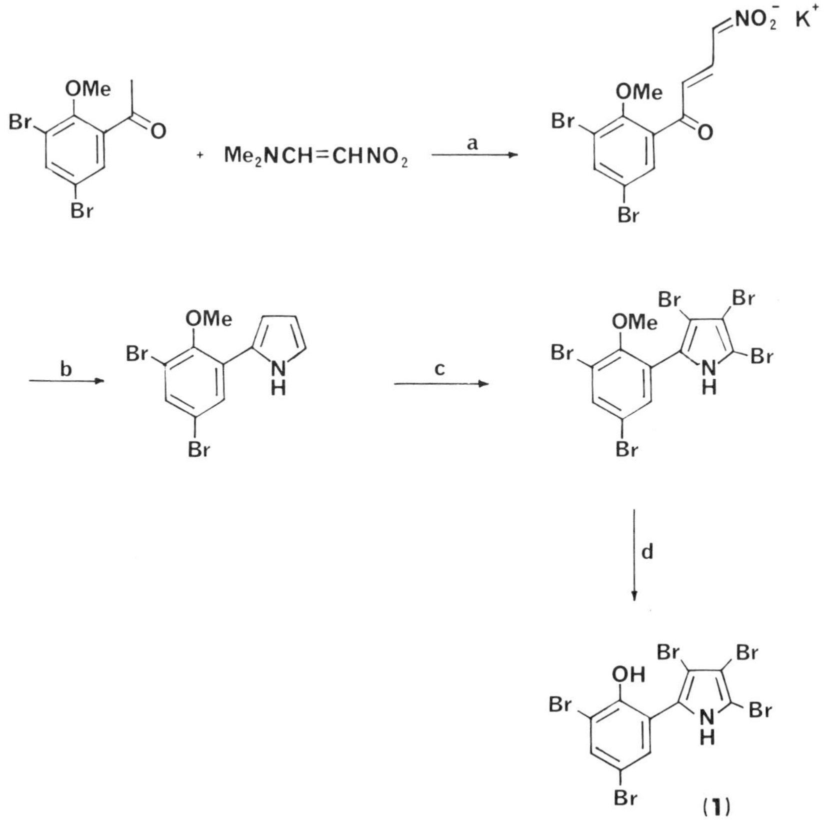

**Scheme 2.1**

Synthesis of 2-(3′,5′-dibromo-2′-hydroxyphenyl)-3,4,5-tribromopyrrole (**1**) [5] a) KOEt, EtOH b) $Na_2S_2O_4$ c) $Br_2$, $CHCl_3$ d) $BCl_3$, $CCl_4$.

We have examined the secondary metabolites of an autotoxic marine bacterium of the genus *Chromobacter* which was isolated from a surface seawater sample taken from the North Pacific Gyre. Together with 2-(3′,5′-dibromo-2′-hydroxyphenyl)-3,4,5-tribromopyrrole (**1**), the same compound isolated by Burkholder *et al.* [3], we isolated tetrabromopyrrole (**2**), hexabromo-2,2′-bipyrrole (**3**), and 4-hydroxybenzaldehyde (**4**) [6]. Both tetrabromopyrrole (**2**) and hexabromo-2,2′-bipyrrole (**3**) were difficult to identify, since the only signals in a $^1$H nmr spectrum were an almost imperceptible hump due to the -NH proton and signals due to impurities. The mass spectrum of each compound showed a molecular ion, allowing structures to be proposed. The compounds were synthesized in a routine manner, and the natural and synthetic materials were shown to be identical. Both compounds were extremely sensitive to light.

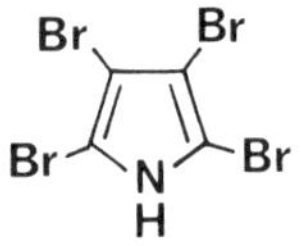

Br Br Br Br N H (2)

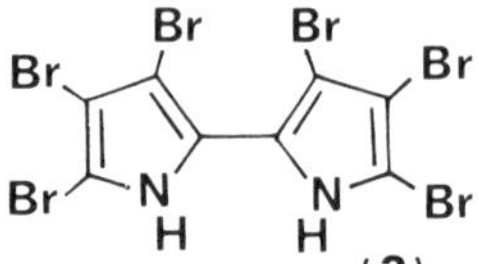

Br Br Br Br Br Br N H N H (3)

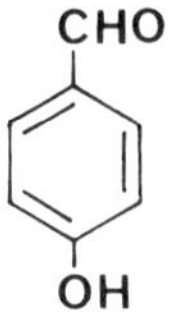

CHO OH (4)

Growing the *Chromobacter* on agar-covered trays allowed separation of the cells from the medium and, hence, separation of the intracellular from the extracellular metabolites. 2-(3′,5′-Dibromo-2′-hydroxyphenyl)-3,4,5-tribromopyrrole (**1**) was found in both cells and medium, while hexabromo-2,2′-bipyrrole (**3**), which was not toxic to *Chromobacter,* was exclusively intracellular and 4-hydroxy-benzaldehyde (**4**) was exclusively extracellular. Tetrabromo-pyrrole (**2**) was not isolated in this experiment. At present it seems advisable to assume that *p*-hydroxybenzaldehyde was produced by partial degradation of tyrosine from the enriched medium. This leaves 2-(3′,5′-dibromo-2′-hydroxyphenyl)-3,4,5-tribromopyrrole (**1**) as the most likely cause of autotoxicity and the metabolite most likely to be of ecological significance.

We have since examined two other antibiotic-producing strains of marine bacteria which were not purple-coloured *Chromobacter* species. Both strains, one yellow and the other off-white, contained 2-(3′,5′-dibromo-2′-hydroxyphenyl)-3,4,5-tribromopyrrole (**1**) as the major antibiotic metabolite. Examination of the literature revealed that the same metabolite could well be responsible for the autotoxicity of *Chromobacter marinum* [7] and other marine bacteria [8].

A yellow marine pseudomonad (designated 102-3) produced three antibiotic compounds: 4-hydroxybenzaldehyde (**4**), 2-*n*-pentyl-4-quinolinol (**5**), and 2-*n*-heptyl-4-quinolinol (**6**) [9]. The latter compound (**6**) had previously been isolated from a terrestrial bacterium, *Pseudomonas aeruginosa* [10]. The two quinolinols (**5**) and (**6**) were active against *Staphylococcus aureus, Vibrio harveyi,* and *Vibrio anguillarum* at 50 μg/disc, using a disc assay technique. There was no indication of autotoxicity. The marine pseudomonad also produced 6-bromoindole-3-carboxaldehyde, but this compound showed no antibiotic activity.

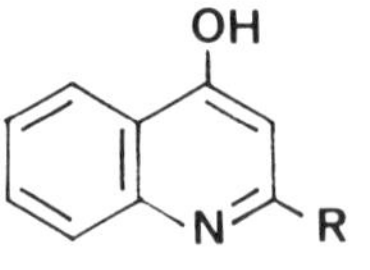

OH N R

(**5**) R = $C_5H_{11}$
(**6**) R = $C_7H_{15}$

There has been very little research on marine fungi. An actinomycete, *Chainia purpurogena* SS-228, later referred to as *Chainia* sp., was shown to produce an antibiotic which inhibited growth of gram positive bacteria [11]. On the basis of spectroscopic data, the antibiotic SS-228V was shown to be a benz(a)anthracene derivative (7) [12]. On exposure to light or heating, the antibiotic rearranged to a naphthacene derivative (8), which was biologically inactive. An ionophore antibiotic, aplasmomycin, has been isolated from *Streptomyces griseus* strain SS-20, found in shallow sea mud [13]. During this study, over 500 strains of marine fungi were isolated from shallow sea mud, but the report did not indicate how many strains showed antiobiotic activity.

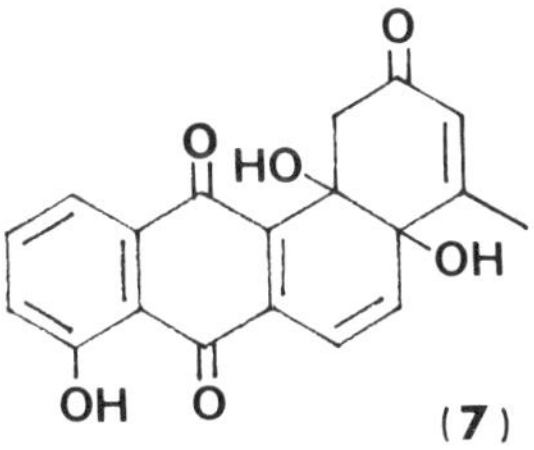

(7) 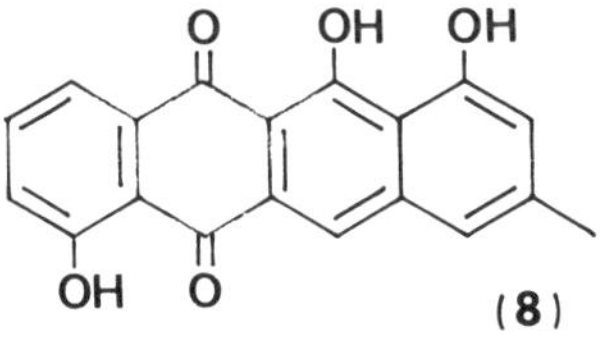 (8)

Two brominated phenols, 3.5-dibromo-4-hydroxybenzyl alcohol (**111**) and 2,3-dibromo-4,5-dihydroxybenzyl alcohol (**112**), have been identified in a marine ascomycete and its culture medium, respectively [14]. The ascomycete was cultured from a brown algae, *Ascophyllum nodosum.* The brominated phenols are generally associated with red algae and will be discussed in greater detail in that section of the review.

## 3 ANTIBIOTICS FROM SPONGES

In the broad surveys of antimicrobial activity in marine phyla, sponges (porifera) have often shown the greatest percentage of active samples. However, the sponges are notoriously difficult to identify, so that many sponges having biological activity remain unidentified. To overcome this problem, many workers seeking antibiotics from sponges have used antimicrobial assays in the field, collecting only those sponges having proven antimicrobial activity. This situation occasionally results in the chemical identification of an antibiotic from an unidentified sponge, but this is probably more useful than the alternative situation.

In compilations of the antimicrobial activity of sponges, the genus *Verongia* is always prominent. Every crude extract of *Verongia* species that we have examined has shown strong antimicrobial activity. Even after studying the metabolites of three *Verongia* species for several years, we have reluctantly reached the conclusion that the most active antibiotics from these sources have not been described. Even though some *Verongia* antibiotics have been isolated and identified, it has always appeared that the strong antimicrobial activity of the crude extracts could not be explained solely on the basis of identified compounds.

Sharma and Burkholder isolated both the dienone (**9**) and the corresponding dimethoxy ketal (**10**) from methanolic extracts of *Verongia fistularis* and *V. cauliformis* [15, 16]. They were able to hydrolyze the ketal (**10**) to the dienone (**9**) under acidic conditions but could not convert the dienone (**9**) to the ketal (**10**). The latter reaction does not occur even under forcing conditions. They therefore proposed that the dienone (**9**) was an artifact caused by hydrolysis of the dimethoxy ketal (**10**), the true sponge metabolite. However, the ketal (**10**) showed little or no antibiotic activity, whereas the dienone (**9**) was highly active. Since it is unlikely that the antibiotic activity of fresh sponge tissue or crude extracts was due entirely to an artifact, one must conclude that the sponges contained other antibiotic substances.

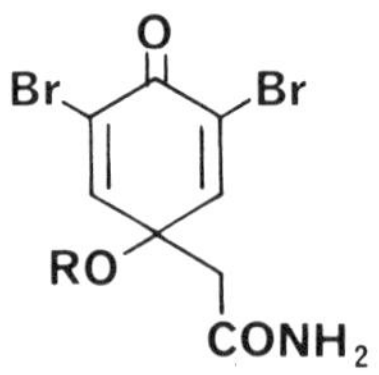

(**9**) R = H (**11**) R = Ac 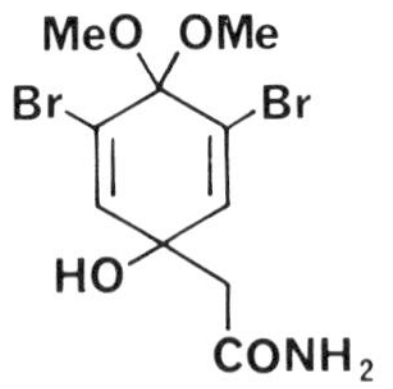 (**10**) 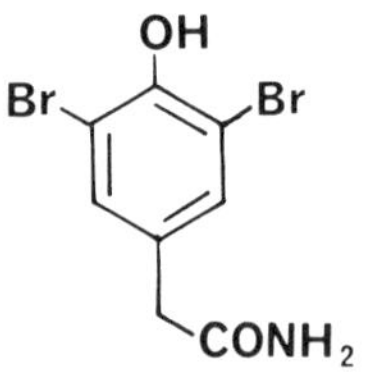 (**12**)

The structure of the dienone (**9**) was elucidated by analysis of the spectral data and by reduction of the corresponding acetate (**11**) with lithium borohydride to obtain 3,5-dibromo-4-hydroxyphenylacetamide (**12**). Oxidation of the phenol (**12**) with nitric acid in acetic acid gave the dienone (**9**). A second synthesis will be presented later (Scheme 5.1).

When an undescribed species of *Verongia* from the Gulf of California was extracted with ethanol, the major halogenated product was an approximately 1:1 mixture of two diastereoisomeric mixed ketals **(13)** and **(14)**, which showed slight antibiotic activity [17]. We have assumed that ethanol had added to a relatively unstable sponge metabolite, thought to be the arene oxide **(15)**.

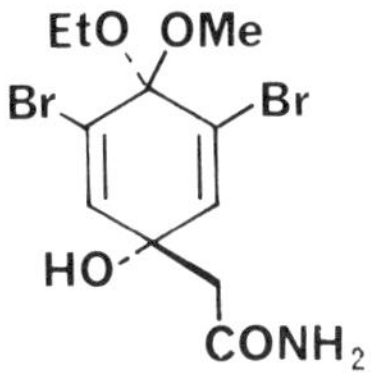

**(13)** 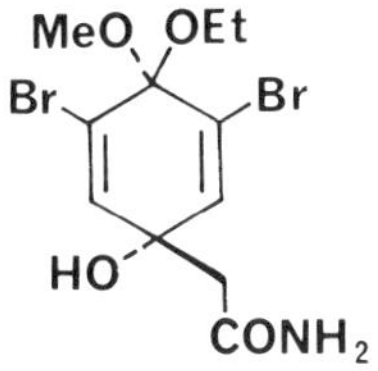 **(14)** 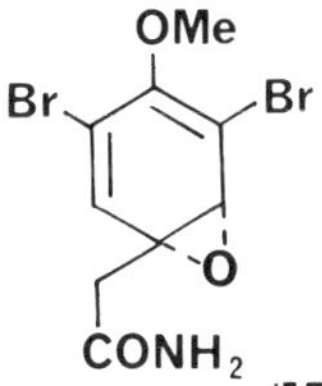 **(15)**

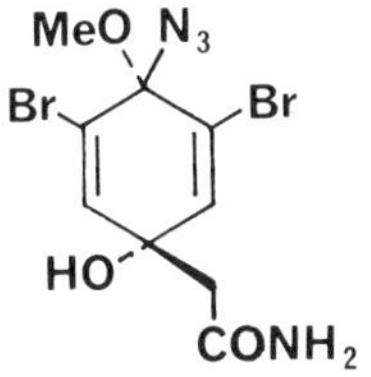

**(16)** 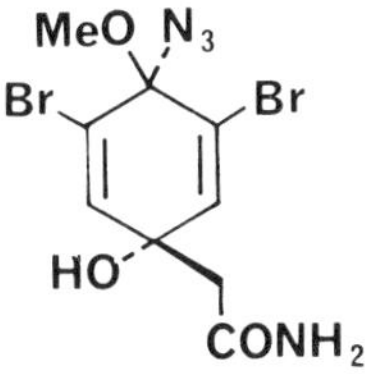 **(17)** 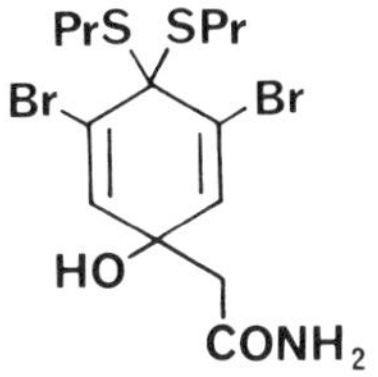 **(18)**

Precedent for the 1,4 addition of methanol to an arene oxide had been demonstrated by Kasperek *et al.* [18]. Addition of sodium azide or propane thiol to an acetone homogenate of the same *Verongia* sp. gave a mixture of azides **(16)** and **(17)** and a dithioketal **(18)**, respectively [19]. Whatever the structure of the unknown metabolite, whether arene oxide **(15)** or an alternative structure, the fact that it irreversibly adds a thiol suggests that this metabolite may derive biological activity in a manner similar to α-methylene lactones and other molecules which act by reaction with mercaptan residues [20].

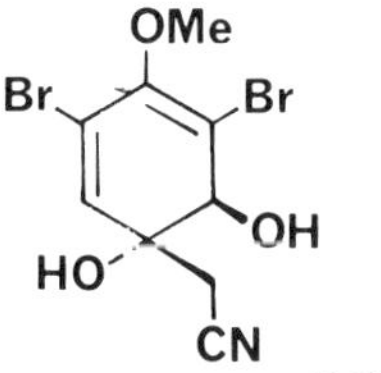

**(19)** 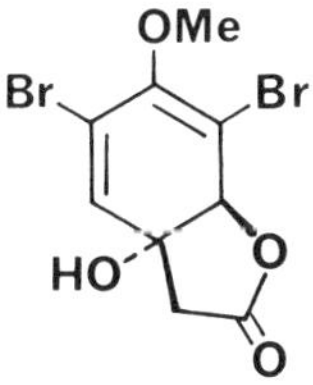 **(20)**

Both optical antipodes of aeroplysinin-1 **(19)** have been isolated from sponges. The dextrorotary isomer, (+)-aeroplysinin-1 **(19)** was isolated from an acetone extract of *Verongia aerophoba,* which also contained the lactone **(20)**, aerothionin-1 **(21)**, and aerothionin-2 **(22)** [21]. The structure of (+)-aeroplysinin-1 **(19)** was established from spectral data and by conversion of the

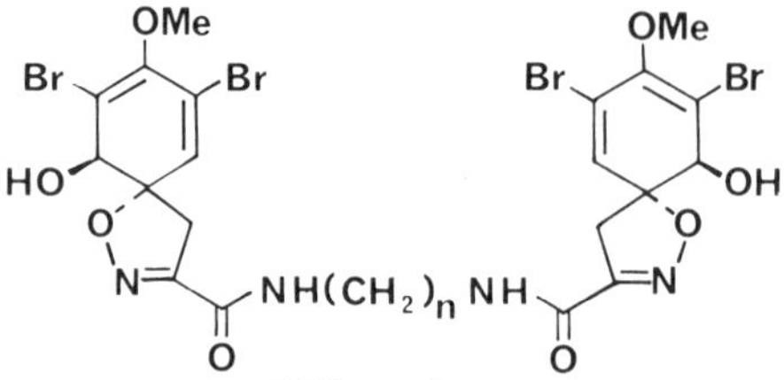

(21) n = 4

(22) n = 5

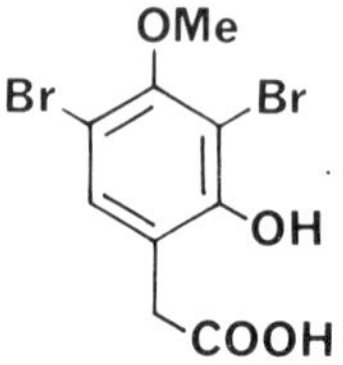

(23)

corresponding diacetate into 3,5-dibromo-2-hydroxy-4-methoxyphenylacetic acid (**23**). The laevorotary isomer (–)-aeroplysinin-1 (**19**) was isolated from *Ianthella ardis* [22], now known as *Pseudoceratina crassa* [23]. The absolute configurations of both antipodes have been independently determined by X-ray studies and show the two hydroxyl groups to be *trans* quasi-diaxial [24]. The absolute configuration could also be predicted from the CD curve, which indicated a left-handed helicity for the (–) isomer. Racemic aeroplysinin-1 has been synthesized from 3,5-dibromo-2-hydroxy-4-methoxyphenylacetonitrile (**24**) by a three-step procedure (Scheme 3.1) [25]. The phenol (**24**) was oxidized with an excess of lead tetra-acetate in acetic acid to obtain the acetoxy-ketone (**25**) in 35% yield. The acetoxy-ketone (**25**) was hydrolyzed, using *p*-toluenesulphonic acid in methanol, and the resulting keto-alcohol was reduced with sodium borohydride in absolute ethanol at 0°C to obtain (±)-aeroplysinin-1 (**19**) in 27% yield. The acetoxy-ketone could also be converted into the *cis*-

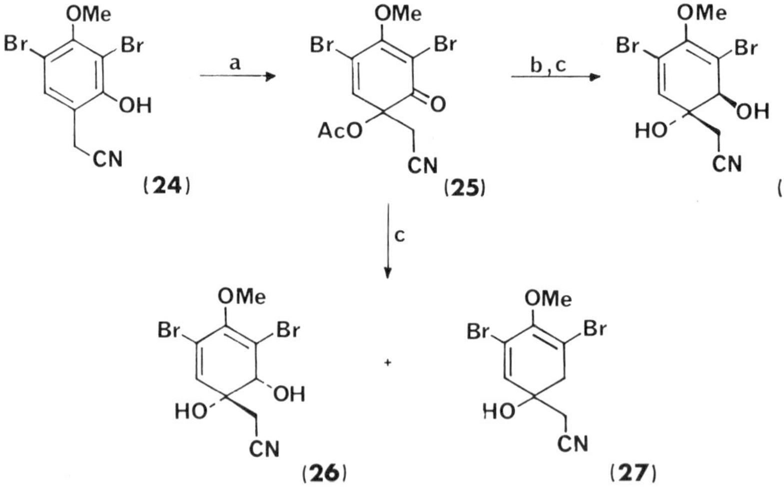

(24) (25) (19)

(26) (27)

**Scheme 3.1**

Synthesis of aeroplysinin-1 (**19**), iso-aeroplysinin-1 (**26**), and 2-desoxyaeroplysinin-1 (**27**) [25] a) $Pb(OAc)_4$, AcOH b) TsOH, MeOH c) $NaBH_4$, EtOH.

glycol, isoaeroplysinin (**26**), and 2-desoxyaeroplysinin (**27**) by reduction with sodium borohydride in ethanol.

Both optical enantiomers of aeroplysinin-1 (**19**) have approximately equal potency for inhibiting gram negative and gram positive bacteria, but neither protected mice from bacterial infections [22]. Aeroplysinin-1 (**19**) showed initial activity in the KB and L-1210 screens established by the National Cancer Institute, but these results have not been repeated with any consistency, possibly because samples had different absolute configurations.

Stempien *et al.* [26] isolated 3,5-dibromo-4-hydroxyphenylacetamide (**28**) from *Verongia archeri*. They showed that the phenol (**28**) inhibited the growth of *E. coli*. As will be shown in a later section, most brominated phenols have some antimicrobial activity, so that this observation was not unexpected. A brominated hydroquinone (**29**) was isolated from *Verongia aurea* [27]. The hydroquinone (**29**), which was identified by X-ray analysis, inhibited the growth of *B. subtilis, E. coli,* and *P. atrovenetum.*

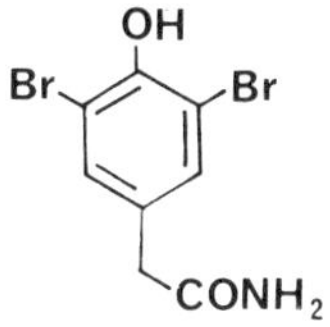

OH Br Br CONH$_2$

**(28)**

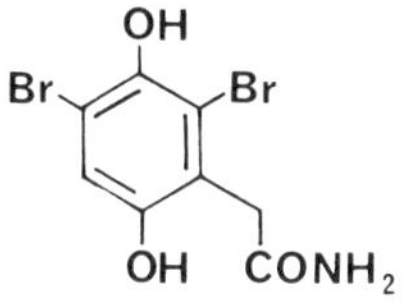

OH Br Br OH CONH$_2$

**(29)**

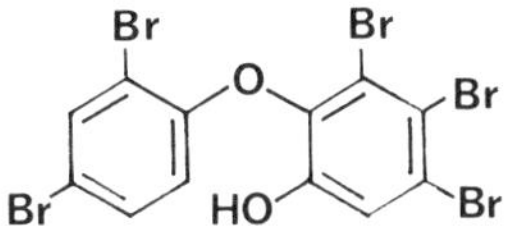

Br Br O Br Br HO Br

**(30)**

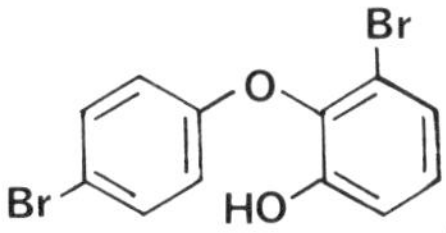

Br O Br HO

**(31)**

Two closely related antimicrobial agents were isolated from *Dysidea herbacea* [28]. The compounds were identified as 2-(2′,4′-dibromophenoxy)-3,4,5-tribromophenol (**30**) and 2-(4′-bromophenoxy)-3-bromophenol (**31**) on the basis of the spectral data, and the structure of (**30**) was confirmed by synthesis of the corresponding methyl ether. The sponge was reported to inhibit the growth of both gram negative and gram positive bacteria, and each compound was shown to be active but detailed screening data were not reported. In a presentation at the 1969 Food-Drugs from the Sea Conference [29], additional bromophenols were reported to contribute to the antimicrobial activity of *D. herbacea,* but detailed structure proofs have not been reported.

Minale and co-workers [30] have reported that 4,5-dibromo-2-cyanopyrrole (**32**) was active against *Streptococcus, Diplococcus, Candida albicans,* and *Trichophyton.* On hydrolysis and subsequent esterification, the known methyl ester (**33**) was formed from the nitrile (**32**) [31]. Since the other compounds described in that paper, the acid (**34**), the amide (**35**), and oroidin (**36**)

[32], were not identified as antibiotics, it is probably reasonable to assume that they showed no antimicrobial activity. In an oral presentation, Stempien *et al.* [33] reported that 4-bromopyrrole-2-carbonylguanidine (**37**) from a Caribbean *Agelas* sp. showed antimicrobial activity.

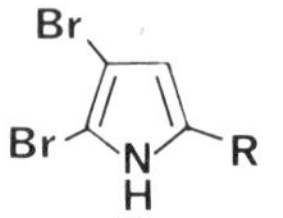

(**32**) R = CN
(**33**) R - COOMe
(**34**) R = COOH
(**35**) R = $CONH_2$

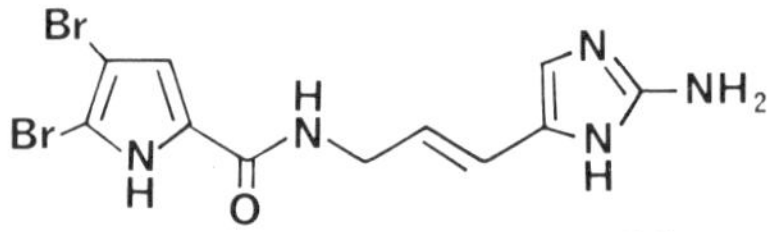

(**36**)

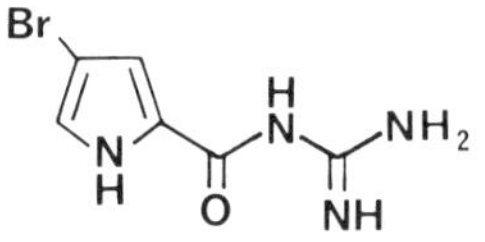

(**37**)

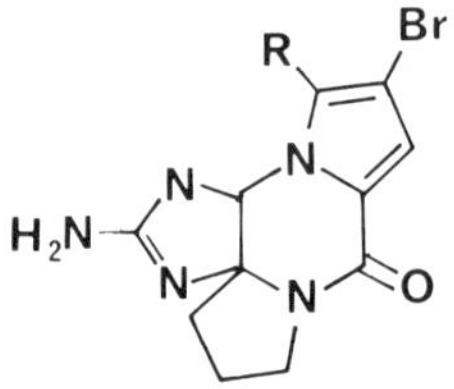

(**38**) R = Br
(**39**) R = H

Both 4,5-dibromophakellin (**38**) and 4-bromophakellin (**39**), from *Phakellia flabellata,* were reported to exhibit an antibacterial action against *E. coli* and *B. subtilis* [29]. The structural elucidation of 4,5-dibromophakellin (**38**) resulted from an X-ray analysis of the mono-acetate of 4,5-dibromophakellin [34]. It is intriguing to note that 4,5-dibromophakellin ($pk_a$ 7.7) does not possess the normal basicity associated with guanidines ($pK_a$ >13.4), so that the possibility of rearrangement during acetylation has been raised [35]. No evidence for the structure of 4-bromophakellin (**39**) was presented.

Two antimicrobial bromoindole metabolites were isolated from *Polyfibrospongia maynardii* [36]. Catalytic hydrogenation of 3-(2-methylaminoethyl)-5,6-dibromoindole (**40**) gave the known compound 3-(2-methylaminoethyl)-indole. The positions of the bromine atoms were deduced from the $^1H$ nmr spectrum. A similar structure proof was employed for 3-(2-aminoethyl)-5,6-dibromoindole (**41**). Both compounds inhibited gram negative and gram positive bacteria at 25-250 $\gamma$/ml in an *in vitro* assay but failed to provide protection against bacterial infection during *in vivo* tests.

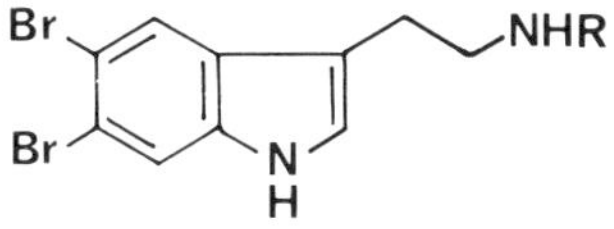

(40) R = Me

(41) R = H

Marine sponges of the order Halichondrida often contain terpenoid isonitriles, some of which have been reported to inhibit bacterial growth. Minale *et al.* [37] isolated acanthellin-1 (**42**) from *Acanthella acuta* and found a minimum inhibitory concentration of 12 $\gamma$/ml against *Mycobacterium* sp. for this isonitrile. The structure of acanthellin-1 was elucidated by analysis of the spectral data and by reduction of (**42**) with lithium in ethylamine to obtain 4-epi-eudesmane (**43**). The pmr spectrum indicated that the isonitrile was at C-6 and that both the isonitrile and isopropylidene groups were equatorial.

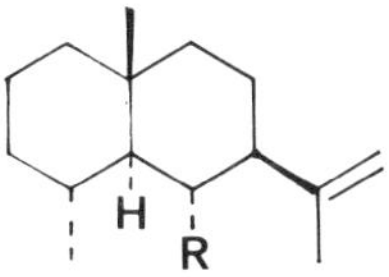

(42) R = $\overset{+}{N}\equiv\overset{-}{C}$

(43) R = H

The spectral properties of isonitriles allow the functionality to be readily identified and located. The ir band at 2140 cm$^{-1}$ is obligatory and, if present, protons on carbon bearing isonitrile occur at ~3.3 ppm in the $^1$H nmr spectrum.

Burreson *et al.* [38] have shown that the antimicrobial activity of *Halichondria* sp. was associated with a mixture of two isonitriles. The two isonitriles were an amorphane derivative (**44**) and a linear diterpene (**45**). The $^1$H nmr spectrum of the amorphane derivative contained a three-proton triplet ($J_{CH_3-{}^{14}N}$ = 1.5 Hz) at $\delta$ 1.42, a signal which was attributed to a methyl group on carbon bearing an isonitrile group. The structure was elucidated by reduction of the isonitrile (**44**) to the corresponding methylamine derivative (**46**), which was converted to zizanene (**47**) by the Hofmann elimination sequence. The structure of the diterpene isonitrile (**45**) was assigned on the basis of spectral data and simple chemical conversions.

Sponges which contain isonitriles usually contain the corresponding formamides and isothiocyanates [38, 39]. We have recently identified two isonitrile dichlorides (**48**) and (**49**) in *Pseudaxinyssa pitys* [40]. The corresponding isonitriles (**50**) and (**51**), which have not yet been found as natural products, both demonstrated antimicrobial activity *in vitro*. It is possible that other isonitriles from sponges may also exhibit antimicrobial activity but have not been tested.

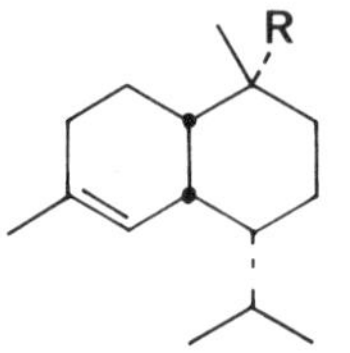

(**44**) R = $\overset{+}{N}\equiv\overset{-}{C}$

(**46**) R = NHMe

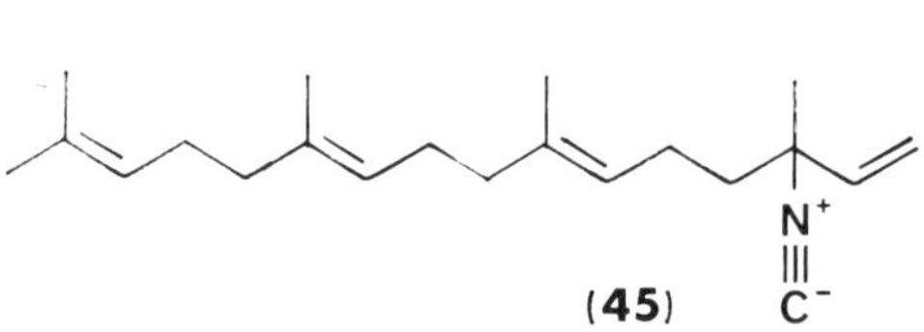

(**45**)

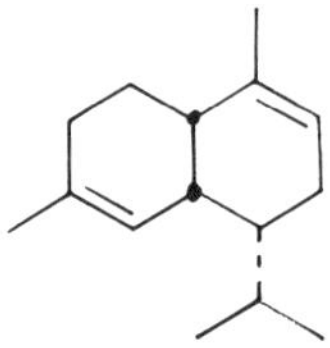

(**47**)

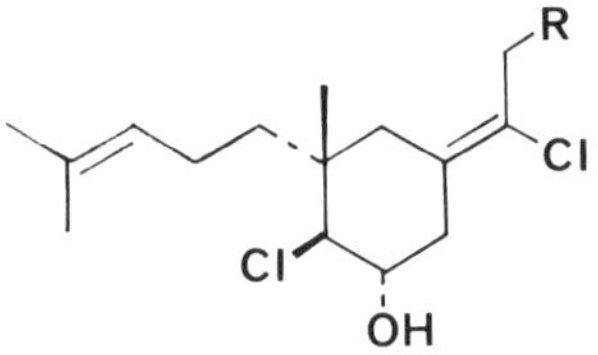

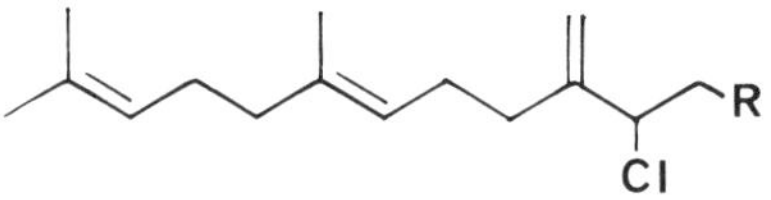

(**48**) R = $N=CCl_2$ (**49**)

(**50**) R = $\overset{+}{N}\equiv\overset{-}{C}$ (**51**)

Linear sesterterpenes containing a tetronic acid moiety have quite pronounced antimicrobial activity. *Ircinia oros* was found to contain a mixture of two sesterterpenes, ircinin-1 (**52a**) and ircinin-2 (**52b**), which inhibited *Diplococcus* sp. (M.I.C. 1 γ/ml) and *S. aureus* (M.I.C. 5 γ/ml). The two isomers, which differed only in the position of the trisubstituted olefinic bond, were not separated. The structures of the two isomers were deduced from spectral and chemical degradation data, particularly from the fragments obtained by ozonolysis [40].

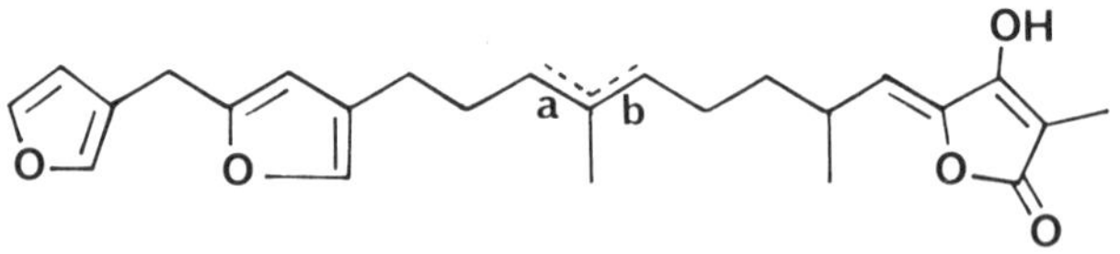

(**52**)

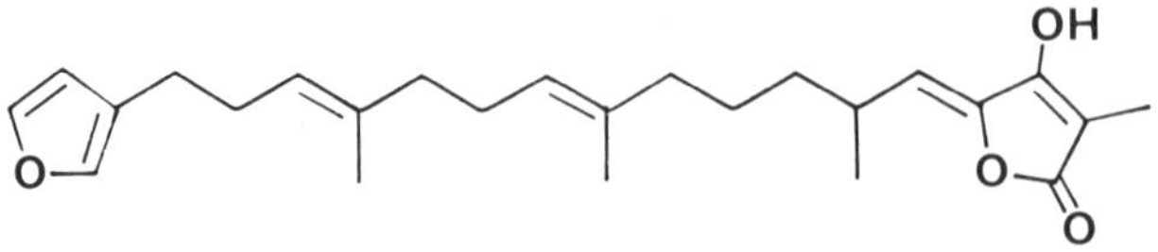

(**53**)

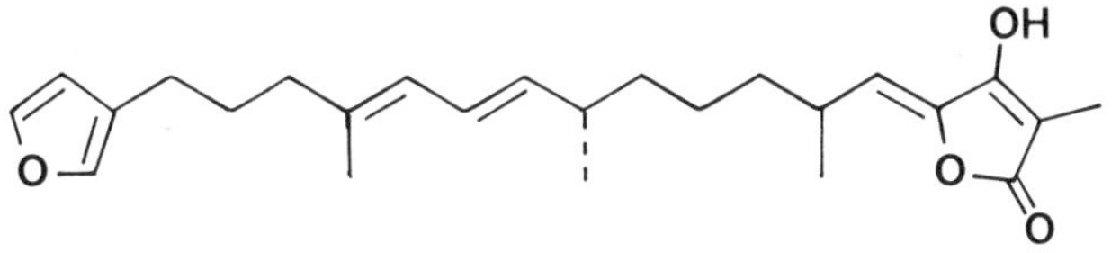

(54)

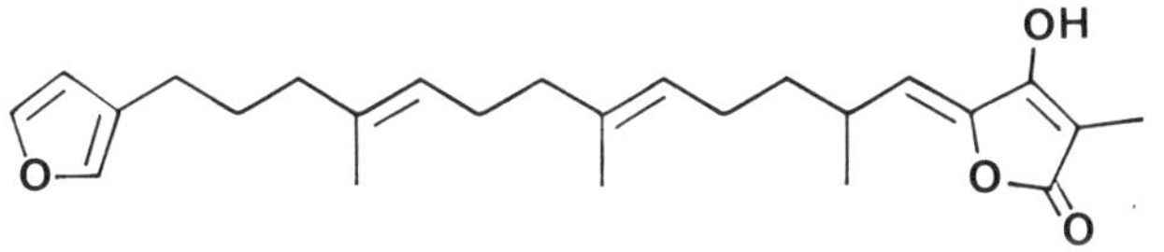

(55)

Sesterterpene tetronic acids have also been reported from *Ircinia fasciculata* [41], *I. variabilis* [42], and *I. strobilina* [43]. The structures of variabilin (**53**), fasciculatin (**54**), and strobilin (**55**) were all determined in the same manner as that of the ircinins (**52a** and **52b**), but in every molecule the stereochemical assignment of the trisubstituted olefinic bonds was not determined. Extracts of *Ircinia variabilis* and *I. strobilina* both inhibit *S. aureus*, but there is no report of antimicrobial activity for *I. fasciculata*. Since strobilin (**55**) occurred in an inseparable mixture with variabilin (**53**) in *I. strobilina*, its biological activity is uncertain. A model tetronic acid (**56**) did not inhibit *S. aureus*.

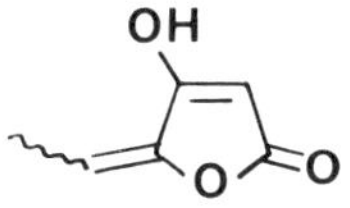

(56)

Nitenin (**57**), a $C_{21}$ metabolite of *Spongia nitens*, has been reported to possess antimicrobial activity against *Mycobacterium* sp. [30]. The structure of nitenin (**57**) was determined by analysis of spectral data and from degradation reactions [44]. The absolute configuration was determined by application of the Horeau method to the diol (**58**). Furospongin-1 (**59**) has been isolated as a major metabolite from *Spongia officinalis* [45], *Hippospongia communis* [45], and five Australian *Spongia* species [35]. Furospongin-1 (**59**) has been reported to show activity at 0.5 γ/ml against *Diplococcus* sp. and 1 γ/ml against *Streptococcus* sp. The structure of furospongin-1 (**59**) was, again, determined by analysis of spectral data and from a degradation sequence. It is interesting that only two of the relatively large group of C-21 difurans, which are thought to be truncated sesterterpenes, have shown any antibiotic activity

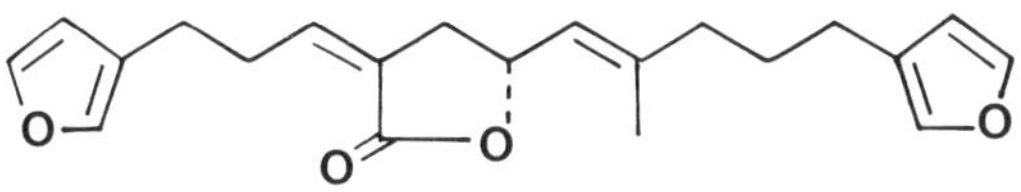

(57)

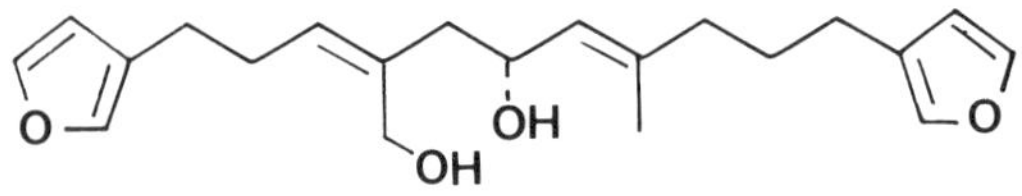

(58)

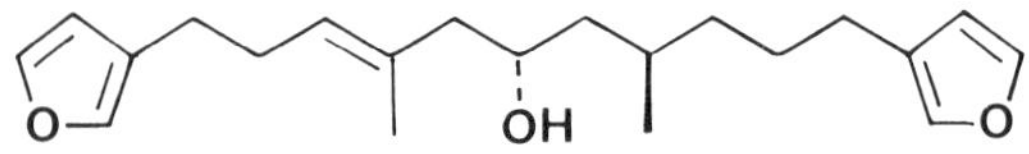

(59)

Although ethanolic extracts of *Halichondria panicae* were reported to show antibiotic activity [46], none of the compounds (**60-64**) isolated from the sponge were recorded as having antibiotic activity [47]. It is not known whether these compounds were screened.

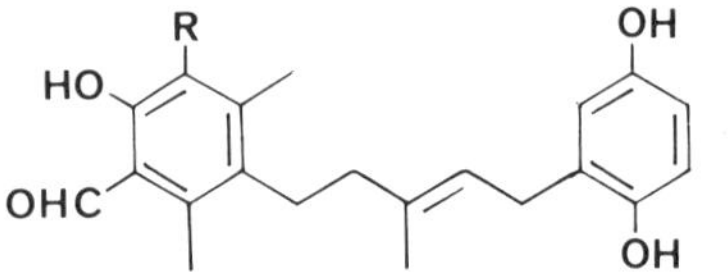

(**60**) R = H
(**61**) R = OH

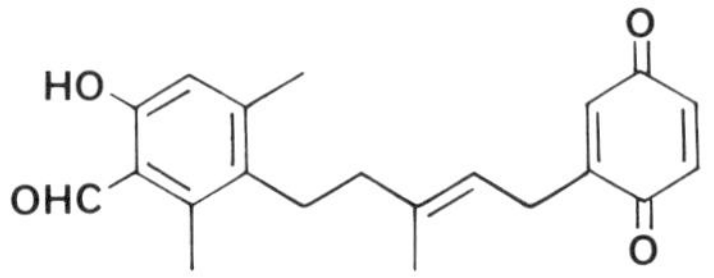

(**62**)

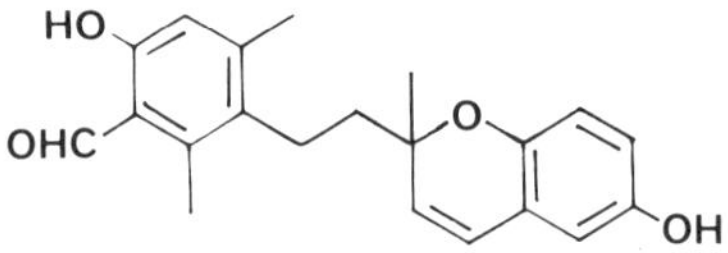

(**63**)

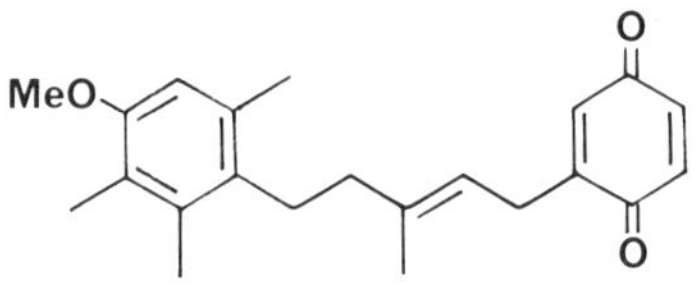

(**64**)

Ravi *et al.* [48] isolated an antimicrobial compound, chondrosione (**65**) from a bright-yellow sponge, *Chondrosia* sp. Some quantitative data for *in vitro* antimicrobial activity was obtained. The structure of chondrosione (**65**) was determined by interpretation of spectral data and by X-ray analysis of an ozonolysis product (**66**) [49].

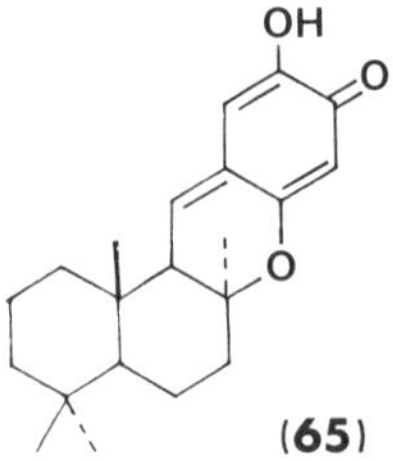

(**65**)

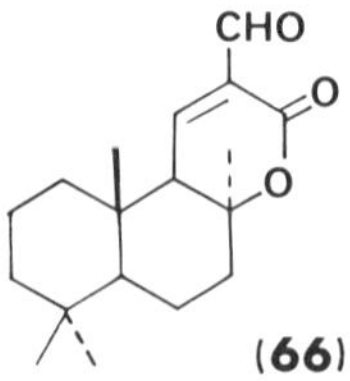

(**66**)

In 1966, Stempien *et al.* [50] reported that the antibiotic metabolite of *Agelas* sp. was either 4,6-dihydroxyindole **(67)** or 6,7-dihydroxyindole **(68)**. In 1974, Stempien *et al.* [51] reported the isolation and partial characterization of an antibiotic from *Haliclona* sp. (CI 207).

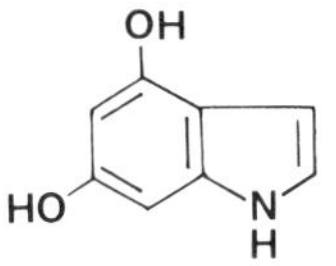

OH HO N H **(67)**

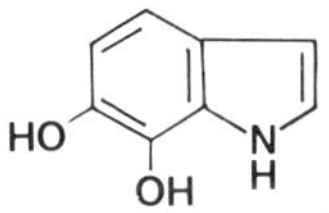

HO N H OH **(68)**

## 4 ANTIBIOTICS FROM COELENTERATES

The coelenterates are a group of invertebrates which include hydroids, sea anemones, jellyfish, soft corals, stony corals, gorgonians and sea pens. It has been difficult to obtain any information concerning the antibiotic activity of coelenterate metabolites because the majority of the chemical studies of coelenterates have been concerned with the toxins and their ecological importance. We have assayed several sea pen toxins for antibiotic activity, with negative results [52].

The majority of marine natural products research on coelenterates has been concerned with Caribbean gorgonians and Indo-Pacific soft corals. The gorgonians have yielded a series of diterpenoid α-methylene lactones which were described as mildly antibiotic [53]. Crassin acetate **(69)**, which may be isolated from *Pseudoplexaura porosa, P. flagellosa* and *P. wagenaari* [54], was active against *Endamoeba histolytica* at 20 μg/ml. However, more than one antimicrobial compound must be present in *P. porosa*, since the volatile oils (probably sesquiterpenes) inhibited growth of *S. aureus* and *Clostridium feseri*. The structure of crassin acetate was determined by X-ray analysis [55]. Crassin acetate was also found to be toxic to fish, to barnacle larvae, and to *Tetrahymena*, as well as demonstrating cytotoxic activity in the KB system. Asperdiol **(70)**, isolated from *Eunicea asperula* and *E. tourneforti*, also showed anticancer activity against the KB (24 μg/ml), PS (6 μg/ml) and LE (6 μg/ml) cell lines *in vitro* [56]. Eunicin **(71)**, isolated from *E. mammosa* [57], was reported to inhibit the growth of *S. aureus* and *C. feseri*.

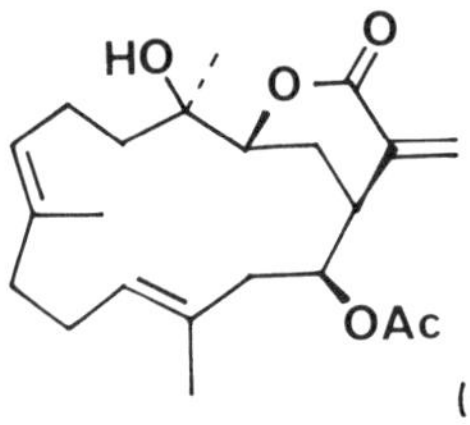

HO O O OAc

**(69)**

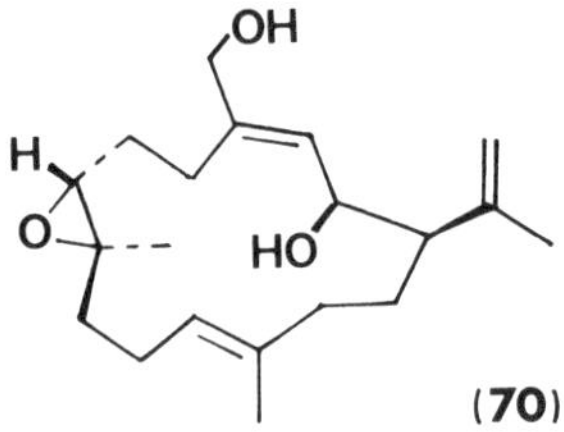

OH H O HO

**(70)**

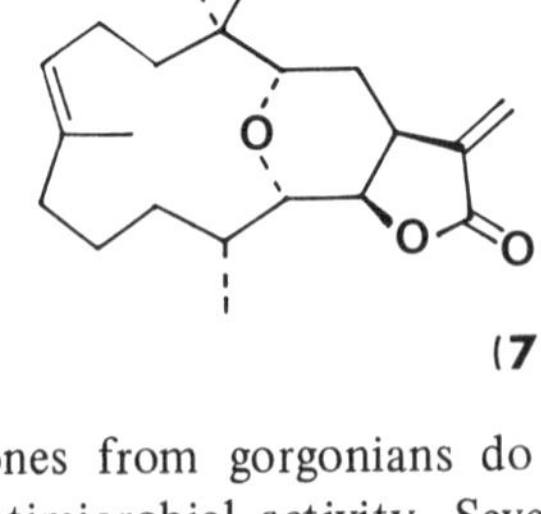

OH O O O

**(71)**

The diterpenoid lactones from gorgonians do not appear to have been adequately screened for antimicrobial activity. Several additional α-methylene lactones have been isolated from *E. mammosa*, according to the location from which it was isolated. However, no biological activity data were reported for jeunicin (72) and ceunicin (73).

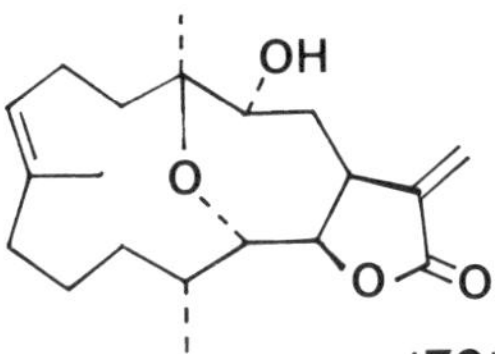

(72)

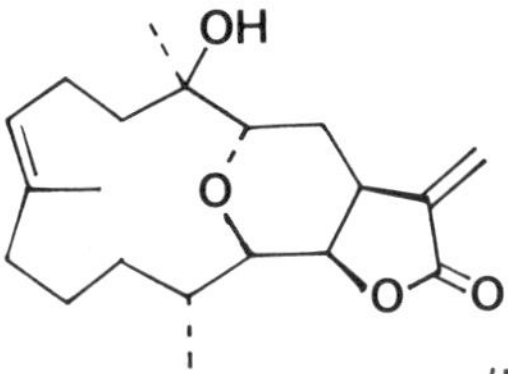

(73)

There are no reports of biologically active molecules from the volatile oils of *P. porosa*, yet this fraction was reported to be active against *S. aureus* and *C. feseri* [53]. The sesquiterpene fraction of *Pseudopterogorgia rigida* contained a phenol (**74**), a hydroquinone (**75**) and a quinone (**76**), all of which showed mild antibiotic activity. The phenol (**74**) inhibited the growth of *S. aureus* at 7 μg/disc and was the most active of the three compounds [6].

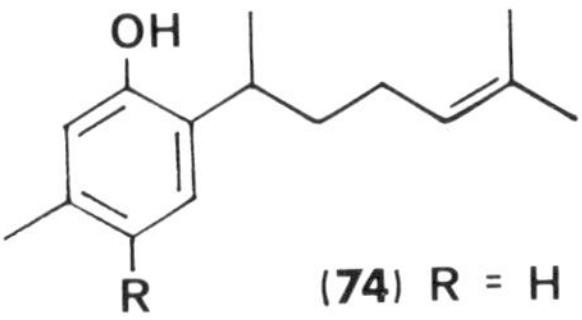

(74) R = H

(75) R = OH

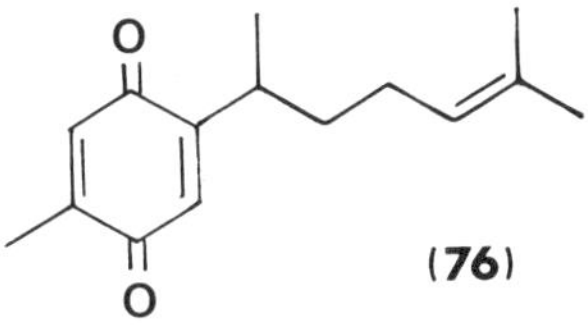

(76)

The gorgonian *Pterogorgia guadalupensis* contains a lactone (77) which exhibited mild antibiotic activity against *S. aureus* and *Mycobacterium smegmatis*. The structural elucidation of (77) was based on spectroscopic data, coupled with its conversion to ancepsenolide (78), which, by inference, has no biological activiy [61].

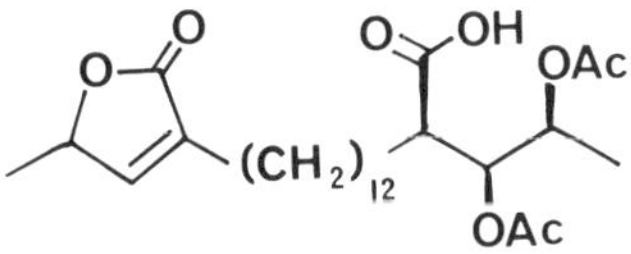

(77)

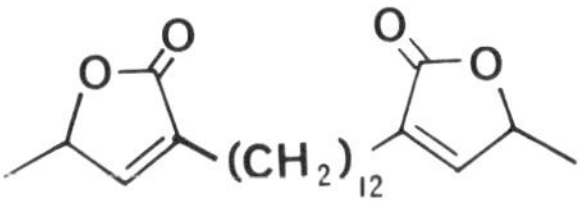

(78)

The chemistry and biological activity of the soft corals (alcyonaceans) has been reviewed by Tursch [62]. From his report, it appears that soft coral metabolites either show no activity against bacteria or have not been tested. However, africanol (**79**), from *Lemnalia africana*, the capnellanes (**80**) and (**81**), from *Capnella imbricata*, and sinulariolide (**82**), from *Sinularia flexibilis*, have been shown to inhibit the growth of the unicellular algae *Chaetoceros septentionalis, Asterionella japonica, Thalaisioscira excentricus, Protocentrum micans,* and *Amphidinium carterae.* It has been suggested that compounds such as these may protect specific coelenterate-zooxanthellae relationships. The structures of africanol (**79**) [63] and sinulariolide (**82**) [64] were obtained by X-ray analysis, while the capnellanes (**80**) and (**81**) were both related to an X-ray-derived structure [65].

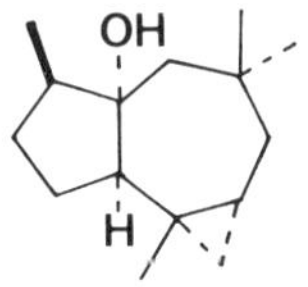

(**79**)

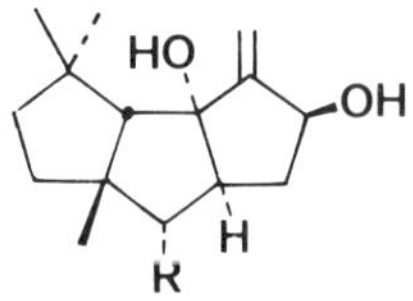

(**80**) R = OH
(**81**) R = H

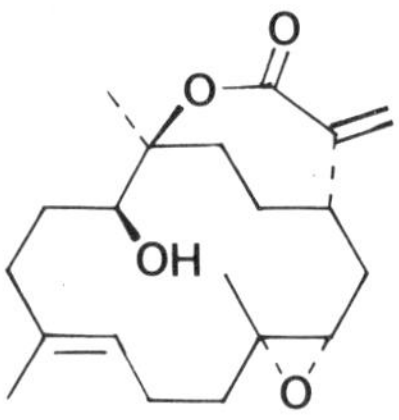

(**82**)

The studies of Burkholder [66] indicate that many gorgonians inhibited the growth of terrestrial and marine microorganisms. Since tropical gorgonians, which harbour symbiotic zooxanthellae, possess antibiotic activity, while the non-symbiotic temperate gorgonians do not, it has been suggested that the antimicrobial compounds may be produced by zooxanthellae or that the gorgonian produces antimicrobial compounds to protect the symbiotic zooxanthellae. The paucity of reports of antimicrobial activity for isolated metabolites suggests either that the pure compounds have not been screened or that the antibiotics are minor metabolites. In either case, more research is required.

## 5 ANTIBIOTICS FROM MOLLUSCS

The marine natural products chemistry of molluscs has been directed almost exclusively toward the opisthobranch molluscs such as the sea hares and nudibranchs [67]. Studies of opisthobranchs have shown that their chemical constituents are predominantly dietary in origin. For instance, the chemical constituents of the digestive gland of the California sea hare *Aplysia californica* were obtained from red algae, such as *Plocamium* and *Laurencia* species, which formed a major portion of the sea hare's diet [68]. Extracts of the digestive gland of *A. californica* inhibited the growth of marine and terrestrial bacteria due to the presence of laurinterol (**83**) and other sesquiterpene phenols, which will be discussed later. Laurinterol (**83**) undergoes rearrangement to aplysin (**84**), an inactive molecule, in the digestive gland of *A. californica* [69]. *Aplysia vaccaria* [70] was shown to contain the mild antibiotic pachydictyol A (**85**) [71].

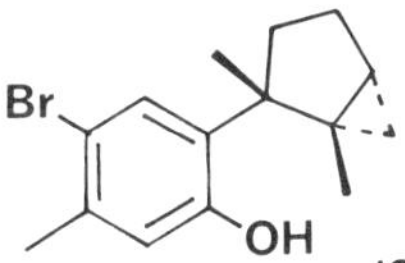

Br OH (**83**)

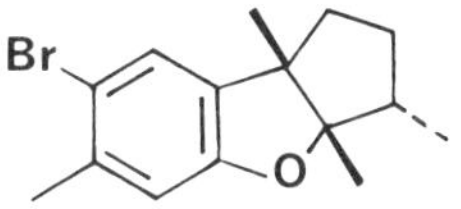

Br O (**84**)

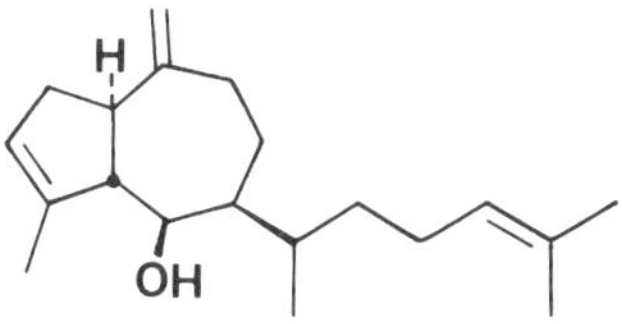

H OH (**85**)

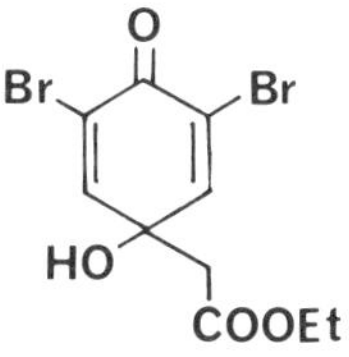

O Br Br HO COOEt (**86**)

The opisthobranch mollusc *Tylodina fungina* lives exclusively on sponges of the genus *Verongia* [72]. Ethanolic extracts of *T. fungina* contained the dienone ester (**86**), which inhibited the growth of *S. aureus* and *E. coli*. The dienone ester (**86**) and the amide (**9**) have been synthesized from 2,6-dibromo-1,4-benzoquinone (**87**) by Evans *et al.* [73] (Scheme 5.1).

When irritated, the opisthobranch mollusc *Onchidella binneyi* secreted a white mucous containing an antibiotic substance [74]. The antimicrobial compound onchidal (**88**), which inhibited the growth of *S. aureus,* could be converted into the corresponding dialdehyde (**89**) and diol (**90**). Ozonolysis of onchidal (**88**), followed by esterification, gave a keto-ester (**91**), which could also be prepared from $\beta$-snyderol (**92**). Onchidal (**88**) appears to be employed by *O. binneyi* as a defensive substance. A dietary source of onchidal (**88**) has not been identified, although green algae seem most likely.

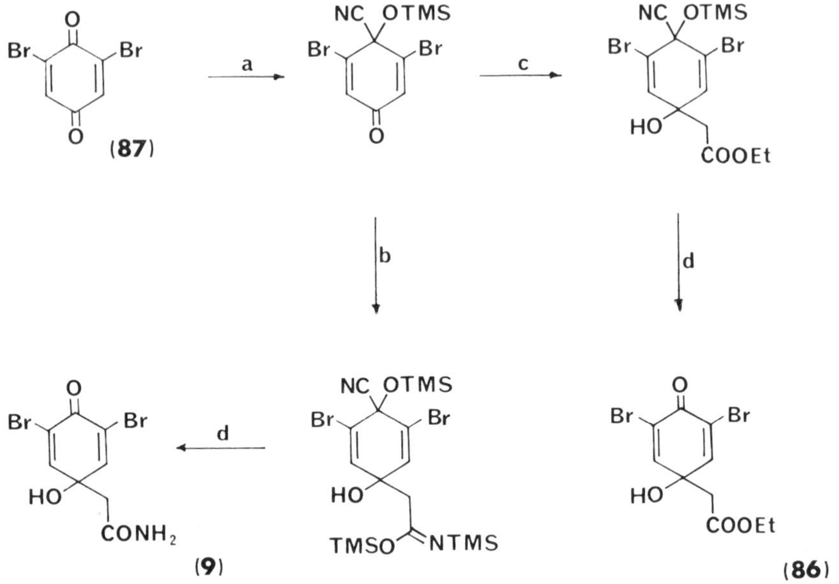


**Scheme 5.1**
Synthesis of dienones (**9**) and (**86**) [73] a) TMSCN, $Ph_3P$, 0°, $CH_3CN$ b) $LiCH_2CON(TMS)_2$, –100°, THF c) $LiCH_2COOEt$, –100°, THF d) AgF, $H_2O$–THF

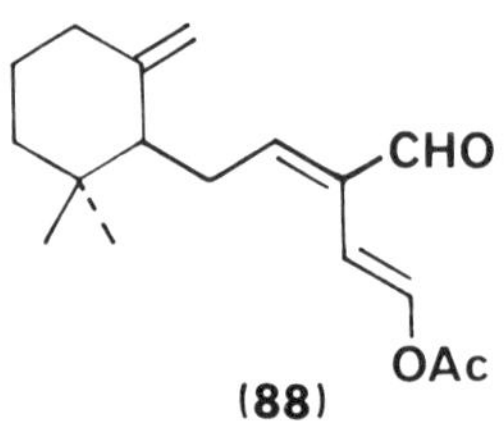


(**88**)

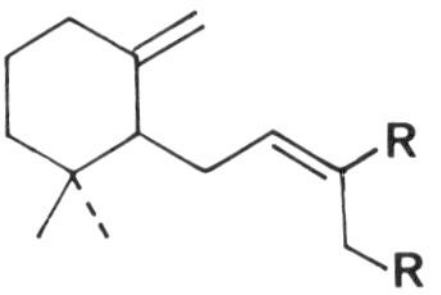


(**89**) R = CHO
(**90**) R = $CH_2OH$

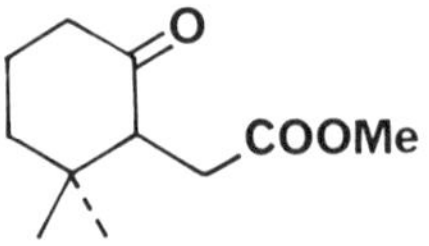


(**91**)

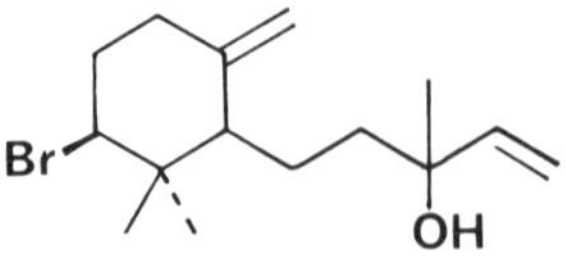


(**92**)

The saccoglossan *Tridachiella diomedea* was found to contain two closely related compounds, one of which showed antibiotic activity against *Vibrio anguillarum* [74]. The structure of the antibiotic (**93**) was determined by X-ray analysis of the ketone (**94**), which was formed on treatment with boron trifluoride in ether.

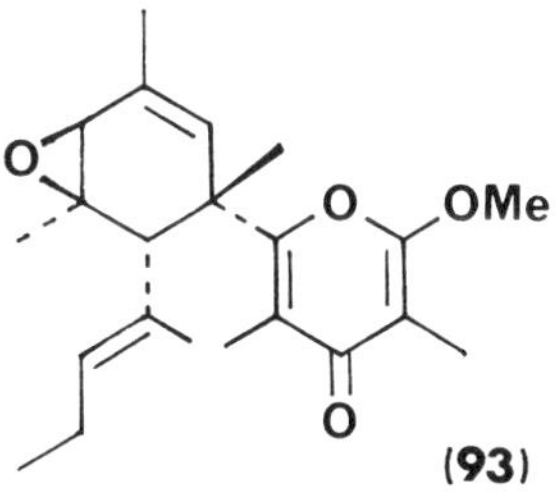

(**93**) 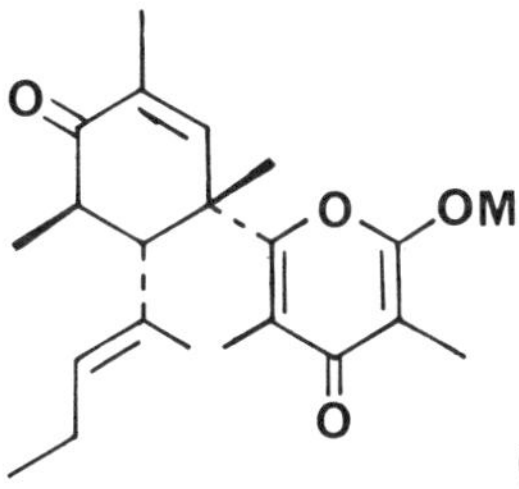 (**94**)

Several other nudibranchs have given extracts having antimicrobial activity. Since most molluscs derive their secondary metabolites from dietary sources, it might be assumed that identification and collection of the primary source might prove most efficient for the chemist. While this is true of small molluscs eating large sponges [75], the reverse is true when the mollusc concentrates interesting molecules from small algae [68].

## 6 ANTIBIOTICS FROM WORMS

For the purposes of this review, I will consider the Annelida (segmented worms), Sipunculida (peanut worms), Platyhelminthes (flatworms), Nemertinea (ribbon worms) and Enteropneusta (acorn worms) under a single heading. While the biologist may consider this practice unacceptable, the chemical constituents isolated from worms may be related to their food supply, which need not be species specific, and not to their biosynthetic capabilities, which should be species or genus specific.

There are relatively few reports of the chemical constituents of worms, but of these few studies, all report the isolation of brominated phenols. Simple brominated phenols are best considered as antiseptic compounds, since their antifungal and antibacterial properties are coupled with toxicity which prevents their use as internal medicines.

In 1967, Ashworth and Cormier [76] isolated 2,6-dibromo-phenol **(95)** from the hemichordate *Balanoglossus biminiensis.* Both 2,6-dibromophenol **(95)** and 2,4,6-tribromophenol **(96)** were subsequently isolated from a mud-dwelling tube worm, *Phoronopsis viridis* [77]. The marine anelid *Thelepus setosus* was shown to contain 3,5-dibromo-4-hydroxybenzyl alcohol **(97)**, 3,5-dibromo-4-hydroxybenzaldehyde **(98)**, *bis*-(3,5-dibromo-4-hydroxyphenyl) methane **(99)**, thelepin **(100)** and thelephenol **(101)**. All are brominated phenols except thelepin **(100)**, which resembles griseofulvin **(102)** in both structure and antifungal activity [78]. Higa and Scheuer [79] have isolated 2,4,6-tribromophenol **(96)** from the hemichordate *Ptychodera flava laysanica,* together with tetrabromohydroquinone **(103)**, tribromohydroquinone **(104)** and dimeric and trimeric ethers derived from **(103)** and **(104)**. Although the latter compounds are all brominated phenols, it is not known whether these compounds have antimicrobial properties.

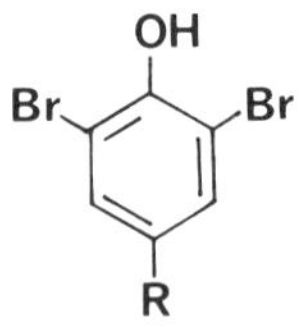

**(95)** R = H
**(96)** R = Br
**(97)** R = $CH_2OH$
**(98)** R = CHO

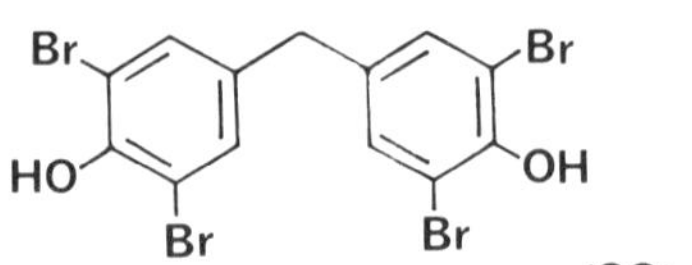

**(99)**

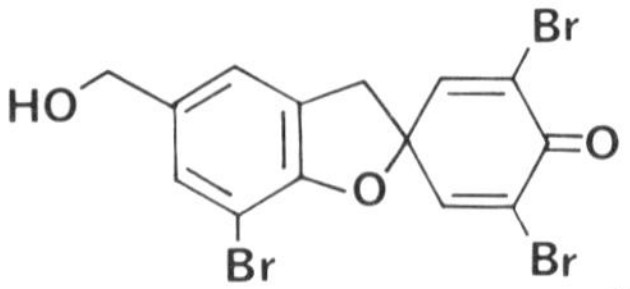

**(100)**

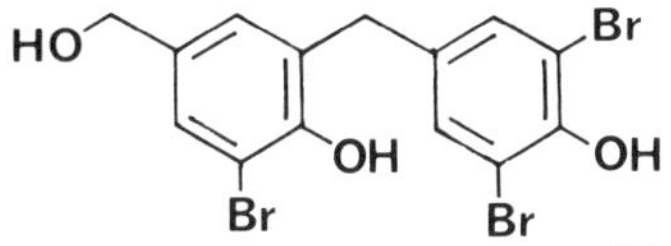

HO Br OH OH Br Br (101)

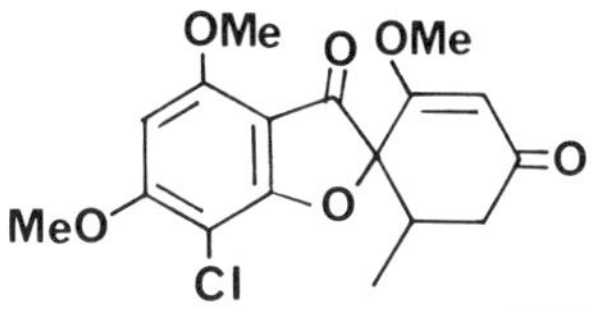

OMe O OMe O MeO O Cl (102)

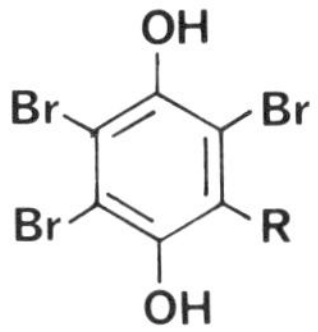

OH Br Br Br R OH

(103) R = Br

(104) R = H

## 7 ANTIBIOTICS FROM TUNICATES

Very few tunicates have been studied by natural products chemists. Fenical [80] found that a tunicate of the genus *Aplidium* contained large quantities of geranyl hydroquinone **(105)**. Geranyl hydroquinone **(105)** has subsequently been found to inhibit the growth of *S. aureus* and *Candida albicans*.

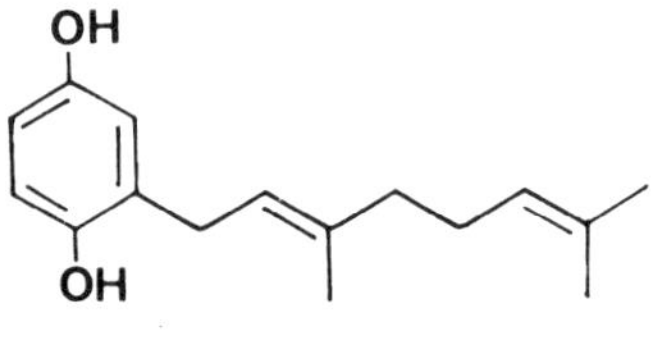

OH

OH

**(105)**

## 8 ANTIBIOTICS FROM ALGAE

The isolation and identification of antibiotics from algae has proceeded more rapidly than similar studies on invertebrates. This is not surprising, since there is a much better background knowledge of algae than of invertebrates. The antibiotic screening data in the literature have been recorded for individual species and may even record results for several extraction solvents. These data, coupled with better collection data for algal species. often allow the chemist to obtain material without resort to screening in the field.

The antibiotic activity of many marine algae can be attributed to the production of brominated phenols. Most, if not all, species of *Polysiphonia* (Rhodomelaceae–red algae) contain brominated phenols which are responsible for antibacterial activity. In 1955, Saito and Ando [81] described the isolation of

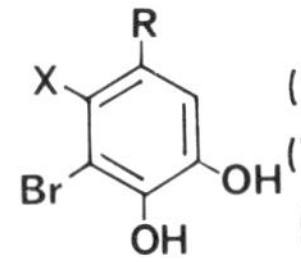

**(106)** R = CHO X = H
**(109)** R = CHO X = Br
**(110)** R = $CH_2OMe$ X = Br
**(112)** R = $CH_2OH$ X = Br
**(117)** R = $CH_2OH$ X = H
**(118)** R = $CH_2OEt$ X = Br
**(119)** R = $CH_2OPr$ X = Br

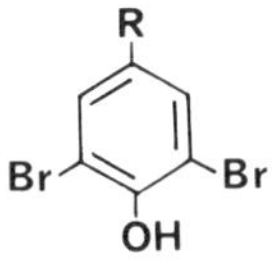

**(111)** R = $CH_2$
**(115)** R = $CH_2COOH$
**(116)** R = $CH_2COCOOH$

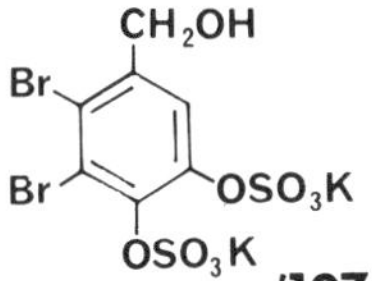

**(107)** 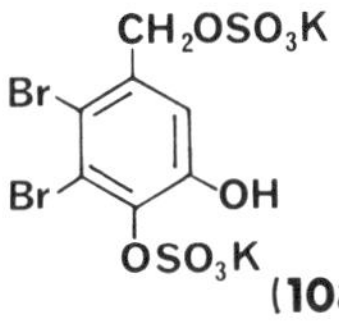 **(108)** 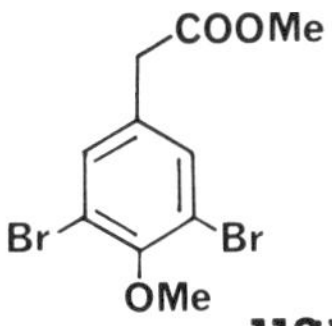 **(113)**

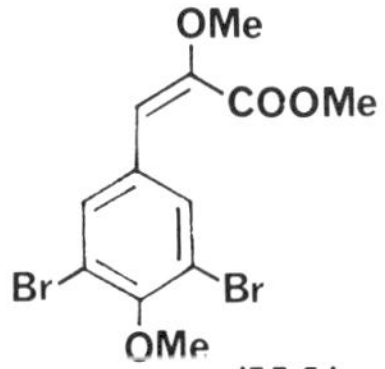

**(114)** 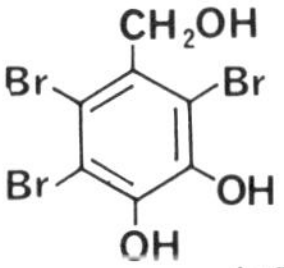 **(120)**

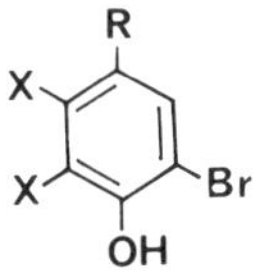

**(121)** R = $CH_2OH$ X = Br
**(122)** R = CHO X = Br
**(123)** R = $CH_2OH$ X = H
**(124)** R = CHO X = H

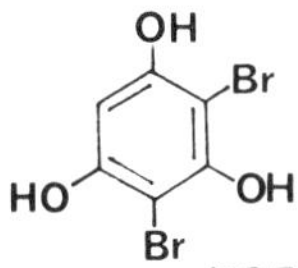

**(125)** 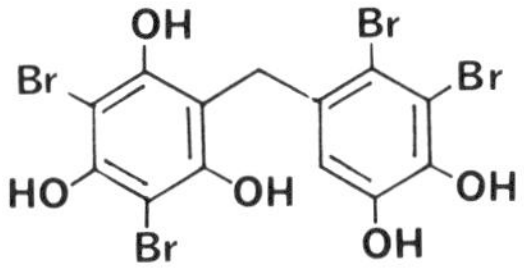 **(126)**

5-bromo-3,4-dihydroxybenzaldehyde (**106**) from *Polysiphonia morrowii.* A report [82] that *P. fastigiata* (syn. *P. lanosa*) contained the dipotassium salt of 2,3-dibromo-4,5-dihydroxybenzyl alcohol 4,5-disulphate (**107**) was later shown to be incorrect, and the structure was reassigned [83] as the dipotassium salt of the 1′,4-disulphate of 2,3-dibromo-4,5-dihydroxybenzyl alcohol (**108**). In 1966, Katsui *et al.* [84] isolated 2,3-dibromo-4,5-dihydroxybenzaldehyde (**109**) and 2,3-dibromo-4,5-dihydroxy-1′-methoxytoluene (**110**) from *Rhodomela larix.* It is significant that the algae had been soaked in methanol for one month, which might have caused the conversion of the corresponding benzyl alcohol to the methyl ether (**110**). Craigie and Greunig [85] identified 3,5-dibromo-4-hydroxybenzyl alcohol (**111**) and 2,3-dibromo-4,5-dihydroxybenzyl alcohol (**112**) in both *Odonthalia dentata* and *Rhodomela confervoides* after treatment of the extracts to hydrolyze any sulphate esters. Kurata *et al.* [86] have found 2,3-dibromo-4,5-dihydroxybenzyl alcohol (**112**), the corresponding 1′-methyl ether (**110**), and the 1′,4-disulphate dipotassium salt (**108**) in *Odonthalia corymbifera.* Examination of the red alga *Halopytis incurvus* resulted in the isolation of methyl 3,5-dibromo-4-methoxyphenylacetate (**113**) and methyl 3,5-dibromo-2′,4-dimethoxycinnamate (**114**), which probably resulted from diazomethane treatment of 3,5-dibromo-4-hydroxyphenyl acetic acid (**115**) and 3,5-dibromo-4-hydroxyphenylpyruvic acid (**116**), respectively [87]. In 1974, two research groups [88, 89] surveyed large numbers of red algae for the presence of simple brominated phenols. The brominated phenols were identified by combined gas chromatography-mass spectrometry of the per-trimethylsilyl ethers. Since each of the extracts was subjected to an extensive work-up procedure prior to silylation, it is not really possible to determine which compounds were originally present in the algae. The ethers are almost certainly artifacts [90], and other bromophenols might well exist as sulphates, rather than free phenols, in the algae [91]. Since the dipotassium-disulphate (**108**) was shown [88] to be inactive and the algae were shown to inhibit bacterial growth, it would seem at first sight that the algae must contain free bromophenols. One cannot, however, discount the possibility that hydrolysis of the sulphate esters occurs as a response to injury, in which case one cannot predict the bromophenol content of the living plant. The antibacterial activities of (**106**), (**109**), (**111**), (**112**) and (**117**) against *B. subtilis, E. coli, Sarcina pelagia, Serratia marinorubra,* and *Vibrio phytoplankton* have been reported [88]. In a recent study, the per-methylated products of (**108**), the corresponding ethyl ether (**118**), 2,4-dibromo-1,3,5-trihydroxybenzene (**125**) and 3,5,5′,6′-tetrabromo-2,4,6,3′,4′-pentahydroxydiphenyl methane (**126**) were obtained from *Rytiphlea tinctoria,* with (**125**) and (**126**) being obtained from a collection from Brittany and (**112**) and (**118**) from a Mediterranean sample. The distribution of simple brominated phenols among the red algae is summarized in Table 8.1.

**Table 8.1**
Brominated phenols from red algae

| Algae | Compound(s) | Reference(s) |
|---|---|---|
| *Antithamnion plumula* | **110, 117** | 89 |
| *Brongniartella byssoides* | **108, 117** | 92 |
| *Calothrix brevissima* | **111, 112, 120-122** | 93 |
| *Ceramium rubrum* | **110, 117** | 89 |
| *Corallina officinalis* | **117** | 89 |
| *Cystoclonium purpureum* | **109** | 89 |
| *Fucus vesiculosus* | **111, 112, 118** | 94 |
| *Halopitys incurvus* | **108, 115-117, 123** | 87 |
| *Odonthalia corymbifera* | **108, 110, 112** | 86 |
| *O. detata* | **106, 109-112, 117, 118, 124** | 89 |
| *O. floccosa* | **110, 117** | 91 |
| *Phycodrys rubens* | **110** | 89 |
| *Polysiphonia brodiaei* | **108-110, 112, 117, 123** | 88 |
| *P. elongata* | **106, 108, 109, 112** | 88 |
| *P. fruticulosa* | **108, 109, 112, 123** | 88 |
| *P. lanosa* | **106, 108-112, 117-120** | 82, 88 |
| *P. morrowii* | **106** | 81 |
| *P. nigra* | **108, 109, 112** | 88 |
| *P. nigrescens* | **106, 108-110, 112, 117, 119, 123** | 88 |
| *P. thuyoides* | **108, 109, 112** | 88 |
| *P. urceolata* | **106, 110, 111, 123** | 88 |
| *P. violacea* | **108, 109, 112** | 88 |
| *Rhodomela confervoides* | **109-112** | 89 |
| *R. larix* | **108-110** | 84, 91 |
| *R. subfusca* | **108, 109, 112, 120** | 88 |
| *Rytiphlea tinctoria* | **112, 118, 125, 126** | 95 |
| *Vidalia volubilis* | **108** | 96 |

Red algae of the genus *Laurencia* contain sesquiterpene phenols and brominated phenols as their antibiotic metabolites. Laurinterol (**83**) and debromolaurinterol (**127**) were first isolated from *Laurencia intermedia* [97] and have subsequently been isolated from *L. nipponica, L. okamurai, L. pacifica, L. johnstonii* and several other *Laurencia* species [98]. Both compounds can also be obtained from the sea hare *Aplysia californica* [68], which grazes on *Laurencia* species. Laurinterol (**83**) and debromolaurinterol (**127**) both inhibit *S. aureus, M. smegmatis* and *C. albicans* [99]. Laurinterol (**83**) is an order of magnitude more active than debromolaurinterol (**127**) against *S. aureus* and *M.*

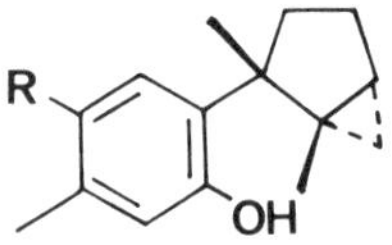

**(83)** R = Br
**(127)** R = H

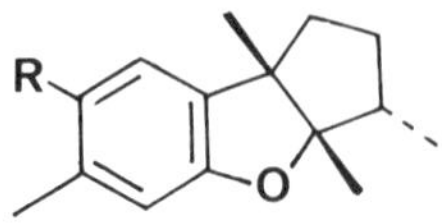

**(84)** R = Br
**(128)** R = H

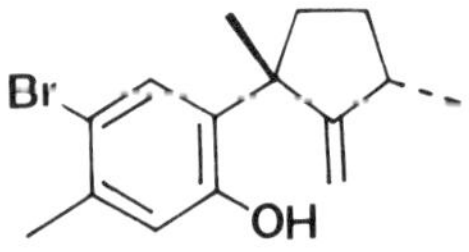

**(129)**

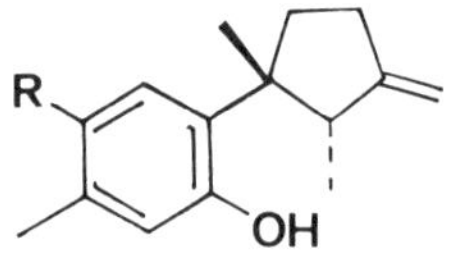

**(130)** R = H
**(131)** R = Br

*smegmatis*, but neither inhibit *E. coli* or *Salmonella choleraesius*. Under mild acid conditions, laurinterol **(83)** and debromolaurinterol **(127)** were converted into aplysin **(84)** and debromoaplysin **(128)**, respectively [100]. Neither cyclic ether inhibits the growth of *S. aureus* [101]. A formal synthesis of (±)-laurinterol in low yield has been reported (Scheme 8.1) [102]. Other related phenols have been isolated and identified. Isolaurinterol **(129)** was found in *L. intermedia* [97]. 7-Hydroxylaurene **(130)** was found to be the major antimicrobial metabolite of *L. subopposita* [103], while 10-bromo-7-hydroxylaurene (or *allo*-laurinterol) **(131)** was found to be a constituent of *L. filiformis* [104] and a minor metabolite of *L. subopposita.* All three compounds form inactive cyclic ethers on treatment with acid.

A number of prenylated bromohydroquinones and corresponding mono-methyl ethers have been isolated from the calcareous green algea *Cymopolia barbata.* An ether extract of the alga inhibited gram positive and gram negative bacteria, yeasts and fungi [105].

The structures of cymopol **(132)** and its mono-methyl ether **(133)** were elucidated from spectral data, and cymopol **(132)** was synthetized in low yield. Cyclocymopol **(134)** and cyclocymopol methyl ether **(135)** may be regarded as derived from cymopol **(132)** and cymopol mono-methyl ether **(133)** by "bromonium-ion"-initiated cyclization of the geranyl sidechain. The structure of cyclocymopol mono-methyl ether acetate **(136)** was determined by X-ray analysis [106]. No antibiotic screening data are available for the pure compounds.

In the absence of screening data for the pure compounds, it is difficult to determine whether the polyphenolic compounds in brown algae are responsible for the antibiotic activity of some of these species. Many brown algae which are shown to inhibit bacterial growth contain polyphenolic compounds [108], but some of the algae known to contain polyphenolic compounds did not demon-

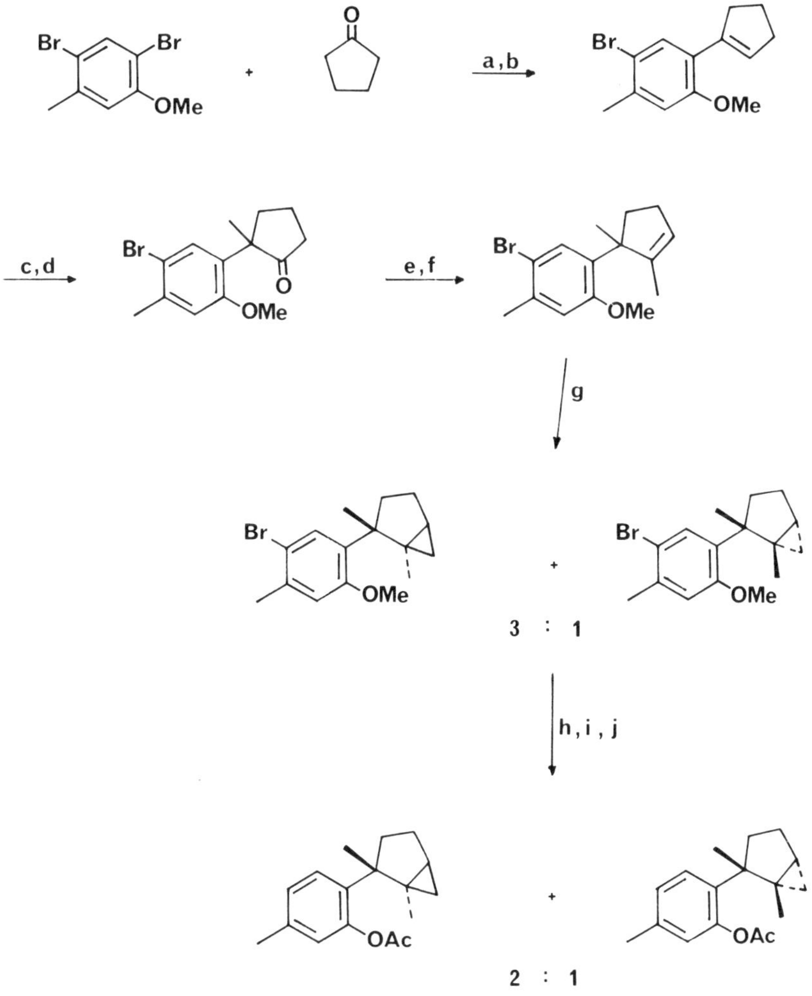

Br Br OMe + O a,b Br OMe

c,d Br O OMe e,f Br OMe

g

Br OMe + Br OMe

3 : 1

h, i, j

OAc + OAc

2 : 1

**Scheme 8.1**

Synthesis of debromolaurinterol acetate – a formal total synthesis of laurinterol **(83)** [102] a) PhLi, $Et_2O$ b) Δ c) $HCO_3H$ d) MeI, NaH, DME e) MeMgI, $Et_2O$ f) $POCl_3$, py g) $Et_2Zn$, $CH_2I_2$, $C_6H_6$ h) $LiAlH_4$, THF i) NaSEt, DMF

strate antibiotic activity. The phenols have also been accorded an antifouling role [109]. The chemical analysis of the phenolic compounds in brown algae has been studied by Craigie in Canada and Glombitza in Germany. The research, which is relatively complex, has recently been reviewed by Glombitza [108].

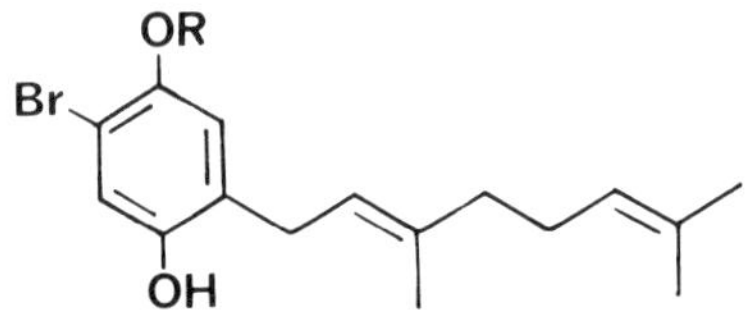

**(132)** R = H

**(133)** R = Me

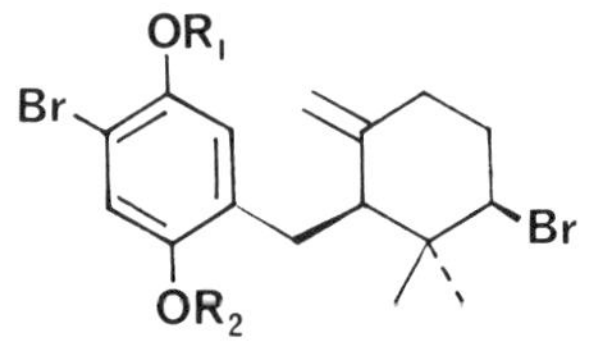

**(134)** $R_1 = R_2 = H$

**(135)** $R_1 = Me$ $R_2 = H$

**(136)** $R_1 = Me$ $R_2 = Ac$

The polyphenols found were phloroglucinol **(137)** [110] and polymers of phloroglucinol alone, or of phloroglucinol and pyrogallol, which may be linked by ether bridges, as in bifuhalol **(138)**, or by direct bonds between two aromatic rings, as in 2,4,6,2′,4′,6′-hexahydroxybiphenyl **(139)**. Dimers, trimers, tetramers and higher polymers too numerous to review in detail have all been described as peracetates.

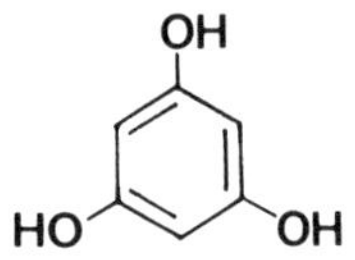

**(137)**

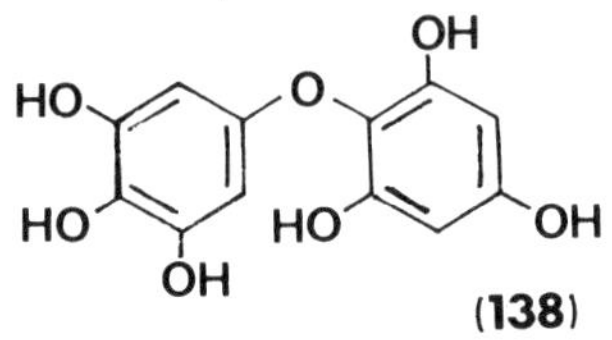

**(138)**

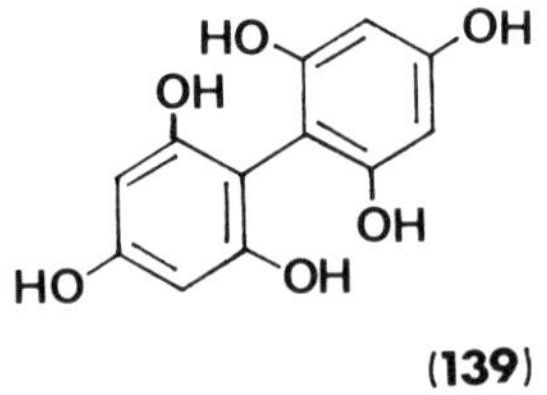

**(139)**

Two fungitoxic hydroquinones, zonarol (**140**) and isozonarol (**141**), were isolated from the brown alga *Dictyopteris zonaroides.* Both compounds inhibited the growth of *Phytophthora cinnamomi, Rhizoctonia solani, Sclerotinia sclerotiorum* and *Sclerotium rolfii,* which are all plant pathogenic fungi. The structures of these compounds were determined by interpretation of spectral data by the conversion of both compounds to an epimeric mixture of dihydrotauranic acids (**142**) [111]. Zonarol (**140**) and isozonarol (**141**) have been synthesized from the ketol (**143**) by a stereoselective route (Scheme 8.2) [112].

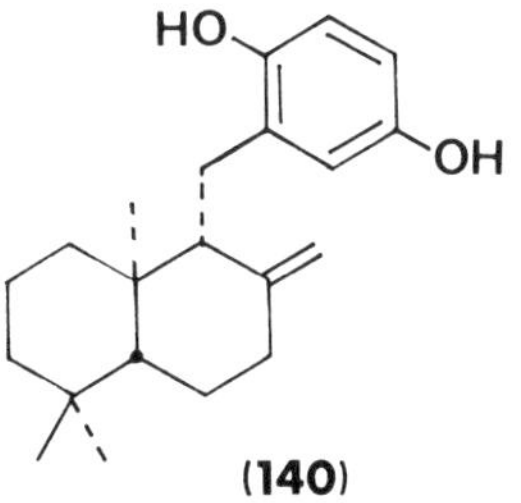

HO, OH

(**140**)

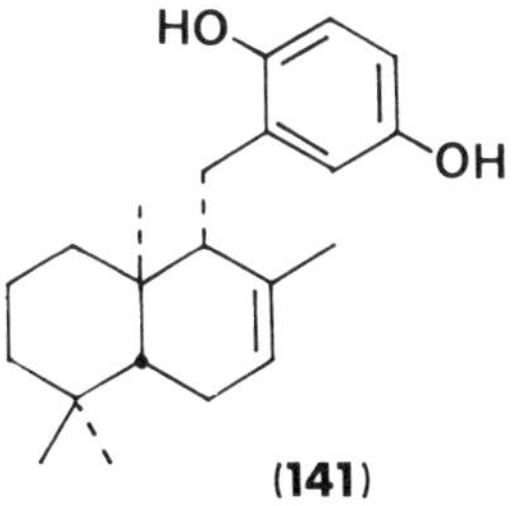

HO, OH

(**141**)

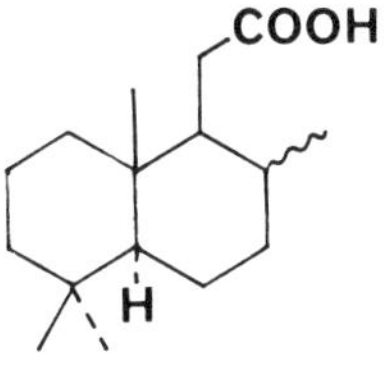

COOH, H

(**142**)

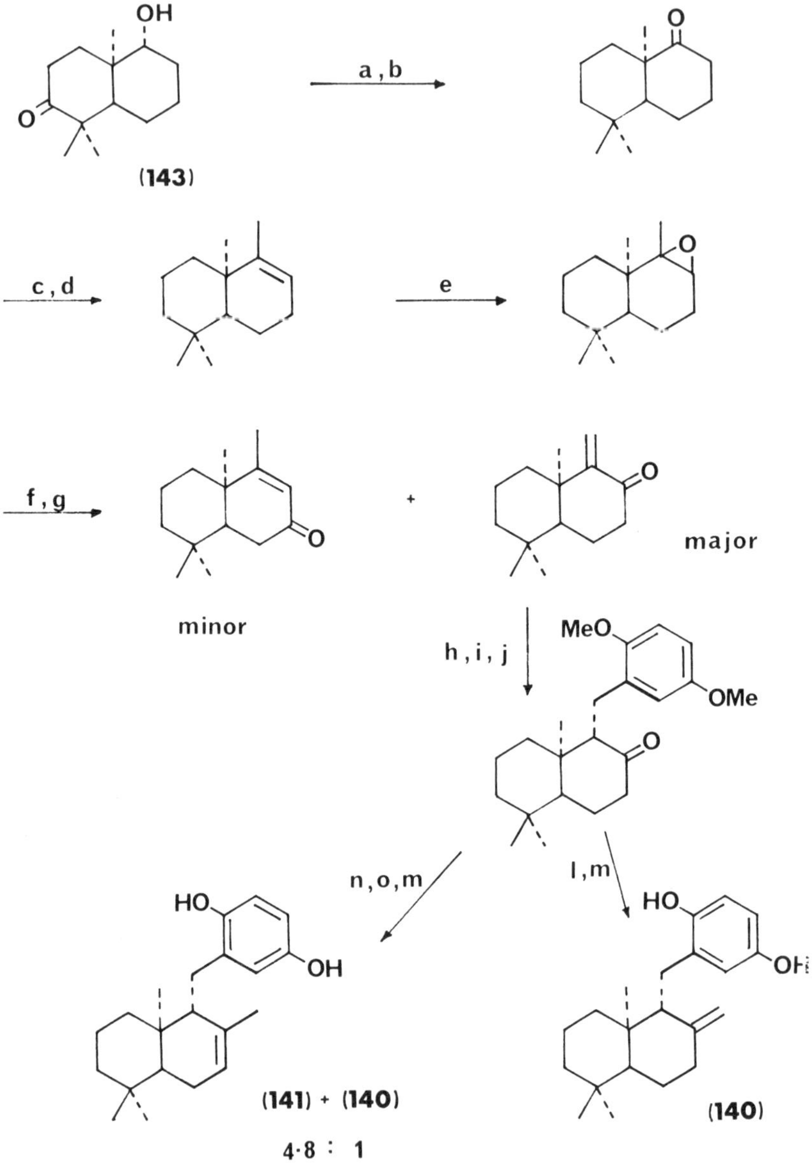

OH

a, b

O

O

(**143**)

c, d

e

O

f, g

O

+

O

major

minor

h, i, j

MeO

OMe

O

n, o, m

l, m

HO

OH

HO

OH

(**141**) + (**140**)

4·8 : 1

(**140**)

Scheme 8.2

Synthesis of zonarol (**140**) and isozonarol (**141**) [112] a) $N_2H_4$, KOH, DEG, Δ b) $CrO_3$ (Jones') c) MeLi, $Et_2O$ d) Δ, DMSO e) MCPBA, $Na_2HPO_4$, $CHCl_3$ f) $LiN(n\text{Pr})_2$, THF, Δ g) $CrO_3.py_2$, $CHCl_3$ h) 2,5-dimethoxyphenyl-magnesium bromide, DME i) $Ac_2O$ j) KOH, MeOH l) $CH_2PPh_3$ m) LiSBu, HMPA n) MeLi, $Et_2O$ o) Δ, DMSO

Pachydictyol A (**85**), isolated from the brown alga *Pachydictyon coriaceum*, was found to have mild antibiotic activity against *S. aureus*. The structure of pachydictyol A (**85**) was determined by X-ray analysis [71].

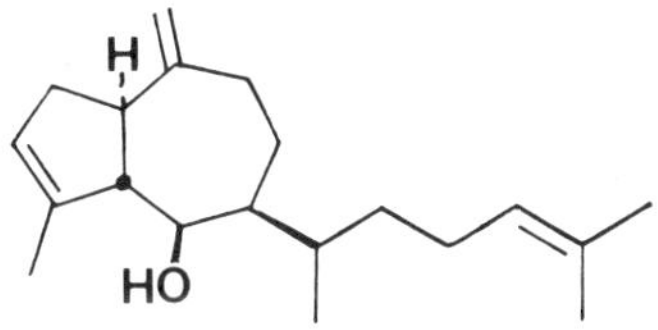

**(85)**

The sesquiterpene cycloeudesmol (**144**) was isolated from *Chondria oppositiclada* [113]. Cycloeudesmol (**144**) inhibited the growth of *Staphylococcus aureus* (10-50 μg/ml), *Mycobacterium smegmatis* (10-50 μg/ml) and *Candida albicans* (10-50 μg/ml). Cycloeudesmol (**144**) was converted into (±)-δ-selinene (**145**) on treatment with *p*-toluene sulphonic acid in benzene.

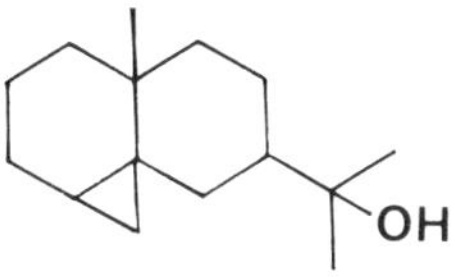

**(144)** 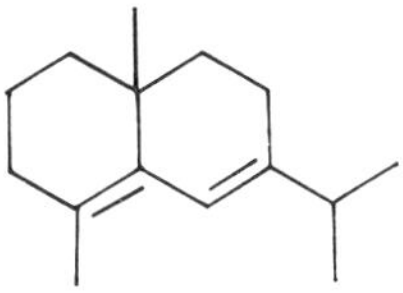 **(145)**

While the brominated phenols are clearly the most active antimicrobial compounds in the *Laurencia* sp., other compounds have been observed to inhibit the growth of microorganisms. 3β-Bromo-8-epicaparrapi oxide (**146**), obtained from *Laurencia obtusa* [114], was mildly active against *S. aureus*. Prepacifenol (**147**), a metabolite of *L. filiformis* [115] and the precursor of pacifenol (**148**) found in *L. pacifica*, inhibited the growth of *S. aureus* (10-100 μg/ml) and *M. smegmatis*. It is interesting to note that neither pacifenol (**148**) [116] nor prepacifenol epoxide (**149**) [117] showed antibiotic activity, suggesting that the activity of prepacifenol was associated with the allylic epoxide functionality.

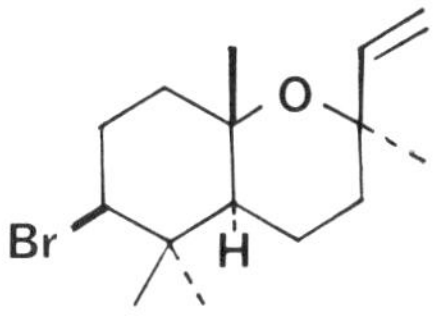

**(146)** 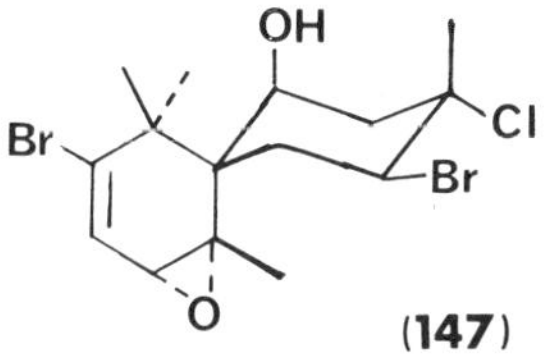 **(147)**

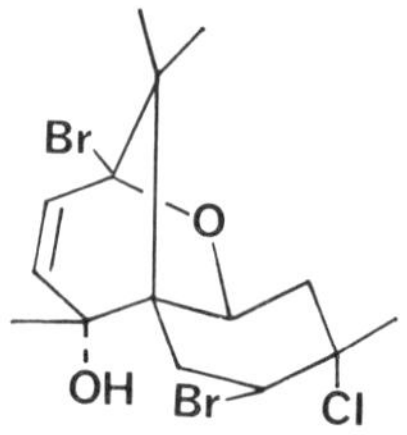

(148) 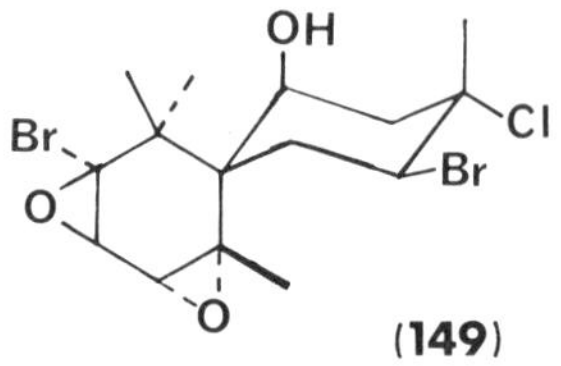 (149)

Chondriol (**150**) exhibited antiviral and mild antibacterial activity against *S. aureus* and *M. smegmatis.* Chondriol (**150**) was isolated from a red alga originally identified as *Chondria oppositiclada* but later reassigned as *Laurencia yamada* [118]. The structure of chondriol was determined by X-ray analysis [119].

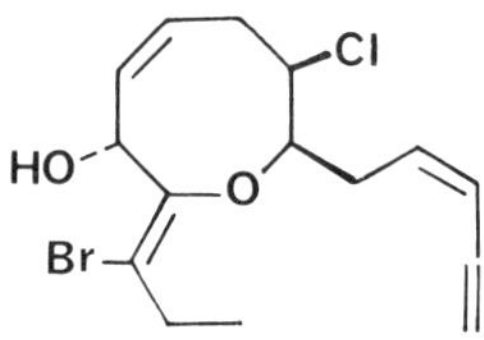

(150)

The red algae of the family Bonnemaisoniaceae all appear to possess strong antimicrobial activity. In these laboratories, it has been found that small quantities of crude extracts of *Asparagopsis taxiformis* inhibited all bacterial growth on an agar plate, since the active compounds were volatile and were distributed across the plate by gaseous diffusion, rather than diffusion through the enriched agar culture medium. Both Fenical and Moore have studied *A. taxiformis* and have shown that the natural products obtained depended on the isolation procedure employed. Fenical obtained seven polyhalogenated acetones and four polyhalogenated 3-buten-2-ones from chloroform extracts of *A. taxiformis*, with 1,1,3-tribromoacetone (**151**) and a tribromo-3-buten-2-one (**152**) as the major constituents [120]. Moore obtained the volatile constituents of *A. taxiformis* and found bromoform to be the major constituent, together with halogenated acroleins, propenes, acetones and 3-buten-2-ones [121]. Moore subsequently identified seventy-four halogenated metabolites of *A. taxiformis* from a dichloromethane extract [122]. Further research by Fenical has shown that halogenated acetic acids were present in aqueous extracts of *A. taxiformis* and that the corresponding ethyl esters were found in ethanolic extracts [123].

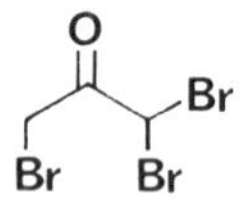

(151) 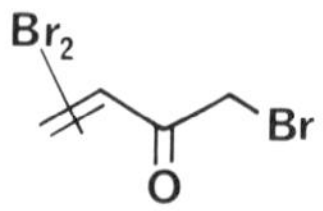 (152) 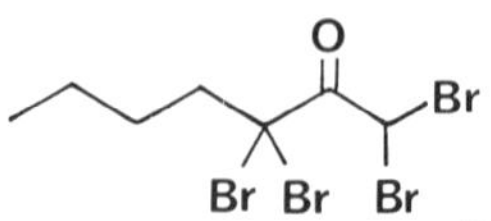 (153)

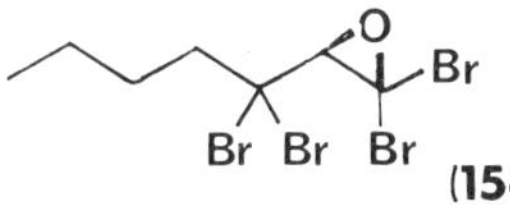

**(154)** 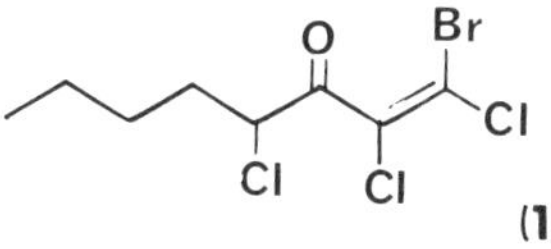 **(155)**

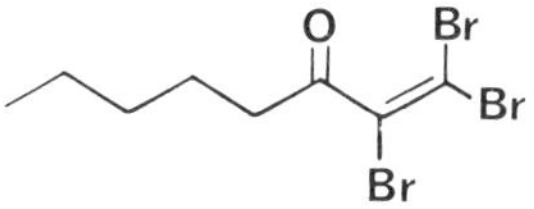

**(156)**

Halogenated methyl alkyl ketones and alkyl vinyl ketones have been described as the major secondary metabolites of *Bonnemaisonia hamifera, Ptilonia australasica, Delisia fimbriata, Bonnemaisonia asparagoides,* and *Bonnemaisonia nootkana.* The major metabolite of *B. hamifera* was shown to be 1,1,3,3-tetrabromo-2-heptanone (**153**), which inhibited the growth of *B. subtilis* and showed low activity against *S. cerevisiae* and *P. atroventum* [124]. The major metabolite of *Bonnemaisonia nootkana* was found to be the epoxide (**154**) [125]. *Bonnemaisonia asparagoides* [126], *Delisia fimbriata* [127] and *Ptilonia australasica* [128] were all shown to contain polyhalogenated l-octen-3-ones. The major constituent of *B. asparagoides* was E-1-bromo-1,2,4-trichloro-1-octen-3-one (**155**), which showed significant antibacterial activity against *S. aureus.* The major linear halogenated ketone in *Delisia fimbriata* was 1,1,2-tribromo-1-octen-3-one (**156**), which showed mild antifungal activity.

Two groups [128, 129] have reported that the antibiotic activity of *Delisia fimbriata* could be traced to a mixture of lactones called "fimbrolides". The structure of the major component (**157**) of the mixture was determined by X-ray analysis of a methanol addition product (**158**). Compounds in which chlorine or iodine replaced bromine at the methylene bond (E or Z) and where the acetoxy group was replaced by hydroxy or hydrogen have also been described.

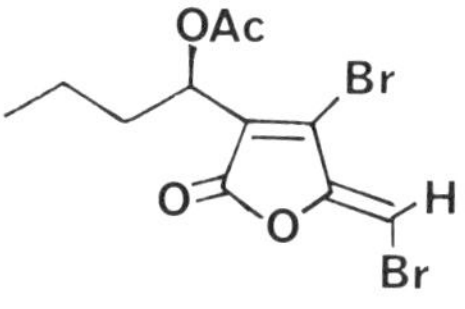

**(157)** 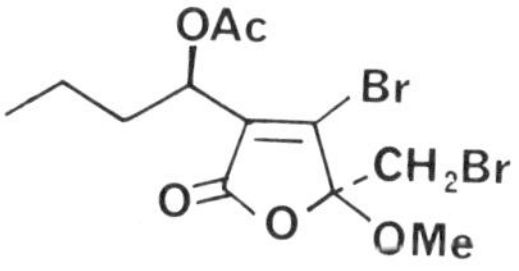 **(158)**

In all of these studies on polyhalogenated metabolites from algae of the family Bonnemaisoniaceae, most compounds were detected by gc-ms and only a few compounds have been purified. Quantitative antimicrobial screening is planned when synthetic materials become available.

The antibiotic activity of some algae has been attributed to simple fatty acids such as capric acid, lauric acid, myristic acid, palmitic acid, stearic acid, oleic acid, linoleic acid and acrylic acid [130]. With the exception of acrylic acid, there seems to be little validity to these results, although it has been suggested that the autoxidation products of fatty acids may have antimicrobial activity. Acrylic acid was detected in *Phaeocystis pouchetti*, which is an organism responsible for phytoplankton blooms in Antartica [131]. The acrylic acid and dimethyl suphide were shown to be produced [153] by enzymatic hydrolysis of dimethyl-β-propiothetin (**159**), so that the smell of dimethyl sulphide may be used as an indication of acrylic acid-producing algae. Glombitza [133] has recently screened a series of algae for their concentrations of acrylic acid and dimethyl-β-propiothetin. The transfer of either acrylic acid or dimethyl-β-propiothetin through the marine food chain to the Antarctic penguins was shown to be the cause of antibacterial activity in the gastrointestinal tract of the penguin [134].

$$Me_2\overset{+}{S}CH_2CH_2COO^-$$

**(159)**

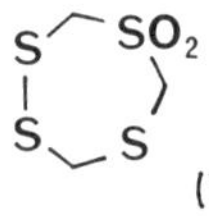

**(160)** 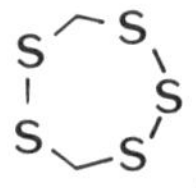 **(161)** 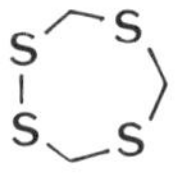 **(162)**

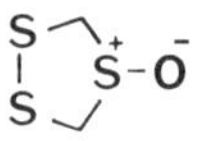

**(163)** 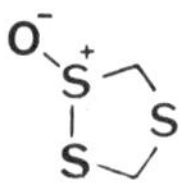 **(164)** 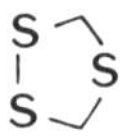 **(165)**

Elemental sulphur was isolated from *Ceramium rubrum* and shown to be the compound responsible for inhibition of the growth of *B.subtilis* [135]. The sulphur content of a number of marine algae was determined, but only the brown alga *Chordaria flagelliformis* contained a significant quantity of sulphur, about one-third that found in *C. rubrum.*

The cyclic polysulphides from *Chondria californica* were isolated and identified by tracing the antibiotic activity of the crude extracts [136]. The compounds would undoubtedly be overlooked in a purely chemical study of the alga, since they appear to be solvent impurities in the $^1H$ nmr spectrum of a crude extract. The major sulphur-containing constituent of *C. californica* was the sulphone (**160**), which was also the most effective antimicrobial agent. Both lenthionine (**161**) and 1,2,4,6-tetrathiepane (**162**) had previously been found in the mushroom *Lentinus edodes.* Two related sulphoxides (**163**) and (**164**), which could be synthesized from 1,2,4-trithiolane (**165**), were also found to be mildly antibiotic. The sulphone (**160**) inhibited the growth of *Vibrio anguillarum, Proteus mirabilis, Salmonella typhimurium* and *E. coli* at 10 μg/ml. Other species of the genus *Chondria* were examined, but they possessed neither antimicrobial activity nor cyclic polysulphides.

## 9 CONCLUSION

In reviewing the antibiotics from marine organisms, many instances have been found where chemists have studied organisms which were reported to show antibiotic activity and have isolated pure compounds which might be the active constituents but which do not appear to have been tested for antibiotic activity. One may therefore confidently suspect that there are many more marine natural products having antimicrobial properties than have been recorded in this review.

## REFERENCES

[1] P. R. Burkholder, *in* 'Biology and Geology of Coral Reefs' (O. A. Jones and R. Endean, eds.) Vol. II, *Biology*, p. 117. Academic Press, 1973.

[2] See references 1 and (a) P. R. Burkholder and G. M. Sharma, *Lloydia*, **32**, 466 (1969); (b) J. Aubert and J. P. Gambarotta, *Rev. Intern. Oceangr. Med.*, **25**, 39 (1972); (c) I. S. Hornsey and D. Hide, *Br. Phycol. J.*, **9**, 353 (1974); (d) P. D. Shaw, W. O. McClure, G. Van Blaricom, J. Sims, W. Fenical and J. Rude, *in* 'Proceedings, Food-Drugs from the Sea 1974' (H. H. Webber and G. D. Ruggieri, eds.), p. 429; Marine Technology Society, Washington, D.C., 1976.

[3] P. R. Burkholder, R. M. Pfister and F. M. Leitz, *Appl. Microbiol.*, **14**, 649 (1966).

[4] F. M. Lovell, *J. Amer. Chem. Soc.*, **88**, 4510 (1966).

[5] S. Hanessian and J. S. Kaltenbronn, *J. Amer. Chem. Soc.*, **88**, 4509 (1966).

[6] R. J. Anderson, M. S. Wolfe and D. J. Faulkner, *Mar. Biol.*, **27**, 281 (1974).

[7] R. D. Hamilton and K. E. Austin, *Antonie van Leeuwenhoek*, **33**, 257 (1967).

[8] M. J. Gauthier, J. M. Shewan, D. M. Gibson and J. V. Lee, *J. Gen. Microbiol.*, **87**, 211 (1975).

[9] S. J. Wratten, M. S. Wolfe, R. J. Andersen and D. J. Faulkner, *Antimicrobial Agents, Chemotherapy*, **11**, 411 (1977).

[10] I. C. Wells, *J. Biol. Chem.*, **196**, 321 (1952).

[11] T. Okazaki, T. Kitahara and Y. Okami, *J. Antibiotics*, **28**, 176 (1975).

[12] T. Kitahara, H. Naganawa, T. Okazaki, Y. Okami and H. Umezawa, *J. Antibiotics*, **28**, 280 (1975).

[13] Y. Okami, T. Okazaki, T. Kitahara and H. Umezawa, *J. Antibiotics*, **29**, 1019 (1976); Y. Okami, personal communication.

[14] M. Pedersen and N. Fries, *Z. fur Pflanzenphysiol.*, **82**, 363 (1977).

[15] G. M. Sharma and P. R. Burkholder, *Tetrahedron Letters*, 4147 (1967).

[16] G. M. Sharma, B. Vig and P. R. Burkholder, *J. Org. Chem.*, **35**, 2823 (1970).

[17] R. J. Andersen and D. J. Faulkner, *Tetrahedron Letters*, 1175 (1973).

[18] G. J. Kasperek, T. C. Bruice, M. Yagi, N. Kaubisch and D. M. Jerina, *J. Amer. Chem. Soc.*, **94**, 7876 (1972).

[19] R. J. Andersen, D. McIntyre and D. J. Faulkner, unpublished results.

[20] S. M. Kupchan, D. C. Fessler, M. A. Eakin and T. J. Giacobbe, *Science*, **168**, 376 (1970).

[21] E. Fattorusso, L. Minale and G. Sodano, *J. Chem. Soc. Perkin*, I, 16 (1972).

[22] W. Fulmore, G. E. Van Lear, G. O. Morton and R. D. Mills, *Tetrahedron Letters,* 4551 (1970).
[23] P. R. Berquist and W. D. Hartman, *Mar. Biol.,* **3**, 247 (1969).
[24] D. B. Cosulich and F. M. Lovell, *Chem. Commun.,* 397 (1971); L. Mazzarella and R. Puliti, *Gazz. Chem. Ital.,* **102**, 391 (1972).
[25] R. J. Andersen and D. J. Faulkner, *J. Amer. Chem. Soc.,* **97**, 936 (1975).
[26] M. F. Stempien, J. S. Chib, R. F. Nigrelli and R. A. Mierzwa, in *Proceedings, Food-Drugs from the Sea Conference,* p. 105. Marine Technology Society, Washington, D.C., 1973.
[27] G. E. Krejcarek, R. H. White, L. P. Hager, W. O. McClure, R. D. Johnson, K. L. Rinehart, Jr., J. A. McMillan, I. C. Paul, P. D. Shaw and R. C. Brusca, *Tetrahedron Letters,* 507 (1975).
[28] G. M. Sharma and B. Vig, *Tetrahedron Letters,* 1715 (1972).
[29] G. M. Sharma, B. Vig and P. R. Burkholder, in *Proceedings, Food-Drugs from the Sea Conference,* p. 307. Marine Technology Society, Washington, D.C., 1970.
[30] L. Minale, G. Cimino, S. de Stefano and G. Sodano, *Prog. Chem. Org. Nat. Prod.,* **33**, 1 (1976).
[31] S. Forenza, L. Minale, R. Riccio and E. Fattorusso, *Chem. Commun.,* 1129 (1971).
[32] See also E. E. Garcia, L. E. Benjamin and R. I. Fryer, *Chem Commun.,* 78 (1973).
[33] M. F. Stempien, Jr., R. F. Nigrelli and J. S. Chib, 164th A.C.S. Meeting, Abstracts, MEDI 21 (1972).
[34] G. M. Sharma and P. R. Burkholder, *Chem. Commun.,* 151 (1971).
[35] J. T. Baker, *Pure Appl. Chem.,* **48**, 35 (1976).
[36] G. E. Van Lear, G. O. Morton and W. Fulmor, *Tetrahedron Letters,* 299 (1973).
[37] L. Minale, R. Riccio and G. Sodano, *Tetrahedron,* **30**, 1341 (1974).
[38] B. J. Burreson, C. Christophersen and P. J. Scheuer, *Tetrahedron,* **31**, 2015 (1975).
[39] F. Cafieri, E. Fattorusso, S. Magno, C. Santacroce and D. Sica, *Tetrahedron,* **29**, 4259 (1973); E. Fattorusso, S. Magno, L. Mayol, C. Santacroce and D. Sica, *Tetrahedron,* **30**, 3911 (1974); E. Fattorusso, S. Magno, L. Mayol, C. Santacroce and D. Sica, *Tetrahedron,* **31**, 269 (1975).
[40] C. Cimino, S. de Stefano, L. Minale and E. Fattorusso, *Tetrahedron,* **28**, 333 (1972).
[41] F. Cafieri, E. Fattorusso, C. Santacroce and L. Minale, *Tetrahedron,* **28**, 1579 (1972).
[42] D. J. Faulkner, *Tetrahedron Letters,* 3821 (1973).
[43] I. Rothberg and P. Shubiak, *Tetrahedron Letters,* 769 (1975).
[44] E. Fattorusso, L. Minale, G. Sodano and E. Trivellone, *Tetrahedron,* **27**, 3909 (1971).

[45] G. Cimino, S. de Stefano, L. Minale and E. Fattorusso, *Tetrahedron,* **27**, 4673 (1971).

[46] S. Jakowska and R. F. Nigrelli, *Ann. N.Y. Acad. Sci.,* **90**, 913 (1960).

[47] G. Cimino, S. de Stefano and L. Minale, *Tetrahedron,* 29, 2565 (1973).

[48] B. N. Ravi, T. R. Erdman and P. J. Scheuer, in *Proceedings, Food-Drugs from the Sea Conference 1974* (H. H. Webber and G. D. Ruggieri, eds.), p. 258. Marine Technology Society, Washington, D.C., 1976.

[49] B. N. Ravi, Ph.D., Thesis, U. of Hawaii (1976).

[50] M. F. Stempien, Jr., *Amer. Zool.,* **6**, 363 (1966).

[51] M. F. Stempien, Jr., J. S. Chib and R. A. Mierzwa, in *Proceedings, Food-Drugs from the Sea Conference 1974,* (H. H. Webber and G. D. Ruggieri, eds.) p. 268. Marine Technology Society, Washington, D.C., 1976.

[52] S. J. Wratten, D. J. Faulkner, K. Hirotsu and J. Clardy, *J. Amer. Chem. Soc.,* **99**, 2824 (1977); S. J. Wratten, W. H. Fenical, D. J. Faulkner and J. C. Wekell, *Tetrahedron Letters,* 1559 (1977).

[53] L. S. Ciereszko, D. H. Sifford and A. J. Weinheimer, *Ann N.Y. Acad. Sci.,* **90**, 917 (1960).

[54] A. J. Weinheimer and J. A. Matson, *Lloydia,* **38**, 378 (1975).

[55] M. Houssain and D. van der Helm, *Rec. Trav. Chim. Pays-Bas,* **88**, 1413 (1969).

[56] A. J. Weinheimer, J. A. Matson, D. van der Helm and M. Poling, *Tetrahedron Letters,* 1295 (1977).

[57] A. J. Weinheimer, R. E. Middlebrook, J. O. Bledsoe, Jr., W. E. Marsico and T. K. B. Karns, *Chem. Commun.,* 384 (1968); M. B. Houssain, A. F. Nicholas and D. van der Helm, *Chem. Commun.,* 385 (1968).

[58] L. S. Ciereszko and T. K. B. Karns, *Biology and Geology of Coral Reefs* (O. A. Jones and R. Endean, eds.). Academic Press, 1973.

[59] L. S. Ciereszko, in *Proceedings, Food-Drugs from the Sea 1974* (H. H. Webber and G. D. Ruggieri, eds.), p. 297. Marine Technology Society, Washington, D.C., 1976.

[60] F. McEnroe and W. H. Fenical, *Tetrahedron,* in press.

[61] F. J. Schmitz and E. D. Lorance, *J. Org. Chem.,* **36**, 719 (1971).

[62] B. Tursch, *Pure and Appl. Chem.,* **48**, 1 (1976).

[63] B. Tursch, J. C. Braekman, D. Daloze, P. Fritz, A. Kelecom, R. Karlsson and D. Losman, *Tetrahedron Letters,* 747 (1974).

[64] B. Tursch, J. C. Braekman, D. Daloze, M. Herin, R. Karlsson and D. Losman, *Tetrahedron,* **31**, 129 (1975).

[65] Y. M. Sheikh, G. Singy, M. Kaisin, H. Eggert, C. Djerassi, B. Tursch, D. Daloze and J. C. Braekman, *Tetrahedron,* **32**, 1171 (1976).

[66] P. R. Burkholder and L. M. Burkholder, *Science,* **127**, 1174 (1958).

[67] D. J. Faulkner and C. Ireland, in *Marine Natural Products Chemistry* (D. J. Faulkner and W. H. Fenical, eds.), p. 23, Plenum Press, 1977.

[68] M. O. Stallard and D. J. Faulkner, *Comp. Biochem. Physiol.,* **49B**, 25 (1974).
[69] M. O. Stallard and D. J. Faulkner, *Comp. Biochem. Physiol.,* **49B**, 37 (1974).
[70] D. J. Vanderah, unpublished observation.
[71] D. R. Hirschfeld, W. Fenical, G. H. Y. Lin, R. M. Wing, P. Radlick and J. J. Sims, *J. Amer. Chem. Soc.,* **95**, 4049 (1973).
[72] R. J. Andersen and D. J. Faulkner, in *Proceedings, Food-Drugs from the Sea Conference,* p. 111. Marine Technology Society, Washington, D.C., 1972.
[73] D. A. Evans, and R. Y. Wong, *J. Org. Chem.,* **42**, 350 (1977).
[74] C. Ireland and D. J. Faulkner, *Bio-org. Chem.* (in press).
[75] B. J. Burreson, P. J. Scheuer, J. Finer and J. Clardy, *J. Amer. Chem. Soc.,* **97**, 4763 (1975).
[76] R. B. Ashworth and M. J. Cromier, *Science,* **155**, 1588 (1967).
[77] Y. M. Sheikh and C. Djerassi, *Experientia,* **31**, 265 (1975).
[78] T. Higa and P. J. Scheuer, *Tetrahedron,* **31**, 2379 (1975).
[79] T. Higa and P. J. Scheuer, in *Marine Natural Chemistry,* (D. J. Faulkner and W. H. Fenical, eds.) p. 35. Plenum Press, New York, 1977.
[80] W. H. Fenical, in *Proceedings, Food-Drugs from the Sea, 1974,* (H. H. Webber and G. D. Ruggieri, eds.), p. 388. Marine Technology Society, Washington, D.C., 1976.
[81] T. Saito and Y. Ando, *Nippon Kaguka Zasshi,* **76**, 478 (1955).
[82] J. M. Hodgkin, J. S. Craigie and A. G. McInnes, *Can. J. Chem.,* **44**, 74 (1966).
[83] K.-W. Glombitza and H. Stoffelen, *Planta Med.,* **22**, 391 (1972).
[84] N. Katsui, Y. Suzuki, S. Kotamura and T. Irie, *Tetrahedron,* **23**, 1185 (1967).
[85] J. S. Craigie and D. E. Gruenig, *Science,* **157**, 1058 (1967).
[86] K. Kurata, T. Amiya and F. Yake, *Bull. Jap. Soc. Sci. Fish.,* **39**, 973 (1973).
[87] J.-M. Chautraine, G. Combaut and J. Teste, *Phytochem.,* **12**, 1793 (1973).
[88] K.-W. Glombitza, H. Stoffelen, U. Murawski, J. Bielaczek and H. Egge, *Planta Med.,* **25**, 105 (1974).
[89] M. Pedersen, P. Saenger and L. Fries, *Phytochem.,* **13**, 2273 (1974).
[90] H. Stoffelen, K.-W. Glombitza, U. Murawski, J. Bielaczek and H. Egge, *Planta Med.,* **22**, 396 (1972).
[91] B. Weinstein, T. L. Rold, C. E. Harrell, Jr., M. W. Burns and J. R. Waaland, *Phytochem.,* **14**, 2667 (1975).
[92] L. Fries, *Experientia,* **29**, 1436 (1973).
[93] M. Pedersen and E. Da Silva, *Planta,* **115**, 83 (1973).
[94] M. Pedersen and L. Fries, *Z. Pflanzen physiol.,* **74**, 272 (1975).

[95] A. M. Chevolet-Magueur, A. Cave, P. Potier, J. Teste, A. Chiaroni and C. Riche, *Phytochem.*, **15**, 767 (1976).

[96] J. Augier and M.-H. Henry, *Bull. Botan. Fr.*, **97**, 29 (1950).

[97] T. Irie, M. Suzuki, E. Kurosawa and T. Masamune, *Tetrahedron,* **26**, 3271 (1970).

[98] W. H. Fenical, personal communication.

[99] J. J. Sims, M. S. Donnell, J. V. Leary and G. H. Lacy, *Antimicrobial Agents and Chemotherapy,* **7**, 320 (1975).

[100] M. Suzuki, Y. Hayakawa and T. Irie, *Bull. Chem. Soc. Japan,* **42**, 3342 (1969).

[101] M. S. Wolfe, this laboratory.

[102] G. I. Feutrill, R. N. Mirrington and R. J. Nichols, *Aust. J. Chem.,* **26**, 345 (1973).

[103] S. J. Wratten and D. J. Faulkner, *J. Org. Chem.,* **42**, 3343 (1977).

[104] R. Kazlauskas, P. T. Murphy, R. J. Quinn and R. J. Wells, *Aust. J. Chem.,* **29**, 2533 (1976).

[105] N. G. Martinez, L. V. Rodriguez and C. Casillas, *Antimicrobial Agents and Chemistry,* 131 (1964).

[106] H.-E. Högberg, R. H. Thomson and T. J. King, *J.C.S., Perkin* I, 1696 (1976).

[107] I. S. Hornsey and D. Hide, *Br. Phycol. J.,* **9**, 353 (1974).

[108] K.-W. Glombitza, in *Marine Natural Products Chemistry* (D. J. Faulkner and W. H. Fenical, eds.), p. 191. Plenum Press, 1977.

[109] S. M. Al-ogily and E. W. Knight-Jones, *Nature,* **265**, 728 (1977).

[110] K.-W. Glombitza, H. U. Rosener, H. Vilter and H. W. Rauwald, *Planta Med.,* **24**, 301 (1973).

[111] W. H. Fenical, J. J. Sims, D. Squatrito, R. M. Wing and P. Radlick, *J. Org. Chem.,* **38**, 2383 (1973).

[112] S. C. Welch and A. S. C. P. Rao, *Tetrahedron Letters,* 505 (1977).

[113] W. Fenical and J. J. Sims, *Tetrahedron Letters,* 1137 (1974).

[114] D. J. Faulkner, *Phytochem.,* **15**, 1993 (1976).

[115] J. J. Sims, W. Fenical, R. M. Wing and P. Radlick, *J. Amer. Chem. Soc.,* **95**, 972 (1973).

[116] J. J. Sims, W. Fenical, R. M. Wing and P. Radlick, *J. Amer. Chem. Soc.,* **93**, 3774 (1971).

[117] D. J. Faulkner, M. O. Stallard and C. Ireland, *Tetrahedron Letters,* 3571 (1974).

[118] W. Fenical and J. N. Norris, *J. Phycol.,* **11**, 104 (1975).

[119] W. Fenical, K. B. Gifkins and J. Clardy, *Tetrahedron Letters,* 1507 (1974).

[120] W. Fenical, *Tetrahedron Letters,* 4463 (1974).

[121] B. J. Burreson, R. E. Moore and P. P. Roller, *Tetrahedron Letters,* 473 (1975).

[122] B. J. Burreson, R. E. Moore and P. P. Roller, *Agri. Food Cehm.*, **24**, 856 (1976); F. X. Woolard, R. E. Moore and P. P. Roller, *Tetrahedron*, **32**, 2843 (1976).

[123] O. J. McConnell and W. Fenical, *Phytochem*, **16**, 367 (1977).

[124] J. F. Suida, G. R. Van Blaricom, P. D. Shaw, R. D. Johnson, R. H. White, L. P. Hager and K. L. Rinhart, Jr., *J. Amer. Chem. Soc.*, **97**, 937 (1975).

[125] O. J. McConnell and W. Fenical, *Tetrahedron Letters*, 4159 (1977).

[126] O. J. McConnell and W. Fenical, *Tetrahedron Letters*, 1851 (1977).

[127] A. F. Rose, J. A. Pettus, Jr. and J. J. Sims, *Tetrahedron Letters*, 1847 (1977).

[128] R. Kazlauskas, P. T. Murphy, R. J. Quinn and R. J. Wells, *Tetrahedron Letters*, 37 (1977).

[129] J. A. Pettus, Jr., R. M. Wing and J. J. Sims, *Tetrahedron Letters*, 41 (1977).

[130] K. Kamimoto, *Jap J. Bacteriol.*, **10**, 897 (1955); T. Katayama, in *Physiology and Biochemistry in Algae* (R. A. Lewin, ed.), p. 467. Academic Press, 1962.

[131] J. M. Sieburth, *Science*, **132**, 676 (1960).

[132] R. Bywood and R. Challenger, *Biochem. J.*, **53**, 26 (1956).

[133] K.-W. Glombitza, *Planta Med.*, **18**, 210 and 281 (1970).

[134] J. M. Sieburth, *Limnol. Oceanogr.*, **4**, 419 (1959).

[135] M. Ikawa, V. M. Thomas, Jr., L. J. Buckley and J. J. Uebel, *J. Phycol.*, **9**, 302 (1973).

[136] S. J. Wratten and D. J. Faulkner, *J. Org. Chem.*, **41**, 2465 (1976).

# PART B

# OLIGOSACCHARIDE ANTIBIOTICS

by

**ASHIT K. GANGULY**
SCHERING CORPORATION, CHEMICAL RESEARCH DEPARTMENT
BLOOMFIELD, NEW JERSEY

**PART B**

**CONTENTS**

## 1 INTRODUCTION

The oligosaccharide group of antibiotics represent complex structures and possess many centres of asymmetry. So far only four members of this group of antibiotics have been isolated. These are the everninomicins [1], curamycins [2], avilamycins [3], and flambamycins [4]. Extensive chemical degradations and spectroscopic evidence have led to the structural elucidation of everninomicin B [5], C [6] and D [7], the first amongst this class of antibiotics whose structures have been determined. Following the degradation methods established in the above structural studies, the structure of flambamycin has recently been elucidated. Curamycin [8] and avilamycin [9] have been degraded and the structures of some of the constituent monosaccharides have been established.

In this review an emphasis is laid on the methods we have developed for tackling these structures, as exemplified with our work on the everninomicins. The methodology has essentially consisted of selective cleavage of the molecule into fragments and the structural elucidation of these parts before attempting to investigate how the parts are joined together. Since these molecules are sophisticated carbohydrates, a lot of the techniques employed were obtained from this area of chemistry. Because the molecules also contain several unique features and unusual sugar components, some of the methodology used had to be developed during the work. In order to illustrate these the review includes detailed chemical descriptions of how the structures of the fragments were determined. The review also contains brief details on the current state of research on the related oligosaccharide antibiotics. It will be apparent to the reader that much more information is needed on the mode of action and structure-activity relationships of this group of antibiotics. These aspects of study are under active investigation.

## 2. BIOLOGICAL ACTIVITY

The everninomicins have been shown [1] to be active against a wide variety of gram positive aerobes and anaerobes as well as Neiseria and Mycobacteria. Everninomicin B and D are the two main constituents of the antibiotic complex produced by *Micromonospora carbonacea* var. Carbonaceae NRRL 2972 and most of the initial microbiological studies were carried out on them. Both of these compounds were active against a variety of strains of Staphylococcus, Streptococcus, Bacillus, and Mycobacteria, including penicillin-resistant strains. The activities of these antibiotics were inhibited by serum and it was estimated that everninomicin B and D were strongly protein bound to the extent of 75 and 95% respectively. In spite of this high serum protein binding both of these compounds showed [10] excellent *in vivo* activities in experimental mice infections, for example $ED_{50}$'s were less than 5 mg/kg for protection against infection caused by gram positive strains. Recently [11] it has been shown that these antibiotics are, a) bactericidal for group A streptococci and bacteriostatic for other organisms and, b) lack cross-resistance with other antimicrobials. Activities against Mycoplasma [12] and a small group of anaerobes [13] have been reported. Everninomicins and their derivatives have no activity against Enterobacteriacae or Pseudomonas. Serum and urine levels in dogs following i.v. administration were high and indicated a serum half-life of about ninety minutes for everninomicin D. Absorption following i.m. administration of everninomicin D to both man and dogs was slow and erratic. Recent studies with everninomicin B in dogs, rats, and mice showed that it behaved similarly to everninomicin D. Urine recoveries of these antibiotics indicated that one of the ways these antibiotics were eliminated was via urinary excretion.

The *in vitro* microbiological activities of flambamycin, curamycin and avilamycin are similar to those of the everninomicins. Detailed studies in animal experiments have not been reported for flambamycin, curamycin and avilamycin.

## 3 STRUCTURAL STUDIES ON THE EVERNINOMICINS

Since 1960 chemical efforts have been made to elucidate the structures of this group of antibiotics but with very little success until the work on the structural elucidation of the everninomicins began in the author's laboratory in 1968. The everninomicins thus represent the first type of this group of antibiotics, the structures of which have been determined. In the following discussion details of the structural elucidation of everninomicin D will be discussed, followed by a summary of the structural elucidation of everninomicins B and C, and flambamycin.

### 3.1 Structural Studies on Everninomicin D

Everninomicin D [7] is a colourless crystalline solid, $C_{66}H_{99}O_{35}NCl_2$ (M.W. 1537), m.p. 169–171°C, $\lambda_{max}^{methanol}$ 289 nm (22), $\lambda_{max}^{NaOH/methanol}$ 295 nm (80.8), $[\alpha]_D^{26}$ −34.2° (chloroform), neutralization equivalent 1558, pKa 7.3. In the infrared it shows absorption for hydroxyl, ester and nitro (1555 $cm^{-1}$) groups. As everninomicin D and its derivatives do not give molecular ion peaks in their mass spectra, it became necessary to discover a new method for the determination of molecular weights of compounds with high molecular weights and possessing several polar, functional groups. The molecular weight of a compound can be determined [14] by the application of the equation $Mx = \frac{n \times Ar}{Ax}$ wherein Mx is the molecular weight of the unknown compound as its derivative, Ax is radioactivity in $\mu$Ci/mg of the unknown, n is the number of equivalents of the reagent which have reacted with the unknown and Ar is the specific activity of the reagent ($\mu$Ci/mmol).

For example, everninomicin D was monomethylated with tritiated diazomethane in the presence of estrone, a compound of known molecular weight. The specific activity of the tritiated diazomethane was deduced by measuring the activity of the esterone mono-methyl ehter prepared in the above reaction. Knowing the specific activity of the tritiated diazomethane and the activity of the mono-methyl ether of everninomicin D and applying the equation $Mx = \frac{n \times Ar}{Ax}$, the molecular weight of the methyl ether of everninomicin D was found to be 1579 (calculated for $C_{67}H_{101}O_{35}NCl_2$ is 1551).

The structural elucidation of everninomicin D involves (see Chart 1) hydrolysis of the antibiotic into its various components, determining their structures and absolute stereochemistries and finally, finding the sequence in which they are linked.

Everninomicin D (**1**) ($C_{66}H_{99}O_{35}NCl_2$) on hydrolysis with aqueous acid yields everninomicin [7] $D_1$ (**2**) ($C_{66}H_{101}O_{36}NCl_2$). On treatment with diazomethane compound (**2**) undergoes smooth cleavage to the methyl ether of everninonitrose pyranosyl(1 → 4)digitolactone [15] (**3**) and olgose [7] (**4**). Solvolysis of (3) with methanolic toluene-p--sulphonic acid yields the methyl ether of everninonitrose methyl glycoside [16] (**5**) which, on prolonged methanolysis, yields evernitrose methyl glycoside [17] (**6**) (the first example of a naturally occurring nitro sugar) and the methyl ether of everninocin methyl glycoside (7).

Olgose (**4**), on solvolysis, yields evertetrose [16] (**8**) and a hydroxymethyl ester [7] (**9**). Evertetrose (**8**), on further hydrolysis with aqueous acid, yields evermicose [18] (**10**), evertriose [19] (**11**) and everninose [20] (**12**). These results are summarised in Chart 1.

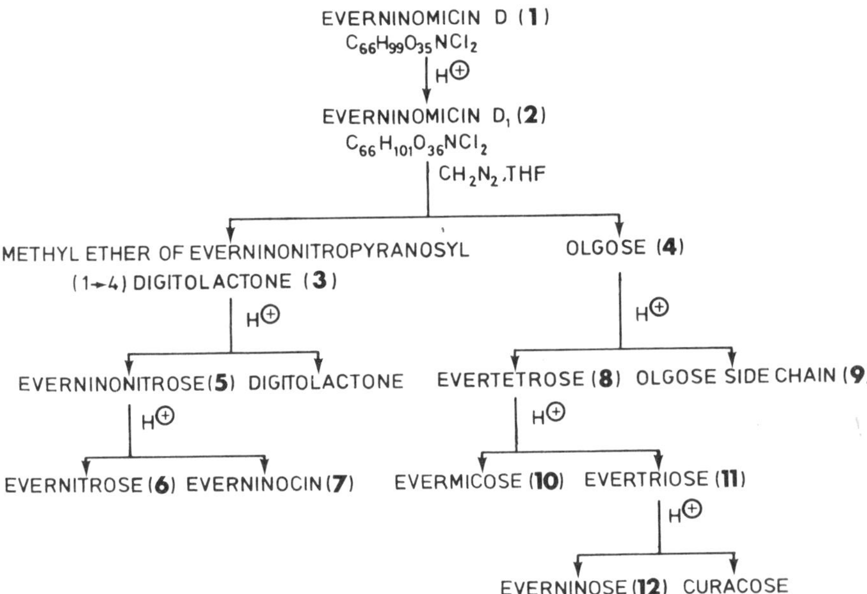

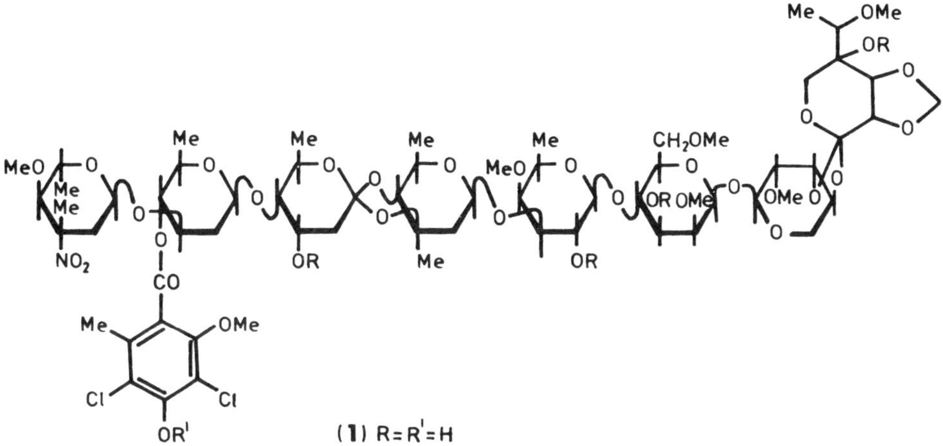

(**1**) R = R' = H

(**1a**) R = H; R' = $CH_3$

(**79**) R = R' = $CH_3$

(**83**) R' = $CH_3$; R = $COCH_3$

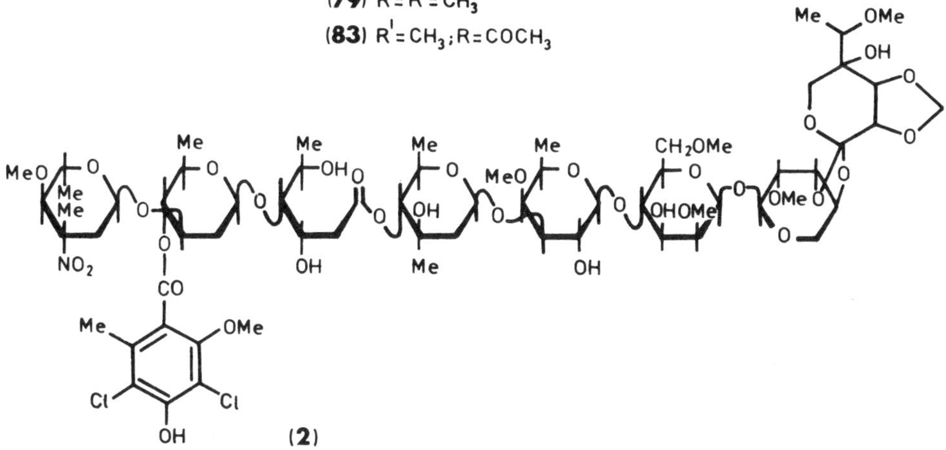

(**2**)

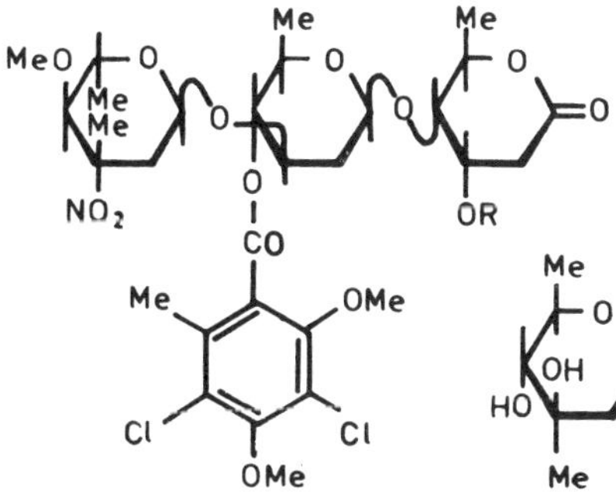

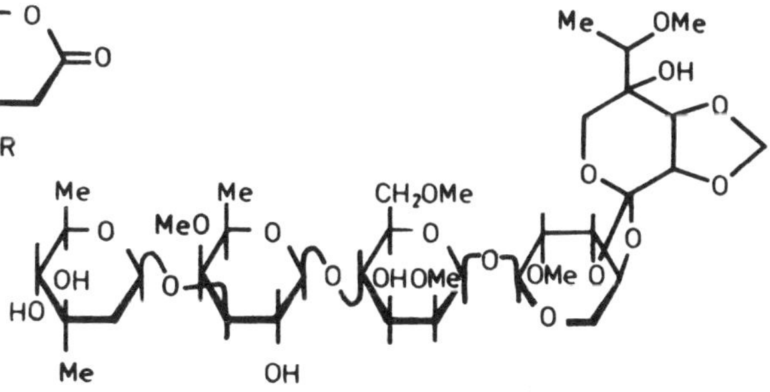

(**3**) R = H

(**80**) R = $CH_3$

(**4**)

(5)

(6)

(7)

(8)

(9)

(10)

(11)

(12)

## 3.2 Structural Studies on component fragments of Everninomicin D

### 3.2.1 *Evernitrose*

Evernitrose [17] (**13**) is a colourless crystalline solid, $C_8H_{15}NO_5$, m.p. 88-93°; $[a]_D$ −49° → −19.4° (ethanol, 24 hrs); $\lambda_{max}^{methanol}$ 283 nm ($\epsilon$ 52.5). In the infrared evernitrose (**13**) shows the presence of hydroxyl and nitro groups at 3344 and 1553 $cm^{-1}$, respectively. Evernitrose forms a mono-acetate (**14**), a colourless crystalline solid, $C_{10}H_{17}NO_6$, m.p. 58-59, $[\alpha]_D$ −20.5°, $\nu$ max 1701 (acetate), 1553 (nitro) $cm^{-1}$ and shows no hydroxyl absorption. In the $^1H$ n.m.r. spectrum the above acetate (**14**) shows the presence of a second methyl group ($\delta$ 1.38, J 7Hz), a tertiary methyl ($\delta$ 1.71), an acetate methyl ($\delta$ 1.95), a methoxyl ($\delta$ 3.88), a one proton multiplet at $\delta$ 3.55, a one proton doublet at $\delta$ 3.38 (J 6Hz) and a one proton quartet at $\delta$ 5.80 for the axial anomeric proton (J 8 and 3Hz).

The presence of a nitro group in evernitrose (**13**) is indicated by the presence of an absorption of 1553 $cm^{-1}$ in the infrared region and also by the presence of a M-$NO_2$ peak in the mass spectrum. As evernitrose was the first example of a naturally-occurring nitrosugar, it was considered important to convert it to an amino-sugar.

Evernitrose (**13**), on treatment with methanolic hydrogen chloride, is converted into the methyl glycoside (**6**; mixture of anomers). Catalytic hydrogenation of (**6**), using 10% palladium on charcoal, yields the amine (**15**), $\nu$ max 3333 $cm^{-1}$ (amino) and no absorption for the nitro group. On acetylation the above amine (**15**) affords the acetamido compound (**16**), $C_{11}H_{21}NO_4$, m.p. 114-115°, $[a]_D$ −30°. In the infrared compound (**16**) shows the presence of —NH (3333 $cm^{-1}$) and amide (1684 $cm^{-1}$) and in the $^1H$ n.m.r. spectrum it shows the presence of an acetamido methyl signal at $\delta$1.95 which agrees well with that of $\delta$1.93-1.86 predicted for an axially oriented acetamido methyl group on a fully substituted carbon atom but lay outside the $\delta$1.87-1.78 range for the corresponding equatorial substituent. It was recognized, however, that such an assignment could not be regarded as being firmly established since there was a lack of any suitable example. This point has been resolved [21] by a single-crystal X-ray analysis of (**16**). Crystals of (**16**) belong to the orthorhombic system, space group p $2_12_12_1$, $a$ = 12.960 (**6**), $b$ = 13.944 (**6**), $c$ = 6.949 (**4**) A°, (Z) = 4. Intensity data to Θ 67°, recorded on an Enraf-Nonius CAD 3 diffractometer (Ni-filtered Cu-K$\alpha$ radiation, $\lambda$ = 1.5418°A; Θ-2Θ scans) yielded 699 statistically significant $[I > 2.0\sigma(I)]$ reflections. The structure was solved by direct methods by use of MULTAN. Full matrix least-squares refinement of atomic positional and thermal (anisotropic, C, N, and O; isotropic H) parameters has converged at $R$ 0.50. The solid-state conformation (see Figure 1) shows that in (**16**) the ring adopts a chair conformation with an equatorially oriented C-3 acetamido function. X-ray structural analysis of (**16**), therefore, demonstrates that the assignment of stereochemistry of an acetamido function on a fully substituted carbon atom could not be made unequivocally by reliance on the predicted chemical shift values of the acetamido methyl group.

Evernitrose (**13**), on oxidation with bromine water, yields a δ-lactone (**17**), $C_8H_{13}NO_5$, m.p. 63-64°, $[\alpha]_D$ −70°. In the infrared spectrum compound (**17**), shows absorption at 1757 (lactone), 1553 $cm^{-1}$ (nitro) and no hydroxyl absorption. The $^1H$ n.m.r. spectrum of (**17**) shows an AB pair of doublets centered at δ3.1 (J 18Hz), a secondary methyl at δ1.50 (J 6.5Hz), a tertiary methyl at δ1.70, a methoxyl at δ3.51, a one proton doublet at δ3.83 (J 9Hz) and a one proton octet at ~δ4.2. On refluxing with methanolic potassium acetate compound (**17**) undergoes smooth conversion to (**18**), $C_8H_{12}O_3$, sublimes at 40° (1 mm), $[\alpha]_D$ −38.6°; $\lambda_{max}$ 205 nm (11200), $\nu_{max}$ 1739 $cm^{-1}$ (α,β-unsaturated δ-lactone) and there is no absorption for a nitro group. An authentic sample of (**18**) was prepared from L-mycarose [22] (**19**), a compound of known absolute geometry, following the above procedure in four steps. Thus, the structure and absolute stereochemistry of evernitrose are represented as (**13**).

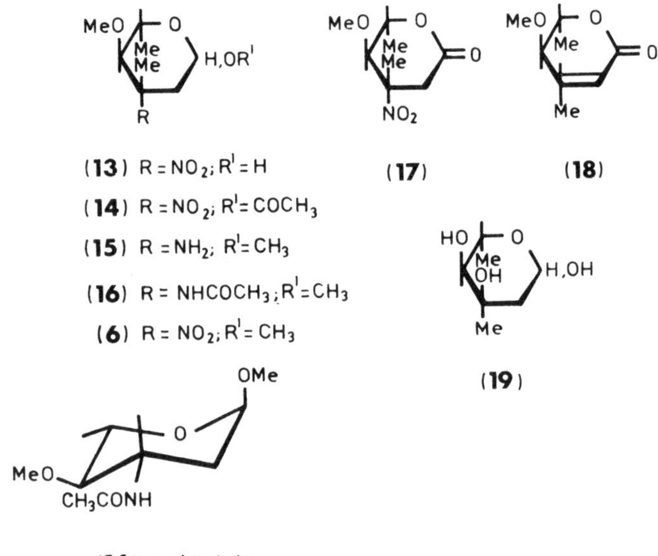


Figure 1

### 3.2.2 *Everninonitrose*

Everninonitrose (**20**) is an amorphous solid $C_{23}H_{31}NO_{11}NCl_2$, $[\alpha]_D$ −65.4°. On hydrolysis everninonitrose (**20**) yields evernitrose (**13**) and everninocin (**21**). The linkage of (**21**) to (**13**) in the structure of (**20**) is shown by the formation of the acetylation product (**22**) of the monomethyl ether of everninonitrose (**23**). Compound (**22**) contains an anomeric acetoxyl group thus showing that evernitrose (**13**) is linked using its anomeric hydroxyl group to the three position of everninocin (**21**). The stereochemistry of the anomeric linkage follows from the $^1$H n.m.r. spectrum of compound (**22**) (δ4.7, q, J 2 and 5Hz; $H_1$) and also by the application of Klyne's rule.

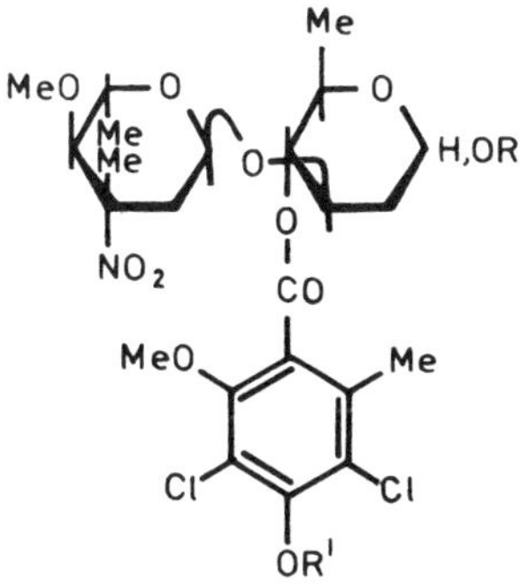

(**20**) R = R' = H

(**22**) R = $COCH_3$; R' = $CH_3$

(**23**) R = H ; R' = $CH_3$

(**5**) R = R' = $CH_3$

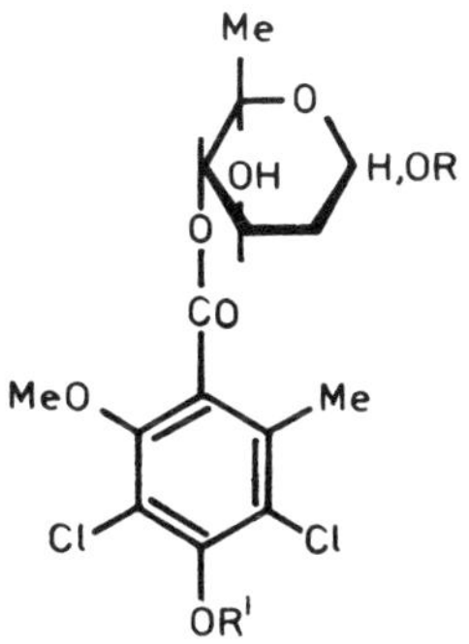

(**21**) R = R' = H

(**7**) R = R' = $CH_3$

A methanolic solution of everninomicin $D_1$ (**2**) on treatment with ethereal diazomethane undergoes smooth cleavage to yield a mixture of two components. The more polar component is olgose (**4**) and the less polar uv absorbing component (**24**) always seems to be transformed, to a small extent, to another, still less polar, component (**3**) on tlc. Component (**24**), on treatment with toluene-p-sulphonic acid in tetrahydrofuran, or when stirred in acetone solution in the presence of silica gel, is quantitatively converted into (**3**). Alternatively, on treatment of compound (**3**) with a methanolic solution of toluene-p-sulphonic acid it is converted completely into (**24**). It is concluded, therefore, that (**24**) is a hydroxy-ester which is easily converted into lactone (**3**).

The methyl ether of everninonitrose pyranosyl(1 → 4)digitolactone (**3**) is a colourless crystalline solid, $C_{30}H_{41}O_{14}NCl_2$ ($M^+$ 709), m.p. 186-188°, $[\alpha]_D$ −57.9°, $\lambda_{max}$ 287 (987) and 210 nm (36159), $\nu_{max}$ 1754 (carbonyl), 1555 (nitro) and 3472 $cm^{-1}$ (hydroxyl). In the infrared spectrum of compound (**3**) the intensity of the nitro absorption is weaker than the carbonyl absorption which is the opposite of what is found in the methyl ether of everninonitrose methyl glycoside (**5**).

In the $^1$H n.m.r. spectrum compound (**3**) shows signals at $\delta$1.42 (d; 3H; J 6.5Hz, $C_6$ methyl, $\delta$2.54 and 3.08 ($J_{AB}$ 17Hz; $H_2'''$), $\delta$3.95 (m; $J_{23}$ 7 and 8Hz; $H_3'''$), $\delta$3.35 (q, J. 9 and 8Hz; $H_4'''$) and $\delta$4.18 (octet; J 6.5 and 9Hz; $H_5'''$). INDOR and spin-spin decoupling experiments confirmed the above assignments. Upon treatment with pyridine and acetic anhydride at room temperature, compound (**3**) forms a monoacetate (**25**), $C_{32}H_{43}NCl_2O_{15}$ ($M^+$ 751), $[\alpha]_D$ −47.9°, $\lambda_{max}$ 287 (924) and 208 nm (35931) and in the infrared spectrum there is no hydroxyl absorption. The $^1$H n.m.r. spectrum of the acetate (**25**) shows the presence of $H_5'''$ at $\delta$4.25 compared to $\delta$4.18 in the case of compound (**3**) thus suggesting that (**3**) is a $\delta$-lactone; $H_3'''$ appeared at $\delta$5.49 (d of t; J 4.8 and 3Hz) and $H_4'''$ at $\delta$3.65 (q; J 8 and 3Hz). The coupling constants of $H_3'''$ with $H_4'''$ and $H_2'''$ protons in (**3**) clearly indicates the presence of an axial acetate in (**25**). The abnormal coupling of these protons in (3) is probably due to the fact that either a) compound (**3**) exists in equilibrium with an open chain hydroxy acid structure or b) that the lactone ring exists in a distorted conformation [23]. The possibility of a hydroxy acid structure is ruled out from its infrared spectrum wherein there is no absorption for the carboxyl group.

The absolute stereochemistry of the sugar lactone part of (**3**) is deduced in the following way. On heating with acetic anhydride and pyridine, compound (**3**) yields an $\alpha,\beta$-unsaturated $\delta$-lactone (**26**), $C_{30}H_{39}NCl_2O_{15}$, $M^+$ 691, m.p. 174-175°, $\lambda_{max}$ 287 (1008) and 208 nm (46066) and it does not show the presence of any hydroxyl group in the infrared. The $^1$H n.m.r. spectrum of (**26**) is consistent with the assigned structure and shows the presence of two vinyl hydrogens at $\delta$5.86 (q, J 1.8 and 10Hz; $H_2'''$) and $\delta$6.9 (q, J 2 and 10Hz; $H_3'''$). In its circular dichroism spectrum, compound (**26**) shows a negative Cotton effect $[\theta]_{280}$ −40900 suggesting [24] the R configuration of $C_5'''$. The methyl ether of everninonitrose (**23**) also shows a negative Cotton effect, $[\theta]_{244}$ −1600. The high resolution mass spectral fragmentation of evernitrose, the methyl ether of everninonitrose and of the lactone (**3**) seems to be initiated by the ready loss of the nitro group.

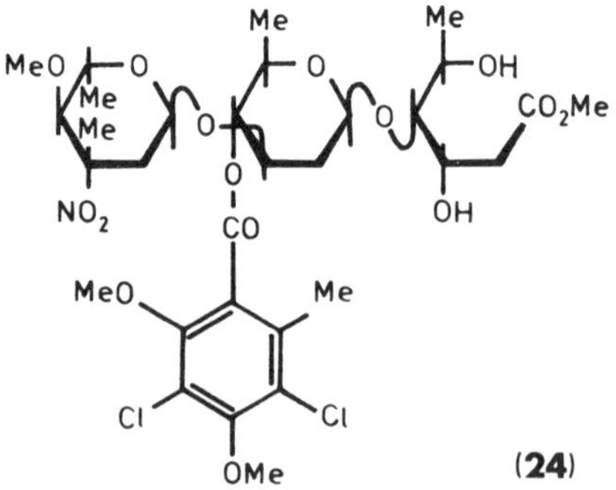

(**24**)

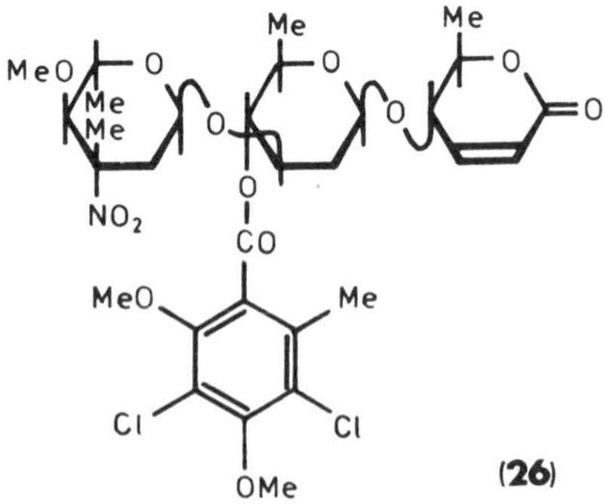

(**26**)

### 3.2.3 *Evertriose*

Evertriose (**11**), $C_{21}H_{38}O_{14} \cdot H_2O$ $[\alpha]_D$ −41.6° ($H_2O$; 24 hours) is an amorphous solid. It is a non-reducing sugar and shows no selective absorption in the u.v. and in the i.r. it does not show any carbonyl absorption. The $^1H$ n.m.r. spectrum ($D_2O$) of evertriose (**11**) shows the presence of four methoxyl groups, a secondary methyl group and three anomeric protons at δ4.31 (J 7Hz), 4.95 (J w/2 1.5Hz) and 5.33 (J2.5Hz). On hydrolysis with aqueous acid, evertriose yields D-curacose (**27**) m.p. 125-127° $[\alpha]_D$ +98.4° → + 86.4° (water) and everninose (**12**). The identity of D-curacose is established by the preparation of a crystalline tosylhydrazone and direct comparison with an authentic sample of D-curacose tosylhydrazone.

Everninose (**12**), $C_{14}H_{26}O_{10}$, m.p. 200-201° $[\alpha]_D$ −74.1° (water) is a non-reducing sugar. It consumes two moles of periodic acid and does not form a trityl derivative. The $^1H$ n.m.r. spectrum (pyridine) of everninose shows the presence of three methoxyl groups and two anomeric protons at δ5.25 (1H; J w/2 1.5Hz) and δ5.7 (1H; J 2.5Hz). Everninose (**12**) forms a tetraacetate (**28**), $C_{22}H_{34}O_{14}$.

The mass spectrum of the tetra-O-trimethyl silyl ether of everninose shows a strong M-15 peak at m/e 627 besides a small molecular ion peak at m/e 642. Other prominent peaks in the mass spectrum could be summarized as follows:

R
O
$Me_3SiO$
$OSiMe_3$ OMe

$\xrightarrow{-90}$ m/e 245 and 201 $\xrightarrow{-90}$ m/e 155 and 111

$\xrightarrow{-32}$ m/e 303 and 259 $\xrightarrow{-90}$ m/e 213 and 169

(**29**) m/e 335; R=$CH_2OMe$

(**30**) m/e 291; R=H

Ions (**29**) and (**30**) indicate that everninose is made up of a dimethoxy hexose and a monomethoxy pentose. As everninose is a non-reducing sugar, the above units must be linked through their anomeric hydroxyl groups.

Everninose (**12**), like trehalose, could be hydrolyzed only on prolonged heating with aqueous acid. The crude hydrolysis product, consisting of a mixture of two monosaccharides, is separated using preparative t.l.c. The structures of the monosaccharides have been shown to be 2:6-di-O-methyl-D-mannose (**31**) and 2-O-methyl-L-lyxose (**32**) in the following way.

Compound (**31**), syrup, $[\alpha]_D$ +7.9° (water; 72 hours) is a reducing sugar. The $^1H$ n.m.r. spectrum of (**31**) shows the presence of two methoxyl groups and an anomeric proton at δ5.3 (J 2 Hz). It forms a triacetate (**33**), syrup, $C_{14}H_{22}O_9$ $[\alpha]_D$ +55.7°. The $^1H$ n.m.r. spectrum of (**33**) agrees well with that published for tri-O-acetyl-2,6-di-O-methyl-D-mannose. The mass spectral fragmentation of the di-n-propyl mercaptal of **(31)**, $C_{14}H_{30}O_5S_2$, m.p. 50°, $[\alpha]_D$ −24.01°, shows, in addition to a molecular ion peak at m/e 342, prominent peaks at m/e 267 **(34)**, 235 **(35)**, 205 **(36)**, 207 **(37)**, 179 **(38)** and 147 **(39)** (see Chart 2).

CHART 2

$R^2-S-\overset{+}{C}H-CHOMe-CHOH-CHOH-CHOH-R^1$

**(34)** ($R^1=CH_2OMe$; m/e 267)

**(42)** ($R^1=H$; m/e 223)

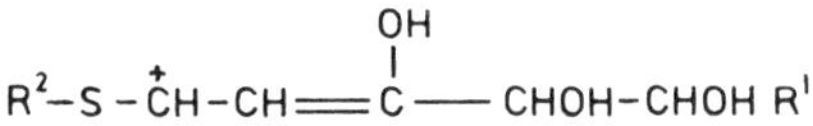

$R^2-S-\overset{+}{C}H-CH{=}C(OH)-CHOH-CHOH\ R^1$

**(35)** ($R^1=CH_2OMe$; m/e 235)

**(43)** ($R^1=H$; m/e 191)

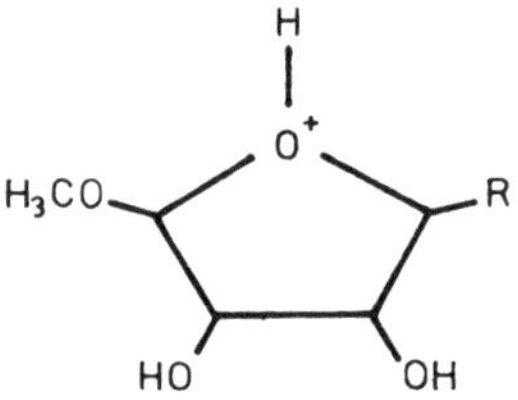

**(38)** ($R=CH_2OMe$; m/e 179)

**(44)** ($R=H$; m/e 135)

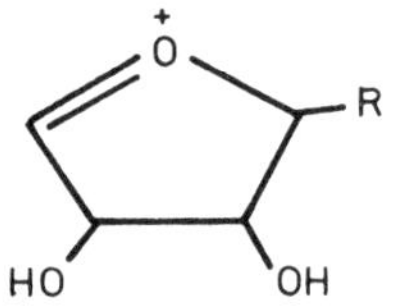

**(39)** ($R=-CH_2OMe$; m/e 147)

**(45)** ($R=H$; m/e 103)

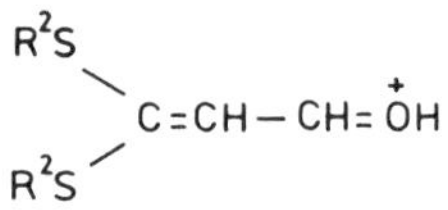

$(R^2S)_2C=CH-CH=\overset{+}{O}H$

**(36)** m/e 205

$(R^2S)_2CH-CH=\overset{+}{O}Me$

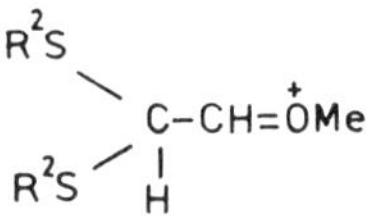

**(37)** m/e 207

In **(34)**, **(35)**, **(36)**, **(37)**, **(42)** and **(43)**, $R^2 = Pr^n$

The methyl glycoside of compound **(31)** on methylation yields **(40)**, which on hydrolysis gave **(41)**, as a syrup, $C_{10}H_{20}O_6$, $[\alpha]_D$ +2.3° (water; 24hr.) identical with an authentic sample of 2,3,4,6-tetra-O-methyl-D-mannose $[\alpha]_D$ +2.3° (water; 24 hr.).

Compound **(32)**, $C_6H_{12}O_5$, is a crystalline solid m.p. 122°, $[\alpha]_D$ +6.2° (water; 72 hr.). It forms a crystalline di-n-propyl mercaptal, $C_{12}H_{26}O_4S_2$, m.p. 49°, $[\alpha]_D$ +19.5°, which in the mass spectrum shows the molecular ion peak at m/e 298 and also peaks at m/e 223 **(42)**, 191 **(43)**, 207 **(37)**, 205 **(36)**, 135 **(44)** and m/e 103 **(45)** (see Chart 2). The above mass spectral fragmentation confirms that compound **(32)** is a 2-methoxy pentose. Compound **(32)** forms a triacetate **(46)**, $C_{12}H_{18}O_8$, $[\alpha]_D$ −10.5°. In the $^1$H n.m.r. spectrum (100 MHz, benzene solution) the triacetate **(46)** shows the presence of three acetyl methyl groups and signals at δ3.88 (1H, q; J 11.5 and 4.5Hz; H-5e), δ3.69 (1H; q; J 11.5 and 7.0Hz; H-5a), δ5.40 (1H, octet, J. 4.5, 7.0 and 8.0Hz, H-4), 5.52 (1H; q; J 8.0 and 2.9Hz; H-3), 3.60 (1H, q; J 2.9 and 4.2Hz; H-2) and 6.29 (1H, d; J 4.2Hz; H-1). The above chemical shifts and coupling constant values are obtained using spin-spin-decoupling experiments. From the above results it is clear that compound **(32)** is 2-methoxylyxose. To prove the absolute stereochemistry of **(32)**, it was converted into **(47)**, $C_8H_{16}O_5$, $[\alpha]_D$ +12.4°. Compound **(47)** proved to be identicle (t.l.c., m.s. and n.m.r.) with an authentic sample of 2,3,4-tri-O-methyl-D-lyxose, except for the opposite sign of rotation $[\alpha]_D$ −21.6°. An interesting feature of the $^1$H n.m.r. spectrum of **(46)** is the higher coupling constants ($J_{1,2}$ 4.2Hz) and comparatively lower value of ($J_{4,5}$ 7.0Hz) and $J_{3,4}$ 8.0Hz) which suggests that 2-O-methyl-1,3,4-tri-O-acetyl-L-lyxose **(46)** exists in a conformational equilibrium between the 1C and C1 conformations, approximately in the ratio of 3:2. C.D. measurement [18] of the cuprammonium complex of the methyl glycosides of **(31)** and **(32)** indicates that they form λ and δ chelates respectively confirming their assigned absolute stereochemistry.

The evidence presented so far establishes that everninose is made up of 2,6-di-O-methyl-D-mannose **(31)** and 2-O-methyl-L-lyxose **(32)** and that they are linked through their anomeric hydroxyl groups. What remains to be proven is the stereochemistry of the anomeric linkages. Everninose **(12)** on methylation yields **(48)**, a syrup, $C_{18}H_{33}O_{10}$, $[M]_D$ −356°. To apply Klyne's [25] rule we have prepared compounds **(49)** to **(52)** in the usual way and determined their molecular rotation values (see Table 3.1).

**Table 3.1**

| | Compound | $[M]_D$ |
|---|---|---|
| **(49)** | Methyl 2,3,4,6-tetra-O-methyl-β-D-mannoside | −218° |
| **(50)** | Methyl 2,3,4,6-tetra-O-methyl-α-D-mannoside | +132° |
| **(51)** | Methyl 2,3,4-tri-O-methyl-β-D-lyxoside | −176° |
| **(52)** | Methyl 2,3,4-tri-O-methyl-α-D-lyxoside | 76° |
| **(48)** | Tetra-O-methyl ether of everninose | −356° |
| **(11)** | Evertriose | −221° |
| **(12)** | Everninose | −262° |
| | Methyl 6-deoxy-α-D-galactopyranoside | +189° |
| | Methyl 6-deoxy-β-D-galactopyranoside | − 14° |

In α,α-trehalose (**53**), the only other example of a naturally occurring disaccharide of this group, Klyne's rule has been successfully applied to determine its stereochemistry. From the table it follows that the structure and absolute stereochemistry of everninose should be represented as (**12**).

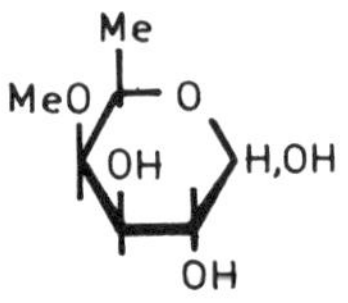

(**27**)

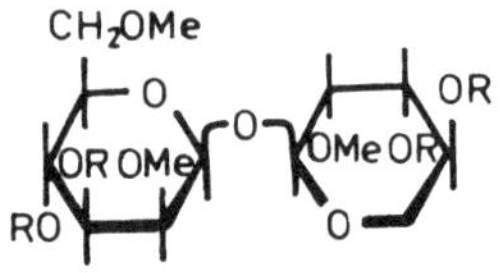

(**28**) $R = COCH_3$

(**48**) $R = CH_3$

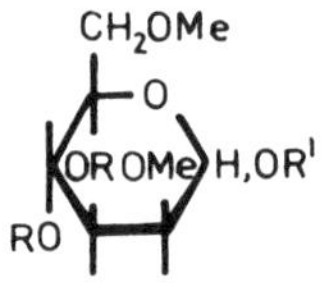

(**31**) $R = R' = H$

(**33**) $R = R' = COCH_3$

(**40**) $R = R' = CH_3$

(**41**) $R = CH_3; R' = H$

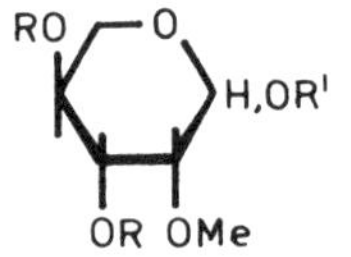

(**32**) $R = R' = H$

(**46**) $R = R' = COCH_3$

(**47**) $R = CH_3; R' = H$

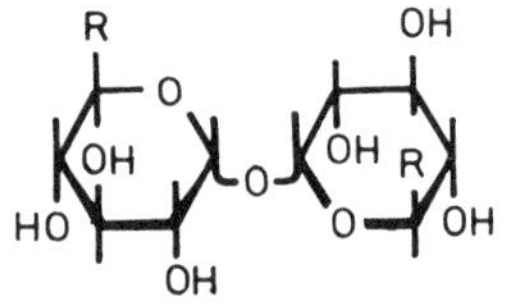

(**53**) $R = CH_2OH$

To establish the structure and stereochemistry of evertriose, it remains now to determine the position and stereochemistry of the linkage of curacose (**27**) to everninose (**12**).

Evertriose on methylation yields a permethylated compound (**54**). $C_{26}H_{48}O_{14}$, $[\alpha]_D$ −47.7°. The $^1H$ n.m.r. spectrum of (**54**) shows nine methoxyl groups, one secondary methyl group and three anomeric protons. Two of the anomeric protons at δ5.30 (d; J 2Hz) and δ4.73 (d; J 1.5Hz) belong to the everninose portion of the molecule and the third one at δ4.36 (d; J 7Hz) is attributed to the curacose part and therefore established the anomeric linkage as β. Besides showing molecular ion peak at m/e 584, compound (**54**) shows peaks at m/e 393, 361, 189, 175, 453, 423.

The probable origin of these ions is summarized in Chart 3.

CHART 3

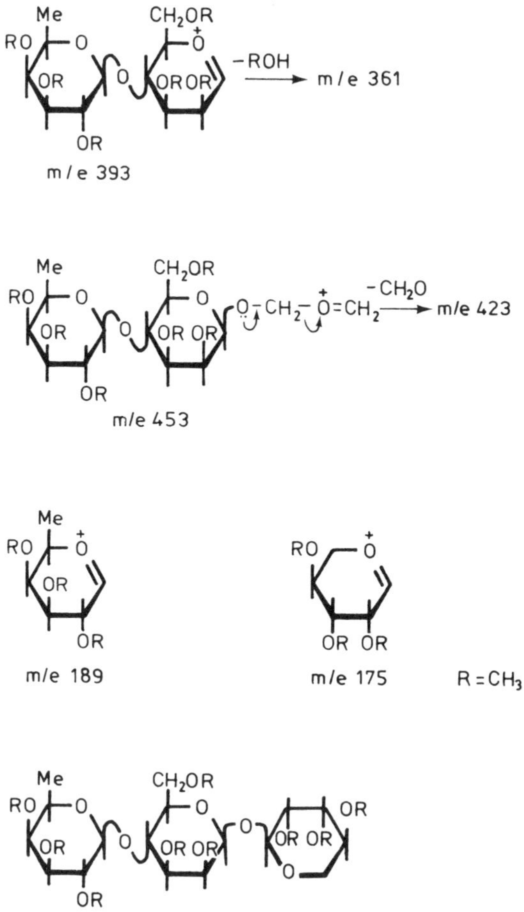

The above mass spectral fragmentation indicates that in evertriose (**11**), D-curacose (**27**) is linked to the 4-position of the hexose moiety of everninose (**12**).

Further proof for the linkage of (**27**) to (**12**) is obtained in the following way. Compound (**54**), on prolonged hydrolysis, yields a mixture which is separated using preparative t.l.c. and the most polar component, syrup, $C_9H_{18}O_6$, $[\alpha]_D$ $+6.9° \rightarrow +5.9°$ is shown to be 2,3,6-tri-O-methyl-D-mannose by acetylation to

1,4-di-O-acetyl-2,3,6-tri-O-methyl-D-mannose, m.p. 95°, $C_{13}H_{22}O_8$, $[\alpha]_D$ +28.4°. Its $^1H$ n.m.r. spectrum shows the presence of three methoxyl groups, two acetoxy groups, an anomeric proton and a one proton triplet at δ5.28 (J 9Hz) ascribed to H-4. The stereochemistry of the anomeric linkage (curacose part) is shown from the $^1H$ n.m.r. spectrum, (anomeric proton at δ4.36 (d; J 7Hz) and is also confirmed by the application of Klyne's rule (see Table 3.1)

The structure and absolute stereochemistry of evertriose is thus established as **(11)**.

3.2.4 *Evermicose*

Evermicose **(10)**, $C_7H_{14}O_4$ is a colourless crystalline solid, m.p. 108-112°, $[\alpha]_D$ +20.7° (water, 24 hr.). It has no selective absorption in the u.v. above 210 nm and in the infrared it does not show the presence of any carbonyl group. Evermicose **(10)** froms a crystalline diacetate **(55)**, $C_{11}H_{18}O_6$, m.p. 73° $[\alpha]_D$ +39.5° and shows absorption for hydroxyl and ester functions in the infrared. The $^1H$ n.m.r. spectrum of **(55)** shows signals at δ1.2 ($C_5$-methyl; d; J 6Hz), 1.3 ($C_3$-methyl; s), 2.1 and 2.13 (two $-OCOCH_3$), 4.6 ($H_4$; d; J 10Hz), 3.63 ($H_5$; octet; J 10 and 6Hz), 5.75 ($H_1$; q; J 9 and 3Hz) and 2.6 (hydroxyl group exchangeable with $D_2O$). It is concluded from the above data that evermicose is 3-epimycarose which is further substantiated by comparison of the $^1H$ n.m.r. spectra of **(55)** with L-mycarose diacetate **(56)**. The $H_1$ and $H_5$ protons in **(56)** are deshielded by the axial hydroxyl group at $C_3$ and appear at δ6.07 and 4.01, respectively. The $C_3$-methyls appear at δ1.3 in compound **(55)** and at δ1.18 in compound **(56)**.

Evermicose **(10)** on oxidation with bromine water yields a mixture of γ- and δ-lactones which on acetylation followed by dehydration affords a mixture of α:β-unsaturated lactones **(57)** and **(58)** which can be separated by preparative t.l.c. Compound **(57)**, a colourless liquid, $C_9H_{12}O_4$, $\nu_{max}$ 1720 cm.$^{-1}$, no hydroxyl group $\lambda_{max}$ 211 nm (13150), $[\alpha]_D$ +97.8°, δ1.4 ($C_5$-methyl; d; J 6.5Hz), 1.95 ($C_3$-vinyl methyl), 2.1 ($-OCOCH_3$), 4.5 ($H_5$; quintet; J 6.5Hz), 5.31 ($H_4$; d; J 6.5Hz) and 5.91 (vinyl hydrogen). The structure of **(58)** is also based on its composition and spectroscopic evidence.

Following the above series of reactions, L-mycarose **(59)** was converted into **(60)** which is identical with compound **(57)** (t.l.c., i.r., n.m.r.) excepting that it has $[\alpha]_D$ −99.8°, Cf $[\alpha]_D$ +97.8° for **(57)** thus proving that evermicose **(10)** is 3-C-methyl-2,6-dideoxy-D-arabinohexose or D-3-epimycarose. (±) 3-Epimycarose has been obtained as a by-product during the synthesis of L-mycarose. The t.l.c. behaviour of evermicose and (±) 3-epimycarose is identical.

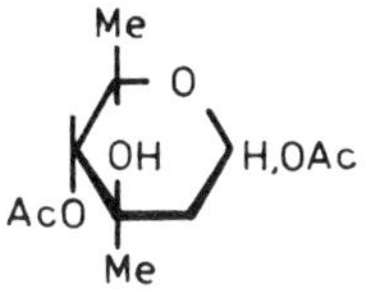

(55) 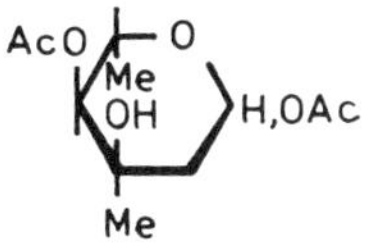 (56) 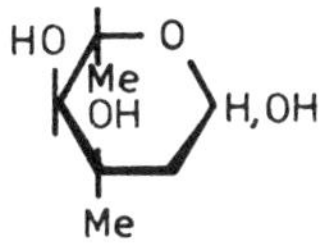 (59)

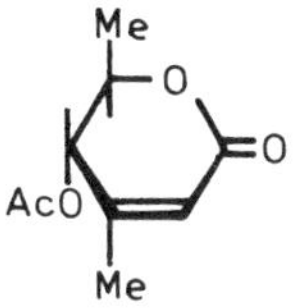

(57) 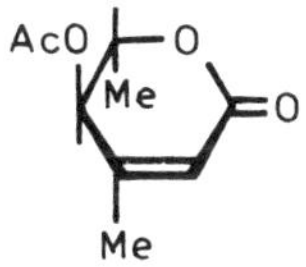 (60)

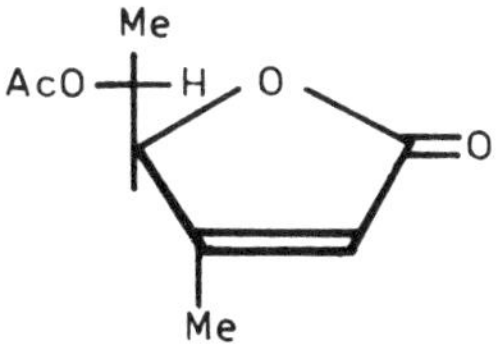

(58)

### 3.2.5 *Evertetrose*

Evertetrose (8) is an amorphous solid, $C_{28}H_{50}O_{17}$, $[\alpha]_D$ $-37.2°$ ($H_2O$, 72 hrs.). It is a non-reducing sugar and does not show any selective absorption in the u.v. and no carbonyl i.r. absorption. The $^1H$ n.m.r. spectrum of evertetrose shows the presence of four methoxyl groups, two secondary methyl groups, a tertiary methyl group and four anomeric protons at $\delta 5.3$ ($H_1''''$ d; J 2Hz), 4.9 ($H_1'''$; broad singlet), 4.25 ($H_1''$; d; J 7Hz) and 4.85 ($H_1'$; q). On hydrolysis with aqueous acid evertetrose (8) yields evertriose (11) and evermicose (10).

The linkage of evertriose (11) to evermicose (10) in the structure of evertetrose (8) is shown in the following way. Methylation of evertetrose (8) yields (60) and (61) which are separated by preparative t.l.c. Besides showing a molecular ion peak at m/e 728, compound (60) shows the presence of ions (62), (63), (64) and (65). In the mass spectrum compound (61) shows the presence of a molecular ion peak at m/e 742 and ions (66) and (67). It is therefore clear that compound (60) possesses the unmethylated tertiary hydroxyl group, whereas in (61) it is methylated. On prolonged hydrolysis compound (60) yields a mixture of products from which the more polar fraction is isolated and then acetylated. The crude mixture of acetates are separated into (68) and (69). Isolation of (69) establishes that in evertetrose (8) the hydroxyl group at $C_3$ of curacose is linked with the anomeric hydroxyl group of evermicose. The stereochemistry of the evermicose part (axial hydrogen) of the anomeric linkage is deduced from the $^1$H n.m.r. spectrum and is also confirmed by the application of Klyne's rule. Based on the above, the structure and absolute stereochemistry of evertetrose is represented as (8).

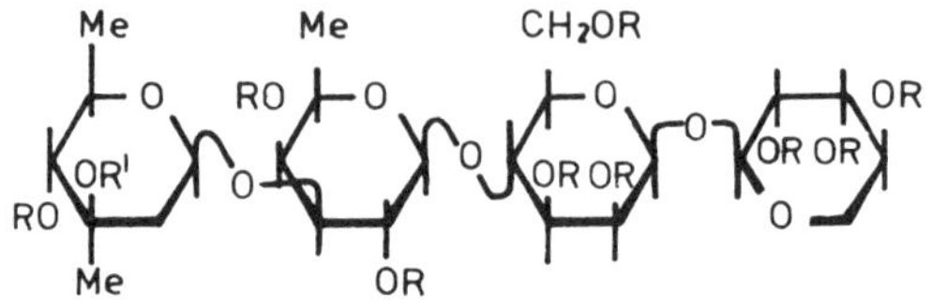

(**60**) R=$CH_3$; R$'$=H
(**61**) R=R$'$=$CH_3$

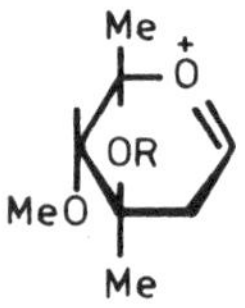

(**62**) R=H
(**66**) R=$CH_3$

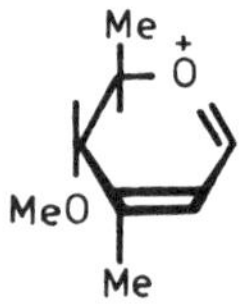

(**63**)

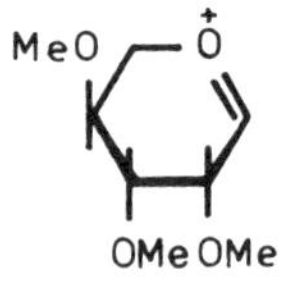

(**64**)

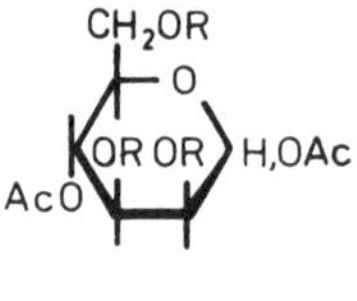

(**68**) R=$CH_3$

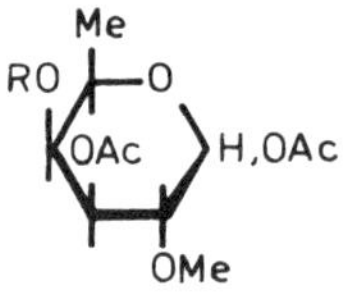

(**69**) R=$CH_3$

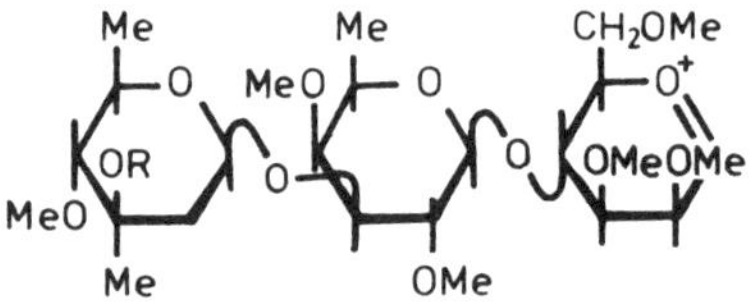

(**65**) R=H; (**67**) R=$CH_3$

3.2.6 *Olgose*

Olgose (**4**) is a colourless crystalline solid, $C_{37}H_{62}O_{22}$, m.p. 212-215°, $[\alpha]_D$ −21.8°. It has no carbonyl absorption in the infrared and in the ultraviolet spectrum it does not show any selective absorption. Although in the electron impact mass spectrum olgose does not show a peak for the molecular ion, it does show the presence of such an ion in the chemical ionization mass spectrum.

Olgose (**4**) when treated with methanolic toluene-p-sulphonic acid undergoes smooth cleavage to evertetrose (**8**) and olgose side chain (**9**).

Compound (**9**) is a colourless liquid, $C_{10}H_{18}O_7$ ($M^+$ 250) $[\alpha]_D$ −28° and shows no selective absorption in the u.v. The i.r. spectrum of (**9**) shows the presence of an ester (1739 cm.$^-$) and a hydroxyl group (3509 $cm^{-1}$). The $^1H$ n.m.r. spectrum showed signals at δ1.25 [d, J 6.5Hz, $CH_3CH(OMe)$], 3.35 (s, 3H, —OMe), 3.81 (s, 3H, —$CO_2Me$), 3.6-3.9 (3H, multiplet), 4.19 (d, 1H, J 5Hz; $H_1$), 4.85 (d, 1H; J 5Hz; $H_2$), 5.0 and 5.21 (s, 1H each, —O-$CH_2$-O-). The apparent absence of vicinal coupling between the methylenedioxy protons is not uncommon as shown [26] in structures (**70**) and (**71**). On treatment with pyridine and acetic anhydride compound (**9**) yielded a monoacetate (**72**), a colourless oil, $C_{12}H_{20}O_8$ ($M^+$ 292). ν max 3546 (hydroxyl) and 1739 $cm^{-1}$ (ester). The $^1H$ n.m.r. spectrum of (**72**) is consistent with the assigned structure and shows signals at δ4.1 and 4.3 (doublets; J 12Hz, —$CH_2OAc$), δ4.88 (d; J 5Hz; $H_1$), δ 4.36 (d; J 5Hz; $H_2$) and δ5.0 and 5.21 (s, 2H, —$OCH_2O$).

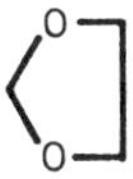

(**71**) 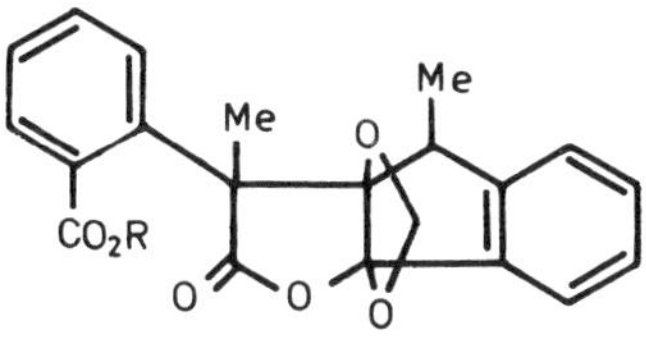 (**70**)

Having established the structure of evertetrose (**8**) and the olgose side chain (**9**) it remained to demonstrate the linkage of (**8**) and (**9**) in the structure of olgose (**4**). Permethylated olgose (**73**) $C_{42}H_{72}O_{22}$ ($M^+$ 928), m.p. 194-195°, $[\alpha]_D$ −13.9° does not show the presence of any hydroxyl or ester function in the i.r. On treatment with methanolic toluene-p-sulphonic acid, compound (**73**) yields (**74**) and (**75**).

Compound (**74**) is a colourless liquid, $C_{11}H_{20}O_7$, $\nu_{max}$ 3448 (hydroxyl) and 1754 $cm^{-1}$ (ester). Acetylation of (**74**) yields (**76**), a colourless liquid, $C_{13}H_{22}O_8$, $\nu_{max}$ 1750 $cm^{-1}$ and no absorption for hydroxyl group. In the $^1H$ n.m.r. spectrum, compound (**76**) shows the presence of —$CH_2OCOCH_3$, δ4.1, 4.3 (doublets; J 12Hz) group and other characteristic features of the molecules eg. —O-$CH_2$-O- at δ5.0 and 5.21 (singlets) and a pair of doublets at δ4.88 ($H_1$; J 5Hz), 4.36 ($H_2$; J 5Hz). Compound (**9**) on periodate oxidation yields (**76a**), which, on treatment with sulphuric acid, yields formaldehyde, thus providing a chemical proof for the presence of a methylenedioxy group in (**9**).

Compound (**75**) is a crystalline solid, $C_{33}H_{58}O_{17}$, m.p. 108-110°, $[\alpha]_D$ −45.1°. The position of the free hydroxyl groups in (**75**) is indicated by measuring the CD of the cuprammonium complex of (**75**), $[\theta]_{288}$ −1250 (suggesting δ chelate). The formation of a δ chelate is possible only if the hydroxyl groups of the 2-O-methyl lyxose moiety in (75) are free. On prolonged acidic hydrolysis compound (75) yields a mixture of products from which 2-O-methyl-L-lyxose (32) is isolated by preparative t.l.c. The formation of (32) from (75) confirms the above conclusion.

As compound (73) has no carbonyl absorption in the i.r. spectrum and on hydrolysis yields (74) and (75), it is evident that the primary hydroxyl group and the carbomethoxy function of (74) and the hydroxyl groups in (75) must be involved in the structure of permethylated olgose (73). Based on all the above observations the structures (4) and (73) are proposed for olgose and its permethylated derivatives. The formation of (74) and (75) from (73) is then easily explained by the opening of the ortho ester function. The $^{13}C$ n.m.r. spectrum of (4) shows a signal at δ119.8 confirming the presence of an ortho ester carbon in olgose (4).

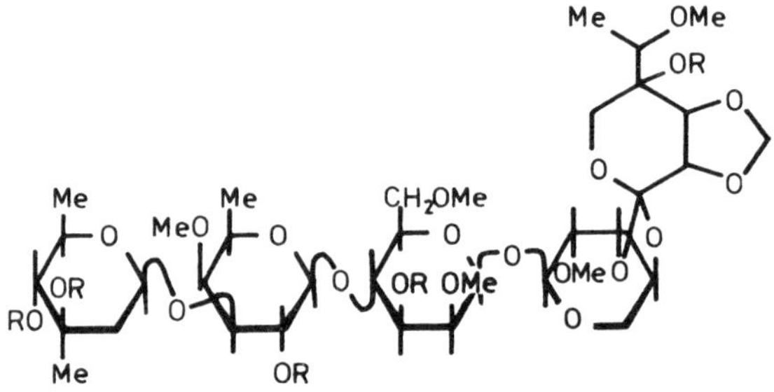

(**73**) R=$CH_3$

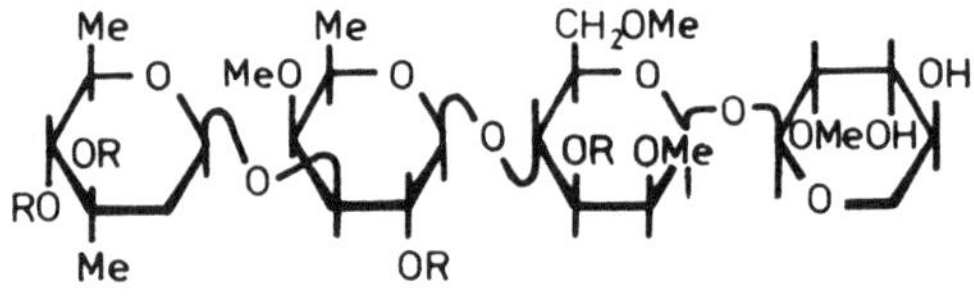

(**75**) R=$CH_3$

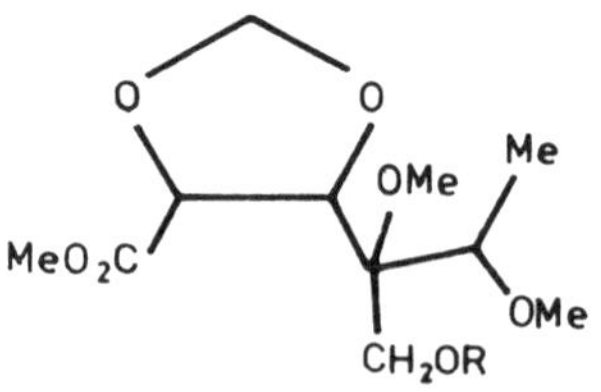

(**74**) R=H

(**76**) R=$COCH_3$

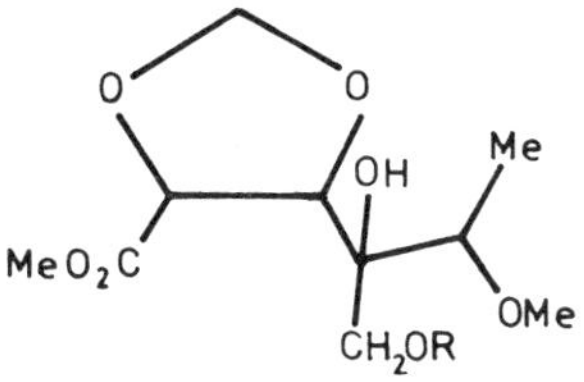

(**9**) R=H
(**72**) R=$COCH_3$

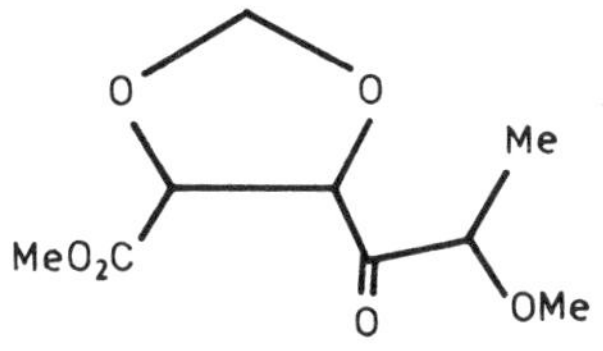

(**77**)

3.2.7 *Everinomicin D*

The linkage of olgose (**4**) to the methyl ether of everninonitrose pyranosyl (1 → 4) digitolactone (**3**) in the structure of the monomethyl ether of everninomicin D (**1a**) follows from the following evidence. Everninomicin D (**1**) on hydrolysis yields a mixture of products from which a tetrasaccharide (**77**) has been isolated, $C_{36}H_{53}O_{18}NCl_2$, 1.5 $H_2O$, $[\alpha]_D$ −44.9°. It forms a tetraacetate (**78**), $C_{44}H_{61}O_{22}NCl_2$, $[\alpha]_D$ −40°. When a solution of (**77**) in tetrahydrofuran is treated with an ethereal solution of diazomethane, it undergoes smooth cleavage to (**3**) and evermicose (**10**). The $^1$H n.m.r. spectrum of (**77**) is consistent with the assigned structure. Elucidation of the structure of compound (**77**) establishes the linkage of evermicose (**10**) to the lactone (**3**). It should be recalled that everninomicin $D_1$ (**2**) on treatment with diazomethane yields (**24**) and olgose (**4**) in a similar way as (**77**) yields (**3**) and (**10**). As we have already established the linkage of evermicose (**10**) in olgose (**4**), the structure of everninomicin $D_1$ should therefore be represented as (**2**).

Everninomicin D (**1**) on exhaustive methylation yields permethylated everninomicin D (**79**), $C_{72}H_{113}O_{36}NCl_2$, $[\alpha]_D$ −27.8°. On solvolysis compound (**79**) yields a mixture of products from which the following compounds are isolated: compound (**80**), $C_{31}H_{43}O_{14}NCl_2$, m.p. 129°, $[\alpha]_D$ −46.1°. Isolation of (**80**) from (**79**) indicates that the hydroxyl group $\beta$ to the ester carbonyl in everninomicin $D_1$ (**2**) is free in everninomicin D (**1**). Compound (**81**), $C_{30}H_{54}O_{17}$, $[\alpha]_D$ −55° yields an amorphous tri-O-acetyl derivative (**82**) which shows besides the other expected features of the molecule a doublet at $\delta$4.6 (J 10Hz) for the $H_4{}'$ proton. As it has been shown earlier in the structure of olgose that the two hydroxyl groups of the 2-O-methyl lyxose portion of the molecule are linked with the olgose side chain (**9**) in the structure of olgose (**4**), it follows, therefore, that the two free hydroxyl groups in the evermicose portion of compound (**82**) must be involved in the linkage in the structure of everninomicin D (**1**).

The n.m.r. spectrum of everninomicin D (**1**) shows the presence of 7-methoxyl groups, nine C-methyl groups and no more anomeric protons than are already accounted for in the structure of everninomicin $D_1$ (**2**). The monomethyl ether of everninomicin D (**1a**) yields a triacetate (**83**), $[\alpha]_D$ −28.1° as evidenced by the $^1$H n.m.r. spectrum. Everninomicin D (**1**) on solvolysis does not yield any products other than those already recognized from the hydrolysis of everninomicin $D_1$(2) (followed by tlc, vpc, etc.). It is therefore concluded that the conversion of everninomicin D (1) to everninomicin $D_1$(2) simply involves the hydrolytic opening of an ortho ester linkage without loss of any component of the molecule.

Based on all the above observations structure (**1**) is proposed for everninomicin D. The hydrolytic opening of one of the ortho ester linkages in everninomicin D (**1**) yields everninomicin $D_1$ (**2**) and hydrolysis of both the ortho ester linkages yields everheptose (**84**). The $^{13}C$ n.m.r. spectrum of everninomicin D shows signals at δ119.6 and 120.0 confirming the presence of two ortho ester carbons in structure (**1**).

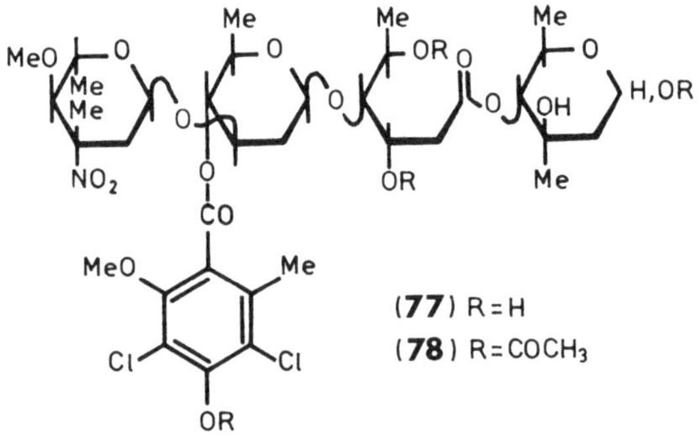

(**77**) R=H
(**78**) R=$COCH_3$

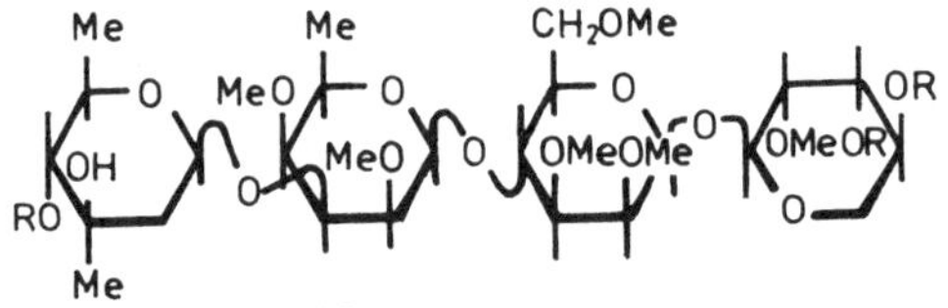

(**81**) R=H
(**82**) R=$COCH_3$

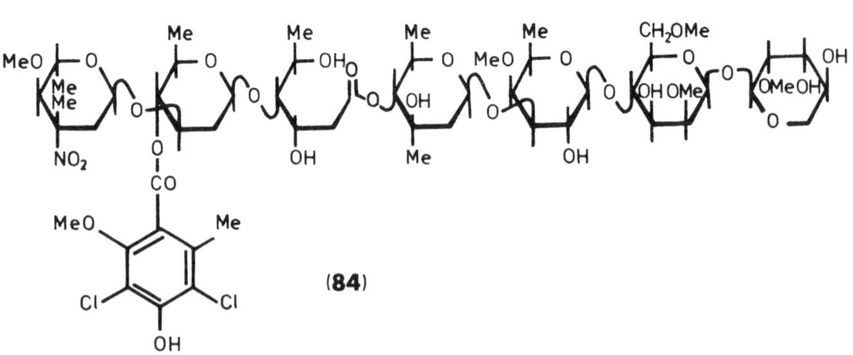

(**84**)

Everninomicin D thus represents the first example of a structural elucidation in this group of complex oligosaccharide antibiotics. Based on similar degradation experiments, structures of everninomicins B, C and flambamycin were elucidated.

### 3.3 Everninomicin B

Everninomicin B [5] (**85**) is a colourless crystalline solid, $C_{66}H_{99}NO_{36}Cl_2$, m.p. 184-185°C, $[\alpha]_D$ −33.1°, $\nu_{max}$ 1732 (ester), 1540 (nitro) $cm.^{-1}$. The monomethyl ether of everninomicin B (**86**) is a colourless crystalline solid, $C_{67}H_{101}NO_{36}Cl_2$, m.p. 187-190°C, $[\alpha]_D$ −34.5°. Its molecular weight is found to be 1587 (calc. for $C_{67}H_{101}NO_{36}Cl_2$, 1567) by the application of the radioactive method [8].

On mild hydrolysis, everninomicin B (**85**) yields everninomicin $B_1$ (**87**), $C_{66}H_{101}NO_{37}Cl_2$, $[\alpha]_D$ −49.1°, $\nu$ max 1730 $cm^{-1}$ (ester), 1540 (nitro) $cm.^{-1}$. As in everheptose (**84**) and everninomicin $D_1$(**2**) compound (**87**) is smoothly cleaved with diazomethane to yield (**3**) and olgose B (**88**).

Solvolysis of olgose B (**88**), $C_{37}H_{62}O_{23}$, $[\alpha]_D$ −23.3° with methanolic p-toluenesulphonic acid at room temperature yields evertetrose B (**89**) and olgose D side chain (**9**).

Evertetrose B (**89**) is a non-reducing crystalline solid, m.p. 276-277°, $[\alpha]_D$ −46.3° (water). It has no selective u.v. absorption and its i.r. spectrum does not show carbonyl absorption. The $^1H$ n.m.r. spectrum of (**89**) shows the presence of four methoxyl groups, one tertiary and two secondary methyl groups and also reveals the presence of four anomeric protons at $\delta$4.7 (d, J 7Hz), 5.19 (s; W 1/2 2.5Hz), 5.68 (d, J 2Hz) and 5.45 (s; W 1/2 2.5Hz). The first three of the above anomeric proton signals have been assigned to the evertriose portion of the molecule which is further confirmed by aqueous hydrolysis of (**89**) to evertriose (**11**) and D-evalose (**90**).

Permethylated evertetrose B (**91**) on prolonged aqueous hydrolysis yields a mixture of products from which 2:3:4-tri-O-methyl D-evalose (**92**) and 2-O-methyl D-curacose are isolated by t.l.c. This establishes that D-evalose is linked through its anomeric oxygen to C-3 of D-curacose.

D-evalose (**90**) is a colourless glass, $[\alpha]_D$ 4.7 → 5.2 (water). The $^1H$ n.m.r. spectrum of (**90**) shows the presence of a secondary methyl doublet, a tertiary methyl singlet and no methoxyl group. On methylation and partial hydrolysis it forms the tri-O-methyl ether (**92**) m.p. 115-120°, $[\alpha]_D$ +18.3 → +6.3°. The n.m.r. spectrum of (**92**) (anomeric mixture) shows the presence of three methoxyl groups, a secondary methyl group ($\delta$1.29; d; J 6.5Hz), a tertiary methyl group ($\delta$1.37) and a one proton doublet at $\delta$3.08 (J 9Hz; $H_4$) corresponding to the major anomer. The stereochemistry at C-2 (axial methoxyl) follows from the coupling constants of the anomeric protons ($\delta$4.7 broad singlet J 3Hz and 5.26, d, J 2.5Hz). These observations establish that compound (**92**) and L-nogalose [27] **(93)** have the same relative stereochemistry at $C_3$, $C_4$ and $C_5$. A direct comparison (i.r., t.l.c., n.m.r.) with an authentic sample establishes the identity of the two compounds. As the absolute stereochemistry of L-nogalose **(93)** has been established by X-ray analysis, it follows that tri-O-methyl D-evalose **(92)** must be D-nogalose. This is confirmed as follows. Jones' oxidation of **(92)** followed by β-elimination yields **(94)**, $[\theta]_{255}$ +3639°; similarly L-nogalose **(93)** gives **(95)**, $[\theta]_{255}$ −4292°. The stereochemistry of the anomeric linkage of D-evalose **(90)** in evertetrose B **(89)** is deduced as β- (equatorial) by application of Klyne's rule and from the n.m.r. spectrum (δ5.45;s;W 1/2 2.5Hz; anomeric proton of D-evalose).

The linkage of evertetrose B **(89)** to olgose D side chain **(9)** is shown in the following way. Permethylated olgose B **(97)** is a colourless crystalline solid, $C_{43}H_{74}O_{23}$, m.p. 182-183°C, $[\alpha]_D$ −26.1°. Solvolysis of **(97)** and isolation of the products show that the two free hydroxyl groups of 2-O-methyl L-lyxose moiety must be linked with the primary hydroxyl group and ester function of **(9)** in the structure of permethylated olgose B **(97)**.

Permethylated everninomicin B **(98)** is an amorphous solid, $C_{72}H_{111}NO_{36}Cl_2$, $[\alpha]_D$ −29.5°. On mild hydrolysis followed by treatment of the reaction product with diazomethane it yields lactone **(80)** and partially methylated olgose B **(99)**, $C_{41}H_{70}O_{23}$, m.p. 167-170°C, $[\alpha]_D$ −35.1°. Compound **(99)** forms a mono-acetate **(96)** which shows $H_4'$ proton at δ4.86 (d, J 10Hz). The position of the free hydroxyl groups in **(99)** is also shown by measuring CD of the cuprammonium complex of **(99)**, $[\theta]_{288}$ + 132° (suggesting λ chelate). It follows therefore that two free hydroxyl groups of **(99)** are linked with the lactone portion of **(80)** in the structure of permethylated everninomicin B **(98)**. Based on all these observations, structure **(85)** is proposed for everninomicin B.

**(85)** R = R' = H
**(86)** R = H; R' = $CH_3$
**(98)** R = R' = $CH_3$

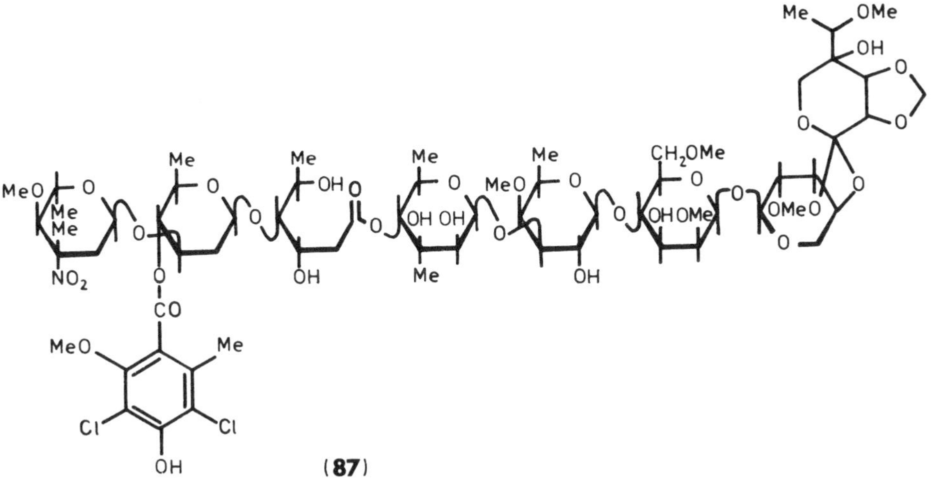

(**87**)

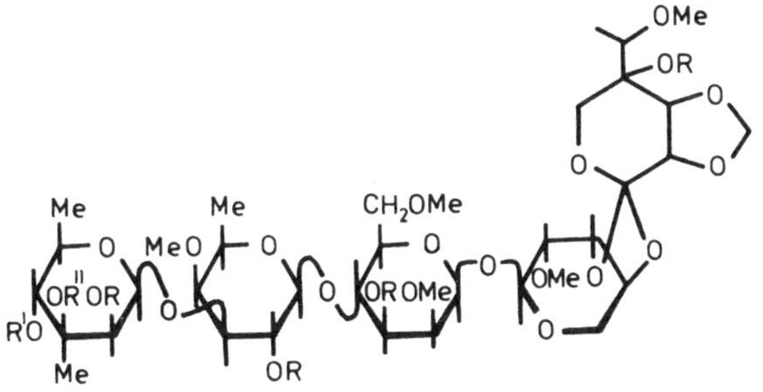

(**88**) R = H ; R' = H ; R'' = H

(**97**) R = $CH_3$ ; R' = $CH_3$ ; R'' = $CH_3$

(**99**) R = $CH_3$ ; R' = R'' = H

(**96**) R = $CH_3$ ; R' = $COCH_3$ ; R'' = H

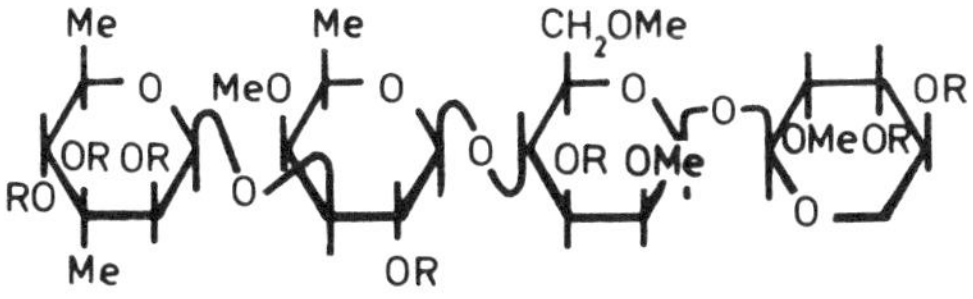

(**89**) R = H

(**91**) R = $CH_3$

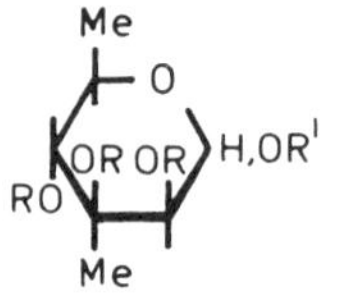

(**90**) R=H; R'=H
(**92**) R=CH ; R'=H

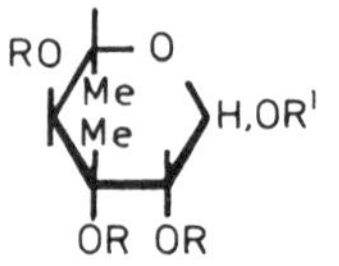

(**93**) R=Me ; R=H

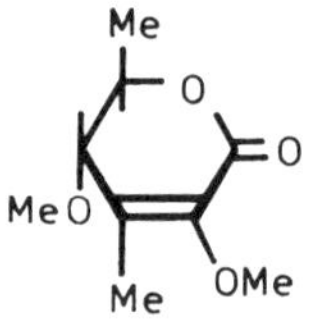

(**94**)

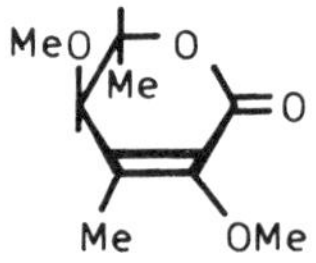

(**95**)

### 3.4 Everninomicin C

Everninomicin C (**100**), $C_{63}H_{93}NO_{34}Cl_2$, m.p. 181-184°C, $[\alpha]_D$ −33.7° shows the presence of an ester function and a nitro group. On hydrolysis everninomicin C (**100**) yields everninomicin $C_1$ (**101**). On treatment with diazomethane (**101**) yields olgose C (**102**) and the lactone (**3**). Solvolysis of (**102**) yields evetetrose (**8**) and the side chain (**103**) which could not be obtained pure because it co-chromatographed with the methyl glycoside of evermicose.

Permethylated olgose C (**104**), $C_{39}H_{66}O_{21}$, m.p. 197-199 °C, $[\alpha]_D$ −8.7° on solvolysis yields partially methylated evertetrose D (**75**) and (**105**). Compound (**105**) is a colourless liquid, $C_8H_{14}O_6$, $\nu_{max}$ 3450, 1754 cm$^{-1}$, δ 3.52, 3.81 ($-OCH_3$ and $-CO_2CH_3$), 3.49 (1H, m; $H_3$), 4.60 (1H; d. J 4.5Hz; $H_1$) 4.25 (1H; t; J 4.5Hz; $H_2$), 5.03, 5.20 (1H each; $-O-CH_2-O-$). The presence of a $-CH_2OH$ group in (**105**) is shown by the formation of acetate (**106**) which shows the presence of $-CH_2-OCOCH_3$ grouping, δ2.1 (3H; s; $-OCOCH_3$), 4.12, 4.47 (1H each; dd; J 4 and 11.5Hz). Based on all the above observations structure (**102**) is proposed for olgose C and (**104**) for permethylated olgose C. The tetraacetate of olgose C (**107**), $C_{42}H_{64}O_{25}$, $[\alpha]_D$ −4.7° shows in the n.m.r. spectrum a signal at δ4.53 ($H_4$; d of t; J 2 and 9Hz) thus indicating that $H_3$ and $H_4$ are axial protons.

The linkage of (**102**) and (**3**) in the structure of the methyl ether of eveninomicin C (**100a**) is shown in the same way as has been demonstrated in the structural elucidation of everninomicin B and D. Permethylated everninomicin C (**108**) is an amorphous solid, $[\alpha]_D$ −25.0° which on hydrolysis yields the lactone

**(80)**, partially methylated evertetrose **(81)** and **(105)**. It has been shown already that the two hydroxyl groups of the 2-O-methyl L-lyxose portion of the molecule are linked with the **(103)** in olgose C **(102)**, it follows therefore that the two free hydroxyl groups in the evermicose portion of **(81)** must be linked with the lactone carbonyl of **(80)** in the structure of permethylated everninomicin C **(108)**.

Based on all the above observations structure **(100)** is proposed for everninomicin C.

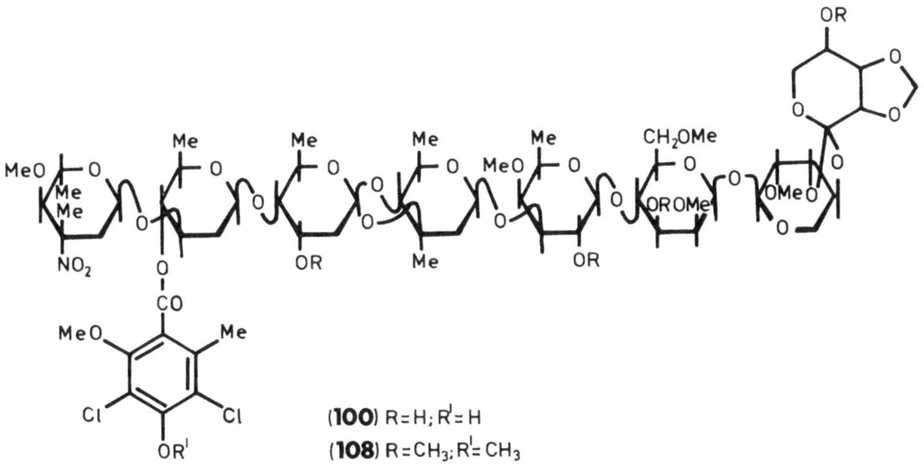

**(100)** R=H; R'=H
**(108)** R=$CH_3$; R'=$CH_3$
**(100a)** R=H ; R'=$CH_3$

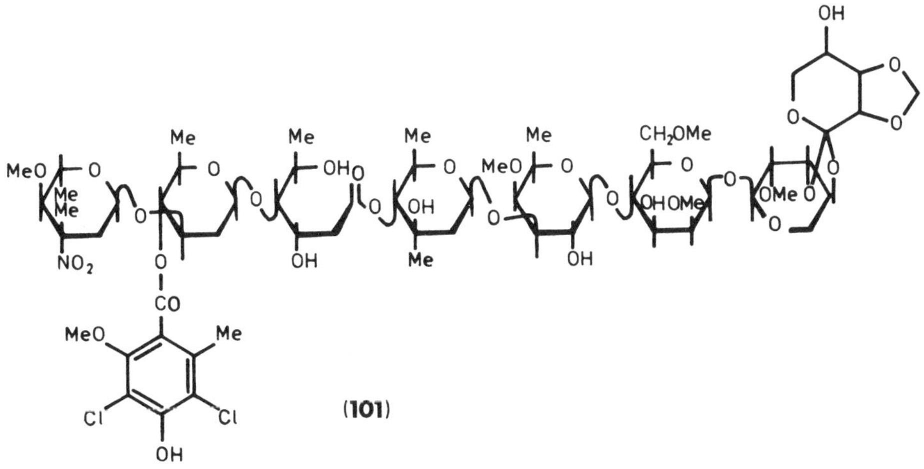

**(101)**

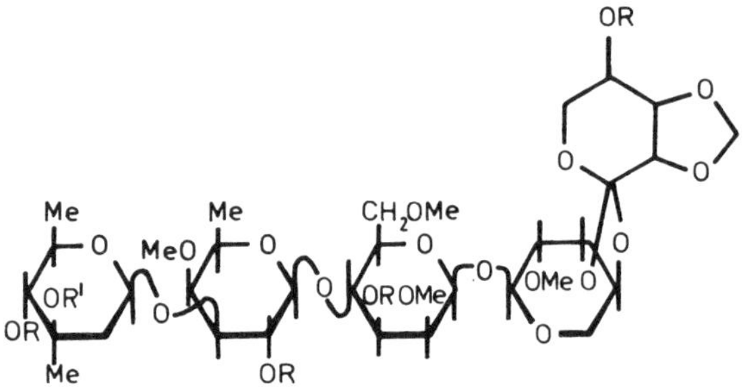

(**102**) R = R' = H
(**104**) R = R' = CH
(**107**) R = $COCH_3$; R' = H

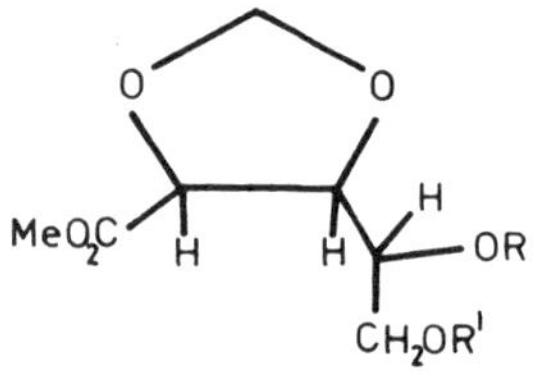

(**103**) R = R' = H
(**105**) R = Me; R' = H
(**106**) R = Me; R' = $COCH_3$

### 3.5 Everninomicin-2

Everninomicin-2 [28] (**109**) is produced by *Micromonospora carbonaceae.* It is highly active against gram positive bacteria and is also active against strains resistant to $\beta$-lactams, tetracycline, lincomycins, ansamycins, macrolides and chloramphenicol.

Everninomicin-2 (**109**) is a colourless crystalline solid, $C_{58}H_{86}Cl_2O_{31}$, m.p. 212-216°C, $[\alpha]_D$ −0.5°, $\nu_{max}$ 3450 (hydroxyl) and 1750 $cm^{-1}$ (ester). The $^{13}C$-n.m.r. spectrum of everninomicin-2 shows signals at $\delta$120.5 and 119.7 ppm indicating the presence of two ortho ester carbon atoms in the molecule as in everninomicin B, C and D. Solvolysis of the monomethyl ether of everninomicin-2 (**110**), $C_{59}H_{88}Cl_2O_{31}$, m.p. 210-212°C, $[\alpha]_D$ +1.2°, yields a mixture of products which could be separated into the hydroxyl-methyl ester (**9**), a lactone (**111**) and evertetrose (**8**). The lactone (**111**) is a colourless crystalline solid, $C_{22}H_{28}Cl_{21}O_{10}$, m.p. 200°C, $[\alpha]_D$ +10.8°, $\nu_{max}$ 3450 (OH) and 1750 $cm.^{-1}$ (ester, lactone). Its $^1H$ n.m.r. spectrum is consistent with the assigned structure and compared well with the n.m.r. spectrum of O-methyl flambolactone. It has been shown earlier that olgose **(4)** on solvolysis yields the hydroxyl methyl ester **(9)** and evertetrose **(8)**. Based on the fact that the monomethyl ether of everninomicin-2 **(110)** on solvolysis yields **(9)**, **(111)** and **(8)** and that the $^{13}C$ n.m.r. spectrum of everninomicin-2 **(109)** shows the presence of two ortho ester carbon atoms, we propose structure **(109)** for everninomicin-2 and structure **(110)** for its monomethyl ether. As the structures of everninomicin-2 **(109)** and everninomicin D **(1)** have identical structures, except for the presence of evernitrose in the latter, it was considered desirable to attempt conversion of **(1)** to **(109)**. It was conceived that nitrosoeverninomicin D **(112)** (preparation of this compound will be described under chemical modifications), on treatment with triethyl phosphite or triphenyl phosphine could be converted into a nitrene (see formulae) which would rearrange with bond migration (one of the three possibilities shown) to an enamine which should, in principle, hydrolyze the required glycosidic bond of everninomicin D **(1)** yielding everninomicin-2 **(109)**. In the event when nitrosoeverninomicin D **(112)** is heated under reflux in benzene solution with triphenyl phosphine for 15 minutes till the blue colour disappears and the reaction mixture worked up in the usual way it yields everninomicin-2 **(109)** in 30% overall yield.

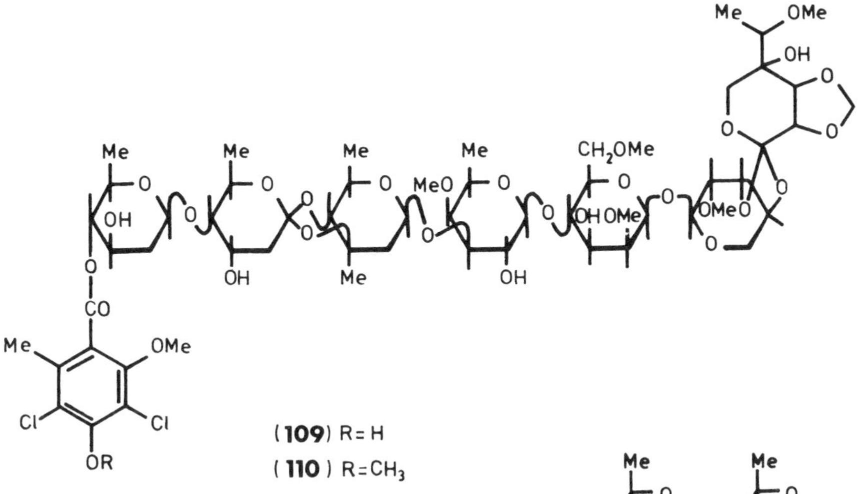

(**109**) R = H
(**110**) R = $CH_3$

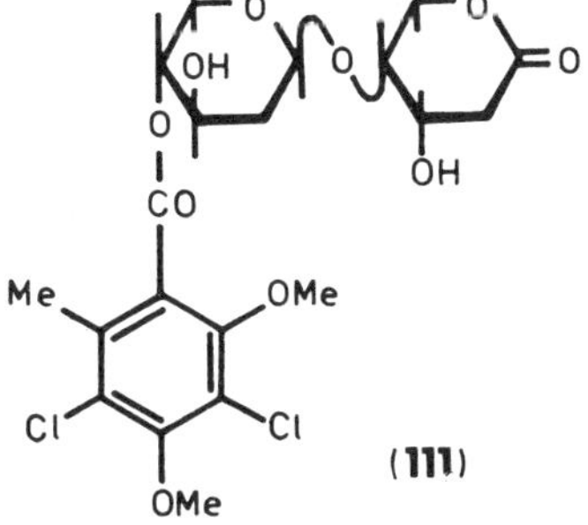

(**111**)

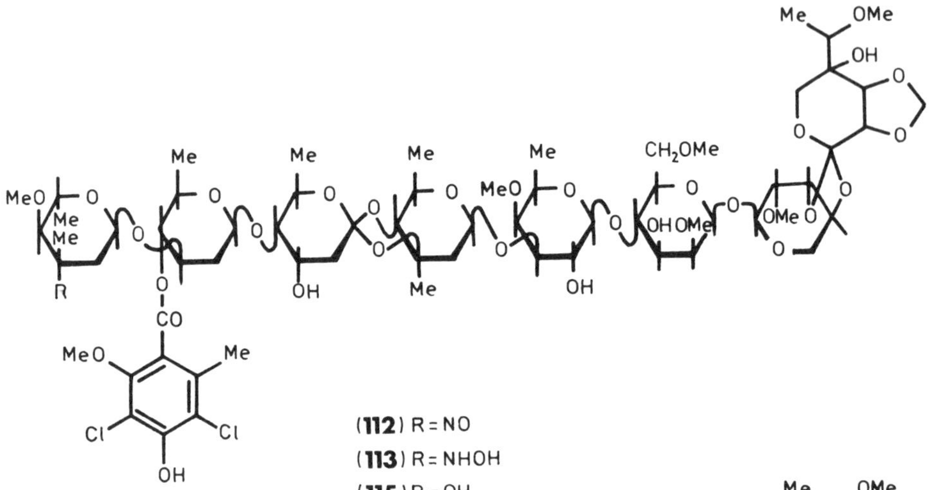

Me OMe OH O O O O Me Me Me Me CH$_2$OMe MeO O O O O O O MeO O O O O Me Me O O O O OH OMe O OMe O O R O OH Me OH CO MeO Me Cl Cl OH

(**112**) R = NO
(**113**) R = NHOH
(**115**) R = OH

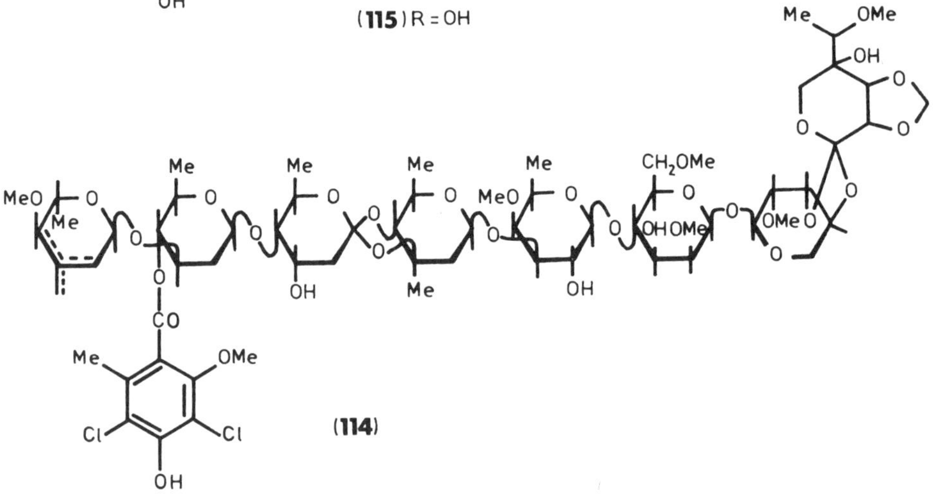

Me OMe OH O O O O Me Me Me Me CH$_2$OMe MeO O O O O O O MeO O O O Me O O O O O OH OMe O OMe O O O OH Me OH CO Me OMe Cl Cl OH

(**114**)

## 4 STRUCTURE-ACTIVITY RELATIONSHIPS

The structure-activity relationship in the everninomicin group of antibiotics is not completely understood. Most of the chemical modifications in this group of antibiotics have been carried out on everninomicin D (**1**), the main constituent of the antibiotic complex produced by *Micromonospora carbonaceae*. Hydrolysis of everninomicin D (**1**) yields everninomicin $D_1$ (**2**) (in which one of the ortho-ester linkages is broken). On further hydrolysis everninomicin $D_1$ (**2**) yields everheptose (**84**) (in which both the ortho ester linkages are cleaved). Although everninomicin D is highly active against gram positive bacteria, compounds (**2**) and (**84**) are essentially devoid of microbiological activity thus indicating that the ortho-ester linkages are necessary for maintaining activity in this group of antibiotics.

The phenolic hydroxyl group in everninomicin D is quite acidic and therefore amenable to selective derivatization to afford phenolic ethers and esters, All the phenolic ethers prepared were inactive and the esters which could not be hydrolyzed easily under the test conditions were inactive. It is obvious, therefore, that the presence of the phenolic hydroxyl group is also associated with the antibacterial activity.

More successful modifications of everninomicins are brought about by changing the nitro function in the evernitrose portion of everninomicin B, C and D. For example, when everninomicin D is reduced with aluminium amalgam, it yields a mixture of products from which hydroxylaminoeverninomicin D (**113**) and nitrosoeverninomicin D (**112**) are isolated by chromatography.

Hydroxylaminoeverninomicin D (**113**) is a colourless crystalline solid, $C_{66}H_{101}Cl_2NO_{34}$, m.p. 185-186°C, $[\theta]_{255}$ (−17400), $\nu_{max}$ 1745 cm.$^{-1}$. It gives a positive colour reaction with triphenyltetrazolium chloride for a hydroxylamino group. Compound (**113**) is unstable to acid and is readily oxidized in air to nitrosoeverninomicin D (**112**). For comparison purposes microbiological activities of everninomicin D and the N-methyl glucamine salt of hydroxylaminoeverninomicin D (**113**) are summarized in Table 4.1

Hydroxylaminoeverninomicin D [29] (**113**) gives the highest blood level, when administered intramuscularly to dogs, compared to other chemically modified derivatives of everninomicin D.

Hydroxylaminoeverninomicin D (**113**) undergoes slow aerial oxidation to nitrosoeverninomicin D (**112**). For preparative purposes hydroxylaminoeverninomycin D (**113**) is oxidized in tetrahydrofuran solution, using sodium hypobromite, to nitrosoeverninomicin D (**112**), a blue amorphous solid, $[\theta]_{255}$ (−15000). It is highly active against gram positive bacteria; minimum inhibitory concentrations against Staphylococci and Streptococci are 0.08–0.8 mcg/ml. *In vivo* studies on nitrosoeverninomicin D (**112**) show similarity to the parent antibiotic, everninomicin D, and it gives a poor peak serum level when administered intramuscularly to dogs.

**Table 4.1**
Dose levels of some everninomicin D compounds

| | | Everninomicin D | Sodium salt and N-methyl-glucamine salt of hydroxylaminoeverninomicin-D |
|---|---|---|---|
| MIC (mcg/ml)[a] | | 0.03-0.3 | 0.08-0.8 |
| MIC (mcg/ml)[b] | | | 0.2-1.0 |
| $PD_{50}$[a] mg/kg | Oral | 15 | 25 |
| | S.C. | 5 | 0.5-5 |
| $LD_{50}$[a] in mice | I.P. | >3800 | 500 |
| (mg/kg) | S.C. | >3800 | 500 |
| | Oral | >3800 | >2000 |
| | I.V. | 125 | 30 |
| Peak serum levels in dogs (mcg/ml) | | | |
| 10 mg/kg | I.M. | 2-3 | 20-30 |
| Peak serum levels in rats (mcg/ml) | | | |
| 25 mg/kg | S.C. | 10-12 | 30-40 |

[a]Staphylococcus and Streptococcus.
[b]N. gonorrhea and N. meningitidis

Hydroxylaminoeverninomicin D (**113**) reacts with aliphatic, aromatic, and heterocyclic aldehydes to yield corresponding nitrones [29]. All the nitrones prepared are highly active against gram positive bacteria. It has been pointed out earlier that nitrosoeverninomicin D on treatment with triethyl phosphite or triphenyl phosphine yields everninomicin-2. The corresponding derivatives of everninomicin-2 from nitrosoeverininomicin B and C have been made and found to be highly active.

Everninomicins are also conveniently reduced electrochemically [30]. When electrolyzed in aqueous solution in the presence of a suitable electrolyte, everninomicin D is reduced to hydroxylaminoeverninomicin D. However, in non-aqueous solvents and in the absence of air, everninomicin D is converted into everninomicin-2 (**109**), everninomicin 3 (**114**) and a small amount of everninomicin 7 (**115**). The yield of everninomicin 7 could be increased by carrying out the electrochemical reaction in the presence of oxygen. The *in vitro* activities of everninomicin 3, 7 and hydroxyaminoeverninomicin D are given in Table 4.2.

**Table 4.2**
Microbiological activity of some Everninomicins

| Microbological Activity (*in vitro*) MIC s mcg/ml | Evernino-micin-3 | Evernino-micin-7 | Hydroxylamino-everninomicin D Sodium salt |
|---|---|---|---|
| *Staphylococcus aureus Strain* | | | |
| 209B | 0.06 | 0.3 | 0.06 |
| Gray | 0.06 | 0.3 | 0.06 |
| 59N | 0.03 | 0.075 | 0.03 |
| Zeigler | 0.03 | 0.75 | 0.06 |
| Wood | 0.06 | 0.75 | 0.06 |
| Microbiological Activity (*in vivo*) | | | |
| $PD_{50}$'s (mg/kg) s.c. Staphylococcus | 0.5 | 1-5 | 0.5-5 |
| Peak Serum Levels in Dogs, 10 mg/kg i.m. | 12-16 | 15-60 | 20-30 |

## 5 OTHER OLIGOSACCHARIDE ANTIBIOTICS

### 5.1 Flambamycin

Flambamycin [31, 32] **(116)** is produced by *Streptomyces hygroscopicus* DS 2320. It shows high activity *in vitro* against gram positive bacteria and Neiserria. Flambamycin, $C_{61}H_{88}Cl_2O_{33} \cdot H_2O$, m.p. 202–203° has been degraded in a similar manner as described in the case of everninomicin D to flambic acid **(117)** and flambeurekanose mono-isobutyrate **(118)**. The structural investigations of **(117** and **(118)** are based on similar logic as established for lactone **(3)** and olgose **(4)**. The linkage of **(117)** to **(118)** in the structure of flambamycin **(116)** is established in the following way. Permethylated flambamycin on acidic methanolysis yields curacin *O*′-methyl ether-3-*O*-methyl ether methyl glycoside, 2-*O*-methyl-D-evalose methyl glycoside, 3,4-di-*O*-methyl-D-fucose methyl glycoside, 2,3,6-tri-O-methyl-D-mannose methyl glycoside and 2-*O*-methyl-L-lyxose methyl glycoside. As in the everninomicins, flambamycin also shows the presence of two ortho-ester carbon atoms at δ119.8 and 120.9 in the $^{13}C$ n.m.r. spectrum.

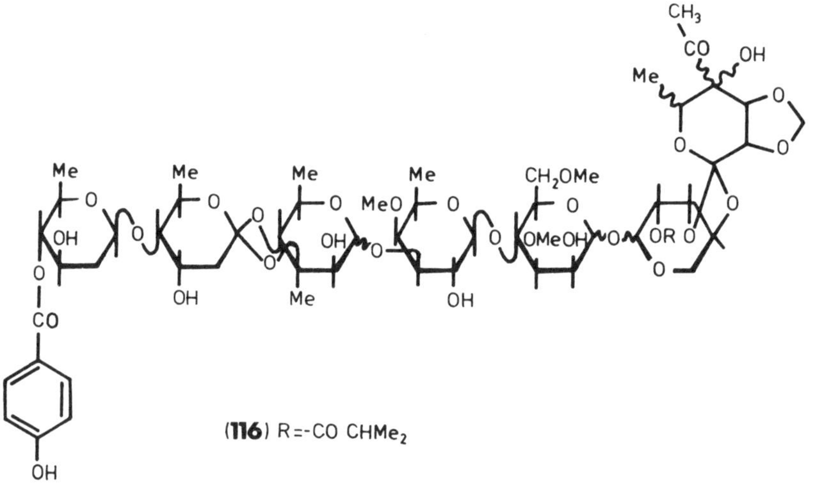

**(116)** R=-CO CHMe$_2$

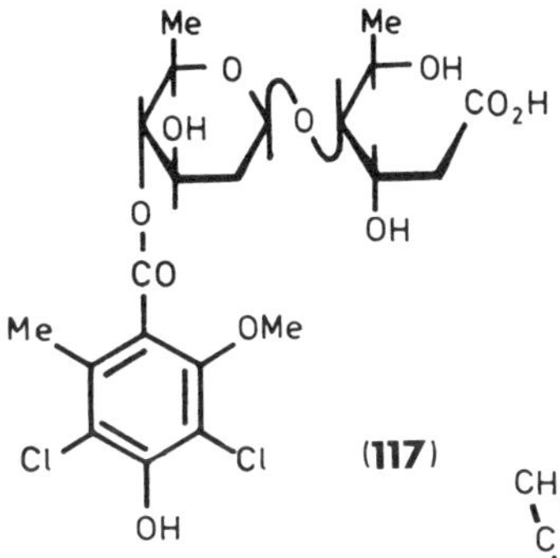

(117)

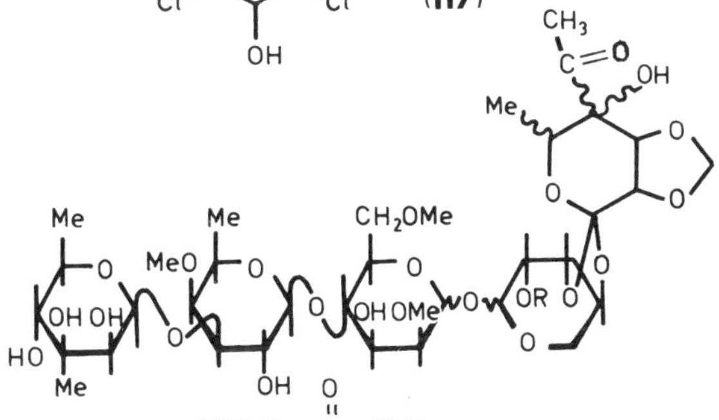

(118) R= $-\overset{O}{\overset{\|}{C}}-CHMe_2$

### 5.2 Curamycin

Curamycin is produced by *Streptomyces Cura-coi* [8]. It is highly active against gram positive bacteria, e.g. it inhibits the growth of *S. aureus* in a concentration of 0.125 mg/ml. Like other antibiotics of this group it is stable at neutral or alkaline pH but very unstable to acidic pH.

#### 5.2.1 *Isolation*

The harvested broth is adjusted to pH 9.5, filtered and the filtrate re-adjusted to pH 7 and then extracted with ethyl acetate. The organic layer is decolourised with charcoal and concentrated to yield a precipitate of curamycin. It crystallizes from a mixture of ethanol, hexane and ether as colourless needles $C_{53-55}H_{82-86}Cl_2O_{32-33}$, m.p. 198°, $[\alpha]_D$ −5.3°, $\lambda_{max}$ 284 nm ($E_1^1$ 9.9), pK 7.48.

#### 5.2.2 *Structural Elucidation*

The work on the structural elucidation has been extremely slow and is far from complete. On acidic hydrolysis curamycin yields a mixture of products from which curacin, L-lyxose and curacose have been isolated.

## 5.3 Avilamycin

Avilamycin is produced by a strain of *Streptomyces viridochromogenes* [9]. It crystallizes from acetone-ether as a colourless crystalline solid, $C_{63}H_{94}O_{35}Cl_2$, 188-189° C, $\lambda_{max}$ 214 (log $\epsilon$ 4.12), 288 nm (log $\epsilon$ 2.89). Its i.r. spectrum is similar but not identical with curamycin. On acidic hydrolysis it yields D-rhamnose, 2,6-di-O-methyl mannose, 4-O-methyl fucose and L-lyxose.

## REFERENCES


[1] M. J. Weinstein, G. M. Luedemann, E. M. Oden and G. H. Wagman, *Antimicrob. Agents Chemotherapy,* 24, (1964).

[2] O. L. Galmarini and V. Deulofeu, *Tetrahedron,* **15**, 76 (1961).

[3] German Patent 1,116,864, Nov. 1961.

[4] L. Ninet, F. Benazet, Y. Charpentie, M. Dubost, J. Flovent, J. Lunel, D. Mancy and J. Preud'homme, *Experentia,* **30**, 1270 (1974).

[5] A. K. Ganguly and A. K. Saksena, *J. Antibiotics,* **28**, 707 (1975).

[6] A. K. Ganguly and S. Szmulewicz, *J. Antibiotics,* **28**, 710 (1975).

[7] A. K. Ganguly, O. Z. Sarre, D. Greeves and J. Morton, *J. Amer. Chem. Soc.,* 1975, **97**, 1982.

[8] E. G. Gros, V. Deulofeu, O. L. Galmarini and B. Flydman, *Experentia,* **24**, 323 (1968); V. Deulofeu and E. G. Gros, *Anales de Quimica,* **68**, 789 (1972).

[9] F. Buzzetti, F. Eisenberg, H. N. Grant, W. Keller-Schierlein, W. Voser and H. Zahner, *Experentia,* **24**, 320 (1968).

[10] J. Black, B. Calesnick, F. G. Falco and M. J. Weinstein, *Antimicrobial Agents and Chemotherapy,* 38 (1964).

[11] W. E. Sanders and C. C. Crowe, *Abs. Proc. 13th Intersciences Conf. Antimicrob. Agents Chemotherapy,* Washington, D.C., 1973, Abs. 139.

[12] J. A. Waitz, E. L. Moss, F. Sabatelli, F. Menzel and C. G. Drube, *Abs. Proc., 13th Intersciences Conf. Antimicrob. Agents Chemotherapy,* Washington, D.C., 1973, Abs. 140.

[13] V. L.Sutter and S. M. Finegold, *Antimicrobial Agents and Chemotherapy,* 736 (1976).

[14] H. P. Faro, A. K. Ganguly and D. H. R. Barton, *J.C.S. Chem. Comm.,* 823 (1971).

[15] A. K. Ganguly, O. Z. Sarre, D. Greeves and J. Morton, *J. Amer. Chem. Soc.,* **95**, 942 (1973).

[16] A. K. Ganguly, O. Z. Sarre and S. Szmulewicz, *J.C.S. Chem. Comm.,* 746 (1971).

[17] A. K. Ganguly, O. Z. Sarre and H. Reimann, *J. Amer. Chem. Soc.,* **90**, 7129 (1968).

[18] A. K. Ganguly and O. Z. Sarre, *J.C.S. Chem. Comm.,* 1149 (1969).

[19] A. K. Ganguly and O. Z. Sarre, *J.C.S. Chem. Comm.,* 911 (1969).

[20] A. K. Ganguly, O. Z. Sarre and J. Morton, *J. C. S. Chem. Comm.,* 1488 (1969).

[21] A. K. Ganguly, O. Z. Sarre, A. T. McPhail and K. D. Onan, *J.C.S. Chem. Comm.,* 313 (1977).

[22] D. M. Lemal, P. D. Pacht and R. B. Woodward, *Tetrahedron,* **18**, 1275 (1962).

[23] R. C. Sheppard and S. Turner, *J.C.S. Chem. Comm.*, 77 (1968); F. L. Carroll and J. T. Blackwell, *Tetrahedron Letters,* 4173 (1970); R. N. Johnson and N. V. Riggs, *Tetrahedron Letters,* 5119 (1967).

[24] R. D. Bucourt, M. Legrand, M. Vignan, J. Tessier and V. Delaroff, *C.R. Acad. Sci.,* 2679 (1963); D. Arigoni, W. Von Daehne, W. O. Godtfredsen, A. Melera and S. Vangedal, *Experentia,* 344 (1964).

[25] W. Klyne, *Biochem. J.,* **47**, XLI, (1950).

[26] P. Yates and R. S. Dewey, *Tetrahedron Letters,* 847 (1962); R. C. Cookson and T. A. Crabb, *Tetrahedron,* **24**, 2385 (1968).

[27] P. F. Wiley, D. J. Duchamp, V. Hsiung and C. C. Chidester, *J. Org. Chem.,* 2670 (1971); P. F. Wiley, F. A. MacKeller, E. L. Caron and R. B. Kelly, *Tetrahedron Letters,* 663 (1968).

[28] A. K. Ganguly, S. Szmulewicz, O. Z. Sarre and V. M. Girijavallabhan, *J.C.S. Chem. Commun.,* 609 (1976).

[29] A. K. Ganguly and O. Z. Sarre, U.S. Patent 3,915,956.

[30] P. Kabasakalian, S. Y. Kalliney, A. K. Ganguly and A. Westcott, U.S. Patent 3,998,708, 1976.

[31] W. D. Ollis, C. Smith and D. E. Wright, *J.C.S. Chem. Comm.,* 882 (1974).

[32] W. D. Ollis, C. Smith, I. O. Sutherland and D. E. Wright, *J.C.S. Chem. Comm.,* 350 (1976).

# PART C

# DAUNOMYCIN AND RELATED ANTIBIOTICS

by

**FEDERICO ARCAMONE**

FARMITALIA-RICERCA CHIMICA

MILAN, ITALY

## PART C

## CONTENTS

## 1 INTRODUCTION

The antitumour anthracyclines are daunomycin, also known as daunorubicin, adriamycin, also known as doxorubicin†, and their derivatives and analogues. Both daunomycin and adriamycin are established useful agents for the chemotherapic treatment of human cancer, and their primary site of action is considered to be at the tumour cell level through an interference with deoxyribonucleic acid (DNA) synthesis and function [1]. Adriamycin is in particular of considerable medical value because of its outstanding activity on a number of solid tumours and it appears to be the most effective, single agent amongst all antitumour drugs presently known. The scientific, clinical, and pharmaceutical importance of adriamycin is well documented in thousands of papers in the biomedical literature. Daunomycin, adriamycin as well as their biosynthetic congeners are all derived from microorganisms of the genus Streptomyces and are obtained following the well known fermentation and recovery techniques generally used in antibiotics technology. The development of the antitumour anthracyclines followed a programme for the screening of new antibiotics, in which the search for antitumour agents was a distinct objective [2].

The isolation of penicillin by Chain and Abraham from *Penicillium chrysogenum* in 1940 and that of streptomycin by Waksman and his co-workers from *Streptomyces griseus* in 1944, indicated the microorganisms as versatile producers of biologically active substances. More specifically the Streptomyces (actinomycetes) appeared to be the most productive genus, and in the following decades they proved to be a practically inexhaustible source of new compounds. Many of the compounds are characterized by varied and complex chemical structures and often endowed with a high inhibitory activity towards different biological systems. Even before the antibiotic era the actinomycetes were known

†Daunorubicin and doxorubicin are the generic names adopted by the W.H.O. The names daunomycin and adriamycin are however more widely used in the scientific literature, especially in the bio-medical papers. Other synonyms for daunomycin are rubidomycin and rubomycin C, see ref. [1].

producers of original coloured compounds and the ability to produce pigments was so typical of this genus that it was used for the naming of a large number of species, and even for classification purposes [3].

Waksman lists the following pigments: (a) anthocyanines and hydroactinochromes, with indicator-like properties, changing from an orange-red colour in acid solution to a blue-violet one with alkalis; (b) green pigments (*e.g.* ferroverdin); (c) lipoactinochromes (*e.g* carotenoids); (d) prodigiosin-like pigments; (e) brown-black pigments (melanines). Practically all known pigments belonging to type (a), notwithstanding the denomination of anthocyanines to some of them, are quinone derivatives, biogenetically derived from acetate and propionate units, and the anthracyclines represent the most important group of such pigments.

The anthracyclines, although endowed with an antibacterial activity, had not found practical application because of their toxicity. They were originally studied in the 'fifties, mainly by Hans Brockmann [4]. Antitumour properties were eventually demonstrated to be associated with a pigment of this type which, however, showed an unfavourable therapeutic index [5]. The product displayed a remarkable inhibition of Ehrlich ascite tumour in mice but did not afford an increase in survival time to treated animals in comparison with the controls. The activity was confirmed with purified preparations of the pigment, which was characterized as a rhodomycin, at very low doses (0.05 to 0.5 mg/Kg body weight) also on other experimental tumours in mice, such as the Ehrlich carcinoma and solid sarcoma 180 [5].

These observations represented the beginning of the history of the antitumour anthracyclines. Shortly afterwards the more selective compound daunomycin was isolated from *Streptomyces peucetius* [6, 7]. The same antibiotic was also isolated in France and named rubidomycin [8]. The compound inhibited the growth of Eirlich ascite tumours and also substantially increased the survival time in treated animals, showing an antitumour activity even higher than those exhibited by known antitumour antibiotics such as mitomycin C and actinomycin C [9]. The early chemical studies carried out on daunomycin [10, 11] were essentially aimed at ascertaining the chemical features of this antibiotic and the structural differences with the pharmacologically less valuable, already known anthracyclines.

Subsequent development of the antitumour anthracyclines involved: (1) the establishment of the clinical efficacy of daunomycin on acute leukemia, reported by different authors, which involved Tan and Di Marco [12] as well as others [13]; (2) the isolation [14] and determination of the chemical structure [15] of adriamycin, which exhibited a more favourable therapeutic index when compared with daunomycin in a number of experimental tumours in laboratory animals [16]; (3) the clinical reports showing that adriamycin was endowed with an impressive broad spectrum of activity on human tumours [17, 18].

The activity of adriamycin has now been established on breast adenocarcinoma, soft tissues and bone sarcomas, bladder adenocarcinoma, bronchogenic carcinoma, testicular carcinoma, pediatric solid tumours, malignant lymphonas, and acute leukemias. Unresponsive tumours are large bowel adenocarcinoma, malignant melanoma,and renal cancer. A number of other human tumour categories show possible responses or inadequacy of data. In present clinical use the drug is generally combined with other active agents to increase the therapeutic efficacy against advanced disease. Additonally, the potential of adriamycin to increase survival when used alone or in combination with other drugs in a combined modality approach with surgery and/or immunotherapy appears of definite clinical interest [19]. Dose limiting side effects are however myelosuppression, stomatitis, nausea and vomiting, alopecia, ECG abnormalities and cardiomyopathy.

The above mentioned facts have in recent years stimulated a wide interest in the chemistry of antitumour anthracyclines. These investigations have as the main objective the development of new derivatives and analogues of daunomycin and adriamycin with improved antitumour efficacy or with reduced toxicity. A characteristic feature of the early development of the biosynthetic antitumour anthracyclines has been the involvement of organic chemistry from the very initial stage. Presently, new potentially clinically useful compounds have been made available by total synthesis and by semi-synthesis. This chapter is aimed at demonstrating the important contribution made by the chemistry of natural products to the control of human cancer.

## 2 THE ANTHRACYCLINE ANTIBIOTICS

Daunomycin (**1**) and its biosynthetic congeners (**2**)–(**8**) represent a structurally defined group of anthracycline antibiotics. These are glycosides of derivatives of 7,8,9,10-tetrahydro-5,12-naphthacenequinone and are a family of pigments, with indicator-like properties (red in acid and blue-violet in alkaline solution), of not rare occurrence in the cultures of strains of the genus *Streptomyces* and related microorganisms. The classical anthracyclines have been reviewed by H. Brockmann [4], to whom most of the early isolation and structure elucidations studies of these compounds are due, by R. H. Thomson [20], and, recently, by Z. Vanek *et al.* [21]. Characteristic features of (**1**), differentiating it from the formerly known anthracyclines, are the methylketone side chain at C-9, the methoxyl group at C-4 and the aminosugar daunosamine, whose occurrence in natural compounds is restricted to the daunomycin group of metabolites. Other structural features, such as the hydroxylation pattern of the aromatic chromophore, the substitution of the A ring and the position of the glycosidic linkage are common to the other anthracyclines. Adriamycin (**2**), the pharmacologically most important component of this group, is the 14-hydroxy-derivative of daunomycin and is therefore, (7S-*cis*) 7-[3-amino-2,3,6-trideoxy-α-L-lyxo-hexopyranosyl)oxy]-9-hydroxyacetyl-4-methoxy-7,8,9,10-tetrahydro-6,9,11-trihydroxy-5,12-naphthacenedione. The numbering system was originally proposed by Brockmann [4] and will be used through this chapter, although not the one followed by the Chemical Abstracts. Rings will be indicated, as also originally proposed [4], by assigning letter A to the non-aromatic ring and D to the aromatic ring bearing the methoxyl group. Other glycosides of this group are carminomycin 1 (**3**) (from *Actinomadura carminata* and from *Streptosporangium sp.*), in which the methoxyl group at C-4 is replaced by a hydroxyl [22], dihydrodaunomycin (**4**), also known as duborimycin or daunorubicinol (from *S. peucetius* and from *S. coeruleoribidus*) [23, 24], its 4-O-demethylanalogue dihydrocarminomycin (**5**) (from *S. peucetius*) [25], the disaccharide derivative daunosaminyldaunomycin (**6**) (from *S. peucetius*) [24] and the baumycins A1, A2 (**7**), B1, B2 (**8**) C1 (N-formyldaunomycin) and C2 (13-dihydro-N-formyldaunomycin, new antibiotics recently isolated from *S. coeruleorubidus* [26]. The following compounds have also been obtained from *S. peucetius* and from related strains: daunomycinone, 7-deoxydaunomycinone, 13-dihydrodaunomycinone, and adriamycinone [1]. A component described as rhodinosyldaunomycin (rubomycin B, RP 13213) has also been reported [27].

Representative compounds belonging to other groups of the anthracycline family antibiotics are rhodomycin A (**9**), rohodomycin B (**10**), citromycin (**11**), pyrromycin (**12**), aklavin (**13**), reticulomycin (**14**), cinerubin (**15**), aclacinomycin A (**16**), steffimycin (**17**), and steffimycin B (**18**) [4, 20 21]. The constituent aglycones (anthracyclinones), display differences in the hydroxylation pattern on the aromatic portion of the molecule, in the presence and the nature

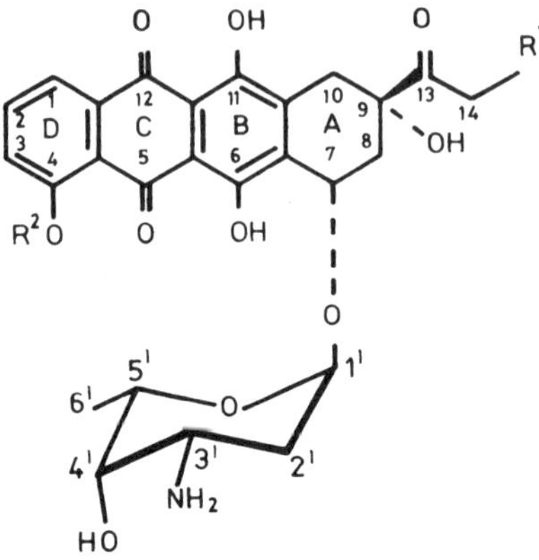

(**1**) $R^1 = H, R^2 = Me$
(**2**) $R^1 = OH, R^2 = Me$
(**3**) $R^1 = R^2 = H$

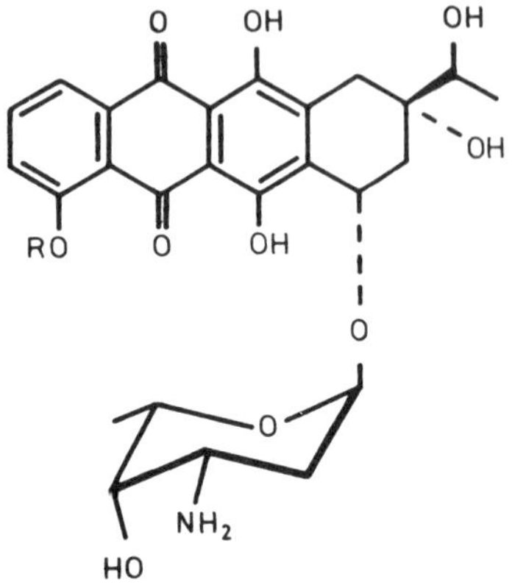

(**4**) R = Me
(**5**) R = H

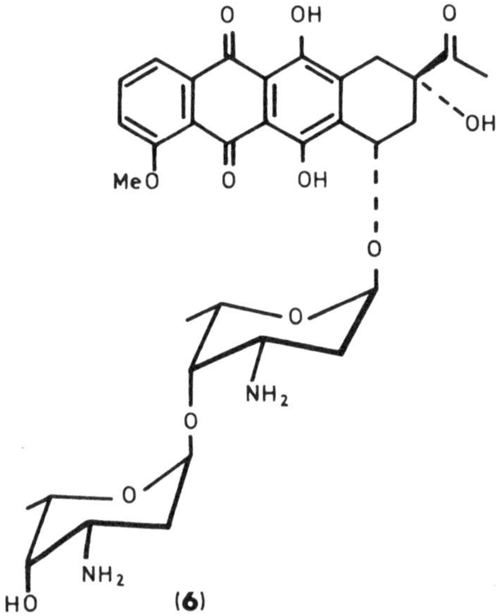

(**6**)

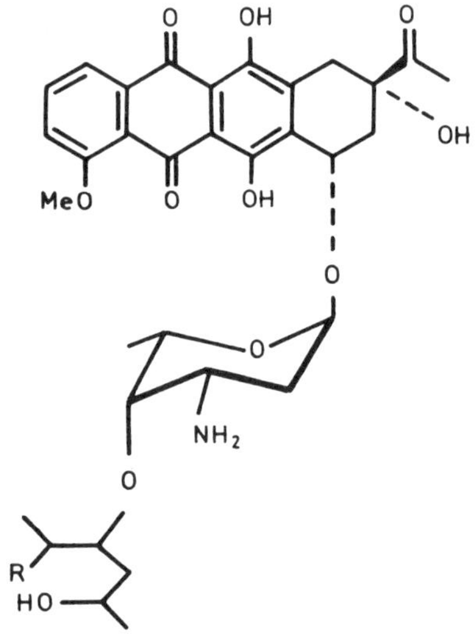

(**7**) $R = CH_2OH$
(**8**) R = COOH

of the substituent at C-10. The C-9 hydroxyl is always present but the C-7 hydroxyl is absent in some cases. This variety of structural features, as well as the modifications concerning oxidation of the side chain typical of the daunomycin group of antibiotics and the presence of methyl groups are considered a consequence of the secondary reactions which take place during their

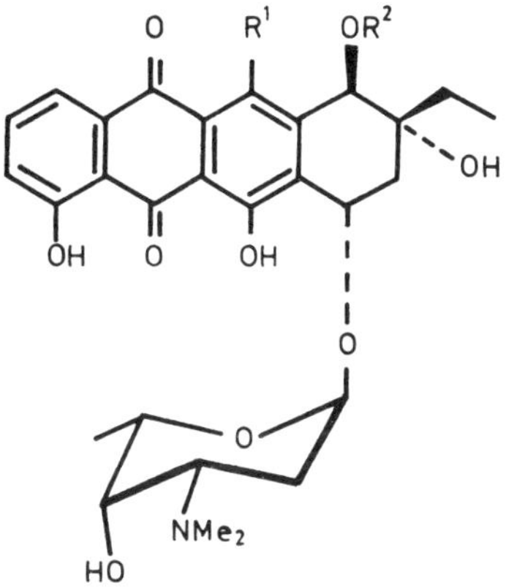

(**9**) $R^1$ = OH, $R^2$ = rhodosaminyl
(**10**) $R^1$ = OH, $R^2$ = H
(**11**) $R^1$ = $R^2$ = H

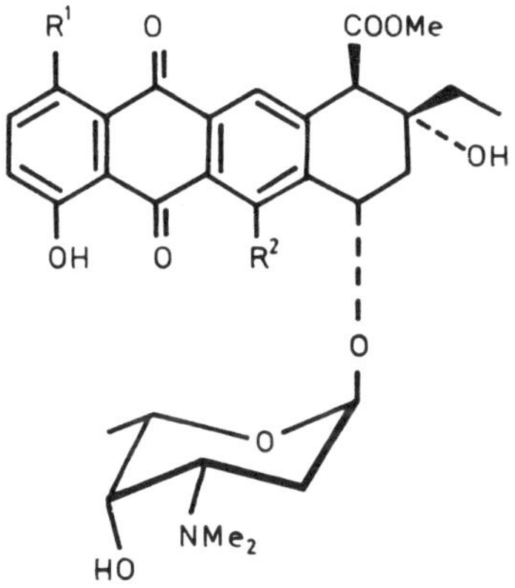

(**12**) $R^1$ = $R^2$ = OH
(**13**) $R^1$ = H, $R^2$ = OH
(**14**) $R^1$ = OH, $R^2$ = H

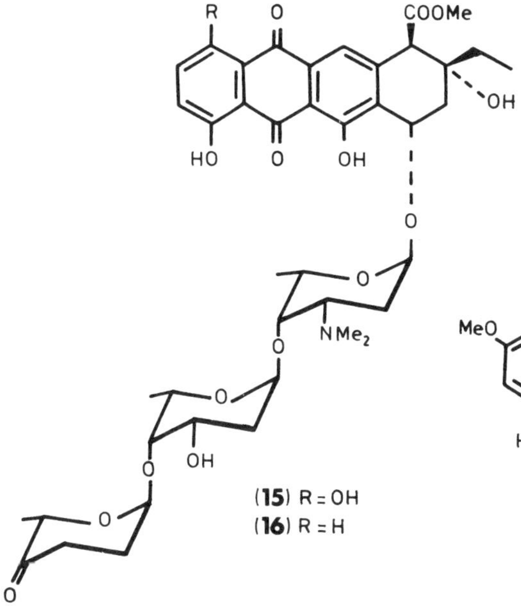

(**15**) R = OH
(**16**) R = H

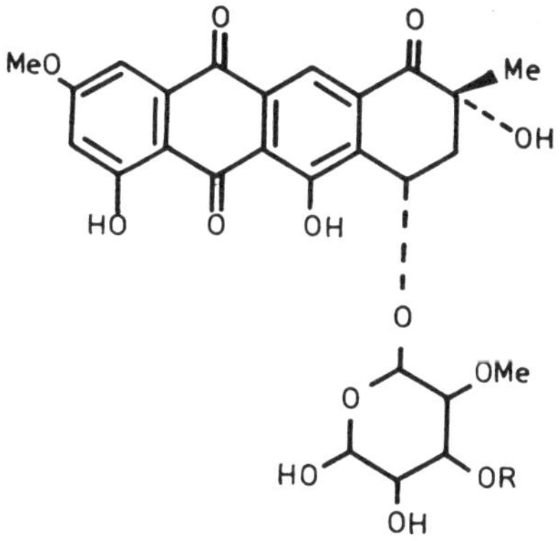

(**17**) R = H
(**18**) R = Me

biogenesis [4, 21]. The closure of a hypothetical decaketide chain (**19**) with concomitant oxidation, decarboxylation, reduction and methylation is exemplified in Scheme 2.1 for ε-rhodomycinone (**20**). The oxygen atoms at C-4 and at C-7 are derived from the original polyketide carbonyls, but only the one at C-4 is present in all anthracyclines, the second being absent in some cases. Methylation of the phenolic hydroxyls, a common feature in many hydroxyanthraquinones of natural origin [18], is restricted to the components of the daunomycin group and to the steffimycins.

SCHEME 2.1

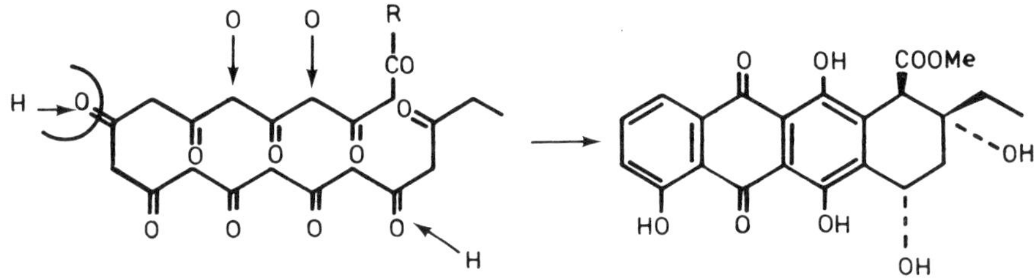

O O R CO H O O O O O O O O O H

O OH COOMe OH HO O OH OH

(**19**) (**20**)

The structure of the amino sugar component is an important feature of the anthracycline antibiotics. As already mentioned, daunosamine (3-amino-2,3,6-trideoxy-L-lyxo-hexopyranose) is present only in (**1**) and related metabolites, while the amino sugar present in other anthracyclines is the N-dimethylderivative, rhodosamine. Other sugars can also be present in the anthracyclines. They include rhodinose (2,3,6-trideoxy-L-threohexopyranose), 2-deoxy-L-fucose, cinerulose (3-oxo-2,3,4,6-tetradeoxy-L-hexopyranose), 6-deoxy-2-O-methylhexose, 6-deoxy-2,3-di-O-methylhexose and nogalose (6-deoxy-3-C-methyl-2,3,4-tri-O-methyl-hexose), the non-aminated sugar present in nogalamycin [28].

## 3 DEGRADATION STUDIES

### 3.1 Daunomycin

Acid hydrolysis of daunomycin afforded the red crystalline aglycone, daunomycinone and the aminosugar, daunosamine. The ultraviolet and visible spectrum of daunomycinone (**21**) ($\lambda$ max. at 234, 252, 290, 480, 495, 532 nm) were similar to those of the antibiotic and indicated the presence of the 1,4,5-trihydroxyanthraquinone chromophore. The formation of naphthacene upon zinc dust distillation showed the presence of the tetracyclic ring system containing 18 of the 21 carbon atoms of (**21**). The remaining carbon atoms were attributed to a methoxyl group (Zeisel determination, singlet at 4.08 $\delta$ in the $^1$H nmr spectrum, see below) and to an acetyl side chain (carbonyl band at 1718 cm$^{-1}$ in the infrared, singlet at 2.43 $\delta$, formation of semicarbazone). The other oxygen functions were attibuted to the quinone groupings (two strong bands in the range 1590-1621 cm$^{-1}$ and behaviour towards reducing agents), four hydroxyl groups (formation of a tetracetate upon treatment with acetic acid anhydride and pyridine), two chelated phenols and two alcoholic functions as deduced from the shifts of the corresponding $^1$H nmr signals at 13.20, 13.90, 2.30 and 2.04 $\delta$.

Scheme 3.1 shows some degradation reactions of daunomycinone [10, 29]. Treatment with dimethyl sulphate allowed the conversion of daunomycinone (**21**) to yellow crystalline trimethyl ether (**23**), which was very useful for the $^1$H n.m.r. studies. Daunomycinone is soluble in dilute alkalis giving a blue-violet solution. When this solution is left standing at room temperature the compound loses two molecules of water to give, after acidification, the fully aromatized bisanhydro derivative (**24**). The reaction can be considered to start with the abstraction of C-10 benzylic proton and is a common feature of all anthracyclinones possessing the hydroxyl group at position 7. A similar process takes place when an acetone solution of (**23**) is treated with sodium hydroxide. This is a very smooth reaction giving rise, after 45 min. at room temperature, to (**26**), which is the result of the elimination of two molecules of methanol from (**23**). Full aromatization of the anthracyclinone ring system follows also after acid treatment (hydrogen bromide in anhydrous acetic acid or p-toluenesulphonic acid in xylene) of (**21**). This reaction, however, requires heating and is likely to follow the formation of a carbocation at C-7, the driving force being represented by the high stability following the aromatization. The formation of (**24**) from (**21**) also takes place upon single heating of the crystals of (**21**), as can be observed on the Kofler hot stage microscope. Oxidative degradation of (**24**) afforded 3-methoxyphthalic acid (**27**) and trimellitic acid (**28**), which gave important information concerning the pattern of substitution on the tetracyclic ring system of (**24**) and, therefore, of (**21**). Alkaline fusion of (**21**) as well as of (**23**) gave salicylic acid.

SCHEME 3.1

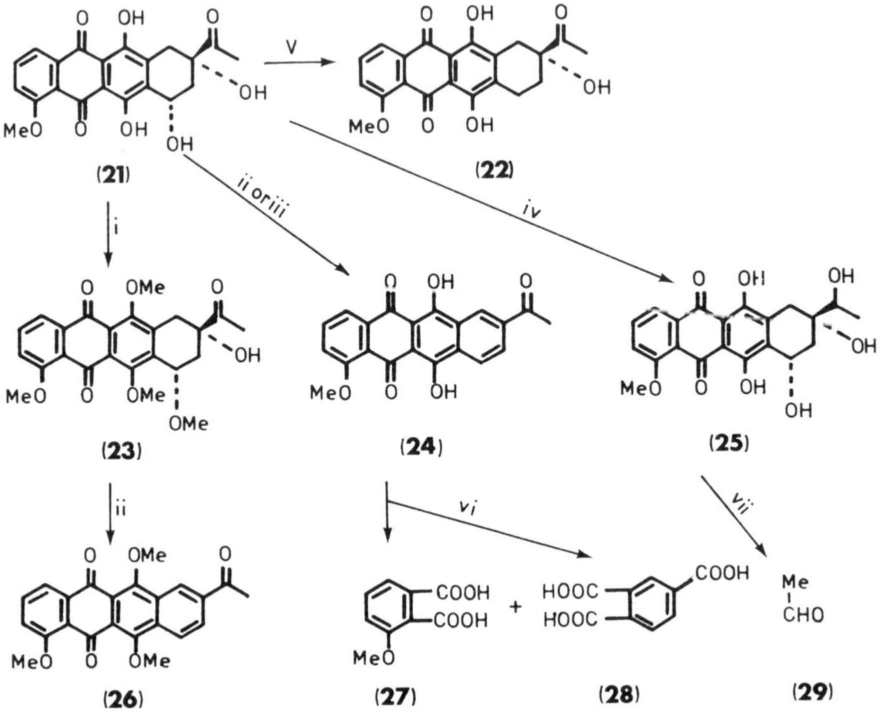

Reagents: i, $Me_2SO_4$, $K_2CO_3$; ii, $OH^-$; iii, $H^+$; iv, $NaBH_4$; v, $H_2$, Pd–$BaSO_4$; vi, $KMnO_4$; vii; $NaIO_4$

Sodium borohydride reduction of **(21)** followed by prompt air reoxidation of the leuco-derivative afforded 13-dihydrodaunomycinone **(25)**, a compound which, aside from the stereochemistry at C-13, is structurally identical to the metabolite of *S. peucetius*, the aglycone of the already mentioned biosynthetic dihydrodaunomycin and of daunorubicinol, the primary metabolic product of daunorubicin in experimental animals and in man [30]. Sodium periodate treatment of **(25)** at pH 4.6 (acetate buffer) gave **(29)**, isolated as the 2,4-dinitrophenylhydrazone. The formation of **(29)** proved the presence of the acetyl side chain in **(21)**. When **(21)** was hydrogenated with palladium on barium sulphate as catalyst and the product was allowed to reoxidize in air, 7-deoxydaunomycinone **(22)** was obtained. The same product was obtained together with daunosamine, from the catalytic hydrogenation of daunomycin, and this proved the attachment of the sugar moiety at C-7 [29].

Acetylation of **(21)** with acetic anhydride and pyridine gave complete substitution of all hydroxyl groups, affording a tetraacetyl-derivative. Similar treatment of (**24**) gave bisanhydro-6,11-diacetyldaunomycinone, of biosynthetic (**25**) gave 13-dihydro-6,7,9,11,13-pentaacetyl daunomycinone, and of (**22**) afforded 7-deoxy-6,9,11-triacetyldaunomycinone. These acetyl derivatives are yellow, crystalline compounds.

Chromic acid oxidation of (**21**) gave 7-deoxy-7-oxodaunomycinone

SCHEME 3.2

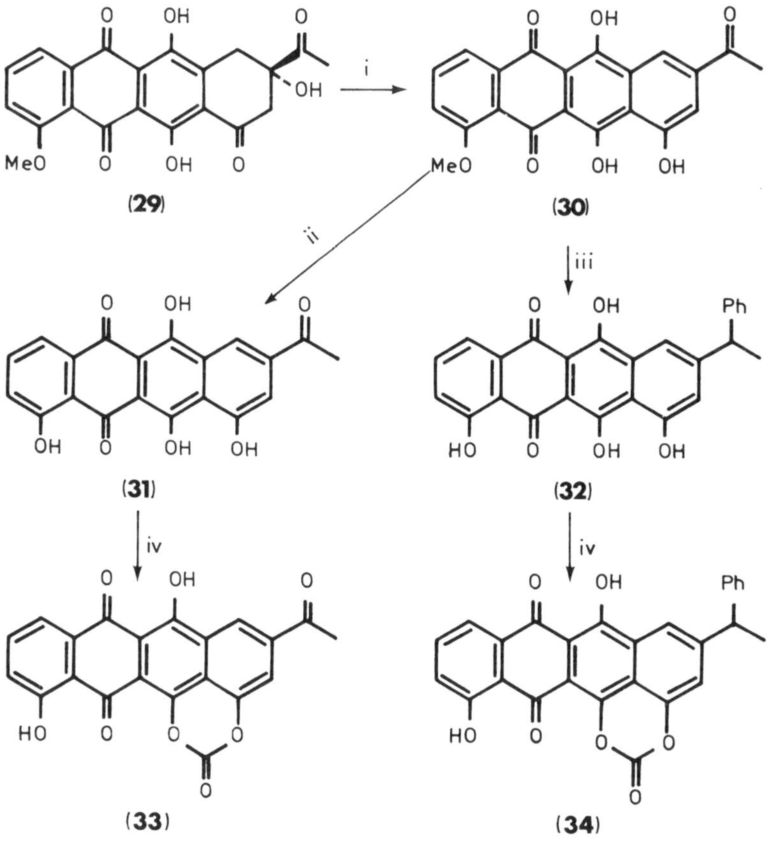

(**29**) (**30**) (**31**) (**32**) (**33**) (**34**)

Reagents: i, $OH^-$; ii, HBr, AcOH; iii, $AlCl_3$, PhH; iv, $COCl_2$, pyridine.

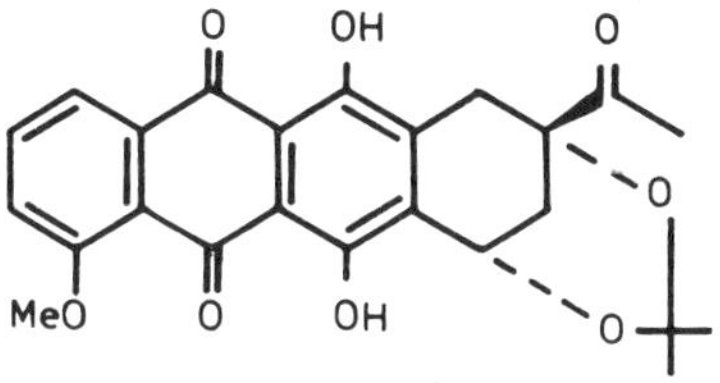

(**35**)

(29). Treatment of (29) with alkali promptly gave 10-hydroxy-bisanhydrodaunomycinone (30) which gave a triacetate with acetic anhydride in pyridine. The presence of a *peri*-hydroxyl group in (30) was also shown by the bathochromic shift of the visible spectrum of (30) when compared with (24) (see Table 8.1). Compound (30) was a useful compound for the demonstration of the presence of the methoxyl group at C-4. O-Demethylation was performed by either heating the solution of (30) in anhydrous acetic acid in the presence of hydrogen bromide or by treatment of (30) with aluminium chloride in benzene at reflux temperature. In the latter reaction concomitant alkylation of the solvent occurred, resulting in the formation of (32). The pattern of hydroxyl substitutions in both (31) and (32) was deduced from the comparison of their visible spectra with those of known tetrahydroxy-5,12-naphthacenequinones as well as from the absence of non-chelated quinone absorption in the two *peri*carbonates (33) and (34) obtained respectively from (31) and (32) with phosgene and pyridine in chloroform and subsequent treatment with aqueous bicarbonate. Owing to the *cis*-relationship of the two hydroxyl groups on ring A, treatment of daunomycinone with 2,2-dimethoxypropane in dioxane and in the presence of p-toluenesulphonic acid afforded (35), the most dextrorotatory of the known daunomycinone derivatives.

SCHEME 3.3

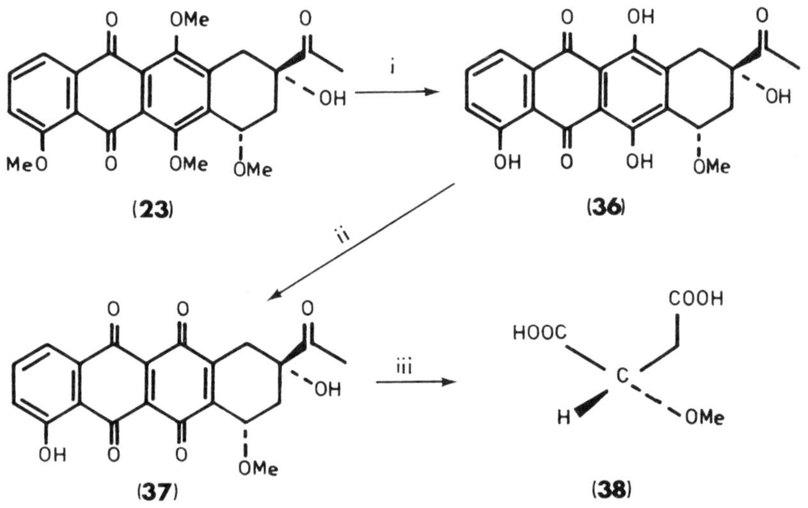

Reagents: i, $AlCl_3$, PhH; ii, $Pb(OAc)_4$, AcOH; iii, $NaIO_4$, $KMnO_4$

Reactions presented in Scheme 3.3 allowed the establishment of the absolute stereochemistry of daunomycinone and related compounds. Aluminium trichloride treatment of daunomycinone trimethyl ether in benzene at 70°

resulted in the selective demethylation of the phenolic methoxyl groups to give 4-O-demethyl-7-O-methyldaunomycinone (**36**). Oxidation of (**36**) with lead tetraacetate in anhydrous acetic acid gave 9-acetyl-4,9-dihydroxy-7-methoxy-7,8,9,10-tetrahydro-5,12:6,11-naphthacenediquinone (**37**), a yellow solid displaying the spectroscopic behaviour of an anthradiquinone [31] and easily revertable to (**36**) upon reduction. Compound (**37**) was oxidatively degraded by the use of the Lemieux reagent [32] to S(-)methoxysuccinic acid.

The aminosugar constituent, daunosamine, was proved to be 3-amino-2,3,6-trideoxy-L-lyxo-hexopyranose (**39**) (Scheme 3.4), a compound not previously found in other natural sources. Its structure was determined on the basis of periodate oxidation studies. Daunosamine itself was converted into malonic dialdehyde and acetaldehyde. The methyl glycoside (**40**) consumed one mole of periodate per mole, indicating the presence of the deoxy group at C-2 and the pyranoside structure. The presence of the aminogroup at C-3 as well as the absolute configuration at this carbon alone were established by means of the periodate oxidation of N-benzoyldainosamine (**43**) affording a non-volatile aldehyde which was in turn converted into N-benzoyl-L-aspartic acid (**44**) upon treatment with hypoiodite. The complete absolute stereochemistry was determined by the comparison of the molar rotations of (**39**) and (**40**) with those of the different known 2,6-dideoxyhexopyranoses and their methyl $\alpha$-glycosides. In addition the $^1$H nmr spectrum of (**41**) indicated the axial orientation of H-3 and the equatorial orientation of H-4, while H-5 had to be axial for reasons related to conformational stability [11, 29].

SCHEME 3.4

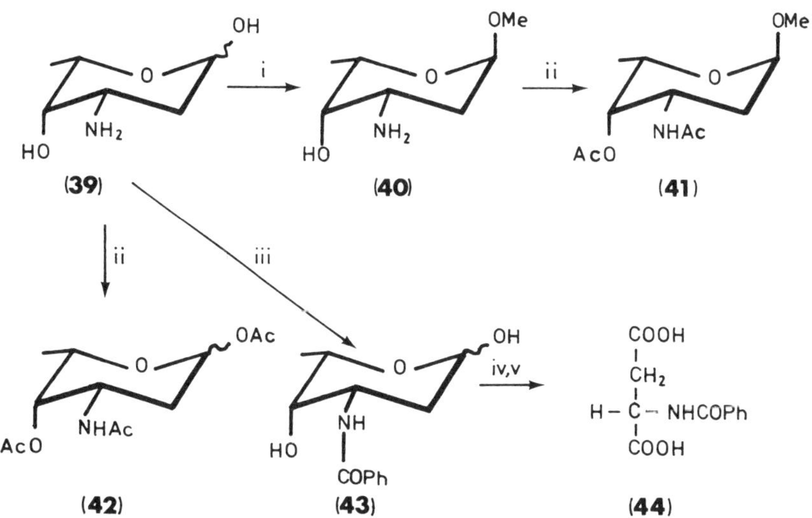


Reagents: i, $H^+$, MeOH; ii, $Ac_2O$, pyr; iii, PhCOCl, $HCO_3^-$; iv, $NaIO_4$; v, NaIO.

### 3.2 Adriamycin and 13-dihydrodaunomycin

The structure of adriamycin was readily established by comparison with previous work on daunomycin [15]. The degradation reactions used for the chemical characterisation of adriamycin are shown in Scheme 3.5. Acid hydrolysis of the antibiotic gave daunosamine and a new aglycone, 14-hydroxydaunomycinone or adriamycinone (**45**). Dehydration of the latter afforded bisanhydroadriamycinone (**47**). Hydrogenolysis of the benzylic glycoside gave daunosamine and 7-deoxyadriamycinone (**46**). Penta-O-acetyladriamycinone was obtained upon treatment of (**45**) with acetic anhydride and pyridine and used for the n.m.r. studies.

SCHEME 3.5

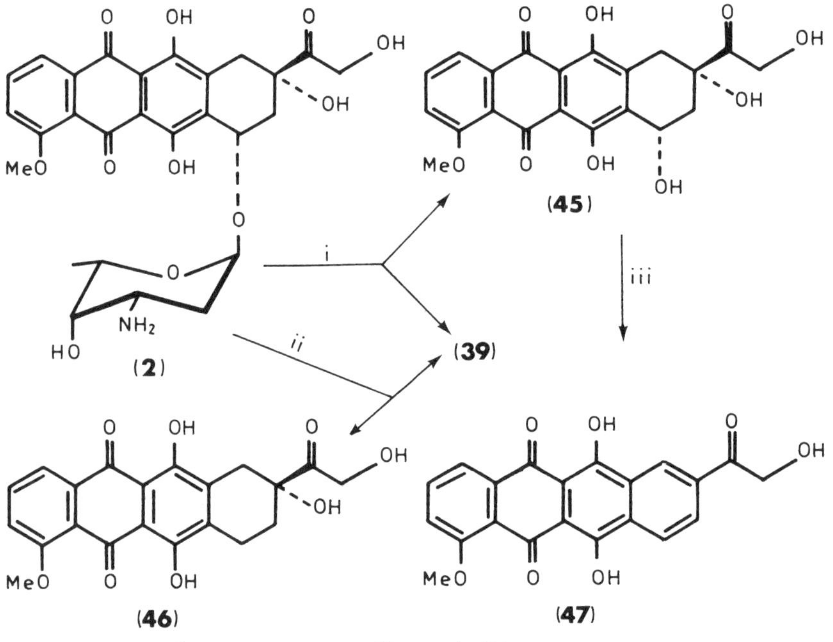

Reagents: i, $H_3O^+$; ii, $H_2$, Pd-Ba$SO_4$; iii, HBr, AcOH.

The aglycone of biosynthetic 13-dihydrodaunomycin was indistinguishable from semisynthetic (**25**) (Scheme 3.1). However dehydration of the biosynthetic aglycone gave (**48**), which displayed an optical rotation value different from the one of the compound prepared starting from daunomycinone. The difference in optical rotation should be attributed to a difference in the stereochemistry at C-13, semisynthetic (**25**) being likely a mixture of diastereoisomers at C-13 (unpublished results from the Author's laboratory).

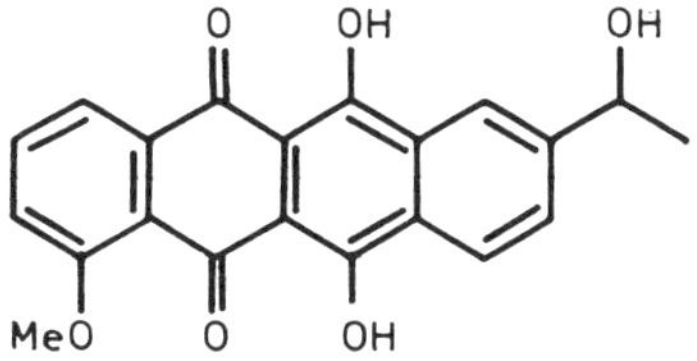

O OH OH

MeO O OH

(**48**)

### 3.3 Carminomycin

Carminomycin (**3**), the biosynthetic congener of daunomycin possessing a hydroxyl group instead of a methoxyl at C-4, gave the aglycone carminomycinone, on hydrolysis with dilute acid. The aglycone was fully acetylated to a pentaacetyl derivative and methylated to a tetramethyl ether, the latter being found identical to daunomycinone trimethyl ether [33].

The structure elucidation was therefore based on analytical data and on physico-chemical studies of carminomycinone and its derivatives. These studies included a X-ray diffractometric determination of the structure as well as of the configurational and conformational features of carminomycin I hydrochloride [22, 34].

## 4 TOTAL SYNTHESIS OF THE AGLYCONES

The outstanding antitumour properties of daunomycin and adriamycin has stimulated a wide interest in the total synthesis of the aglycones. These studies are important for two reasons. First, the total synthesis of the biosynthetic aglycones would furnish an alternative method, possibly competitive with the microbiological process, for the preparation of adriamycin. Second, the establishment of synthetic routes to the anthracyclinones would also make available new analogues with potential antitumour activity. Although the total synthesis of adriamycin has been formally achieved, the former objective appears to be, at the present time, remote. The second line of research has instead already led to important results, as will be shown in this section.

SCHEME 4.1

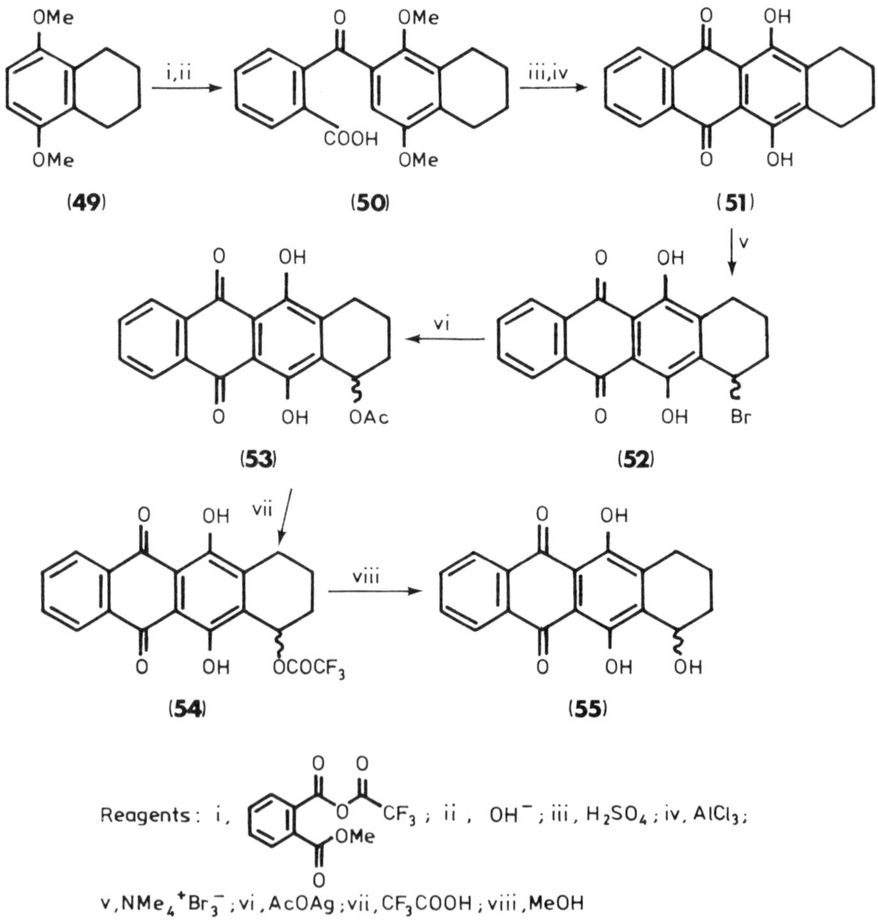

(**49**) —i,ii→ (**50**) —iii,iv→ (**51**) —v→ (**52**) —vi→ (**53**) —vii→ (**54**) —viii→ (**55**)

Reagents: i, [2-(methoxycarbonyl)benzoyl trifluoroacetate, $C_6H_4(CO_2Me)CO\text{-}O\text{-}COCF_3$]; ii, $OH^-$; iii, $H_2SO_4$; iv, $AlCl_3$;
v, $NMe_4^+Br_3^-$; vi, AcOAg; vii, $CF_3COOH$; viii, MeOH

An initial approach to the synthesis of the tetracyclic ring system of the anthracyclinones was based on the classical reaction of a substituted tetralin with a phthalic acid derivative [35, 36]. Following this scheme, Marsh and others [37] carried out the synthesis of the simplified anthracyclinone analogue **(55)** as indicated in Scheme 4.1. Dimethoxytetralin **(49)** was acylated with the mixed anhydride of phthalic acid monomethylester and trifluoroacetic acid to give, after hydrolysis of the ester group, compound **(50)**. Cyclization of **(50)**, followed by demethylation afforded **(51)** which was brominated to **(52)** with tetramethylammonium tribromide. Treatment of **(52)** with silver acetate gave **(53)** which, dissolved in trifluoroacetic acid, was converted into **(54)**. Methanolysis of the latter compound gave racemic 9-deacetyl-4-demethoxy-9-deoxy-daunomycinone **(55)**.

The first published study concerning the synthesis of a daunomycinone

SCHEME 4.2

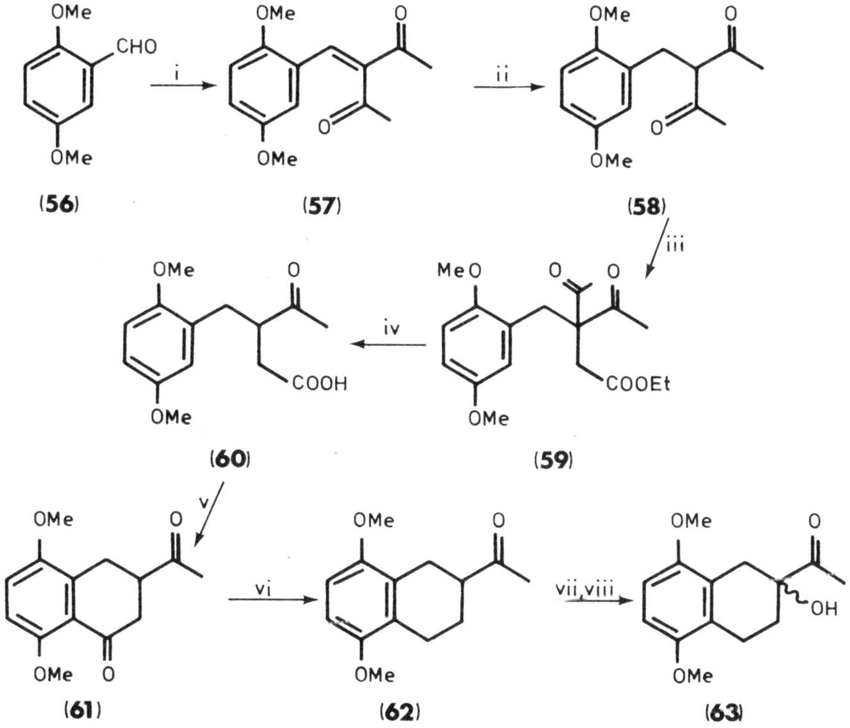

Reagents : i, (acetylacetone), piperidine, AcOH; ii, $H_2$, Pd–C; iii, NaH, $CH_2BrCOOEt$; iv, $OH^-$; v, liq. HF; vi, $H_2$, Pd–C; vii, $Bu^tOK$, $O_2$; viii, AcOH, Zn.

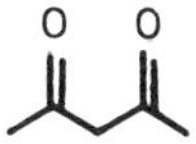

analogue and, in general, of a fully functionalized anthracyclinone analogue is that of Wong and co-workers, dealing with the synthesis of racemic 4-demethoxy-7-O-methyldaunomycinone [38]. This synthesis utilized 1,4-dimethoxy-6-hydroxy-6-acetyltetralin **(63)** as the source of the BA ring moieties. Compound **(63)** was obtained from 2,5-dimethoxybenzaldehyde **(56)** in seven steps as indicated in Scheme 4.2. The Knoevenagel condensation of **(56)** with 2,4-pentanedione in benzene solution gave **(57)**, which was hydrogenated to the diketone **(58)**. Alkylation of **(58)** to **(59)** followed by a reversed Claisen reaction and hydrolysis of the ester gave the ketoacid **(60)**. Cyclization of **(60)** to **(61)** and subsequent hydrogenolysis of the benzylic carbonyl group afforded 1,4-dimethoxy-6-acetyltetralin **(62)**. Oxidation of **(62)** by the Barton reaction afforded the desired **(63)**. In a subsequently published alternative procedure **(56)** was converted into **(62)** according to the reaction sequence in Scheme 4.3. This procedure resulted in an overall yield from **(56)** to **(63)** of about 36%, each step of Scheme 4.3, as well as the conversion of **(62)** to **(63)**, showing a yield in the range from 70% to 100%.

SCHEME 4.3

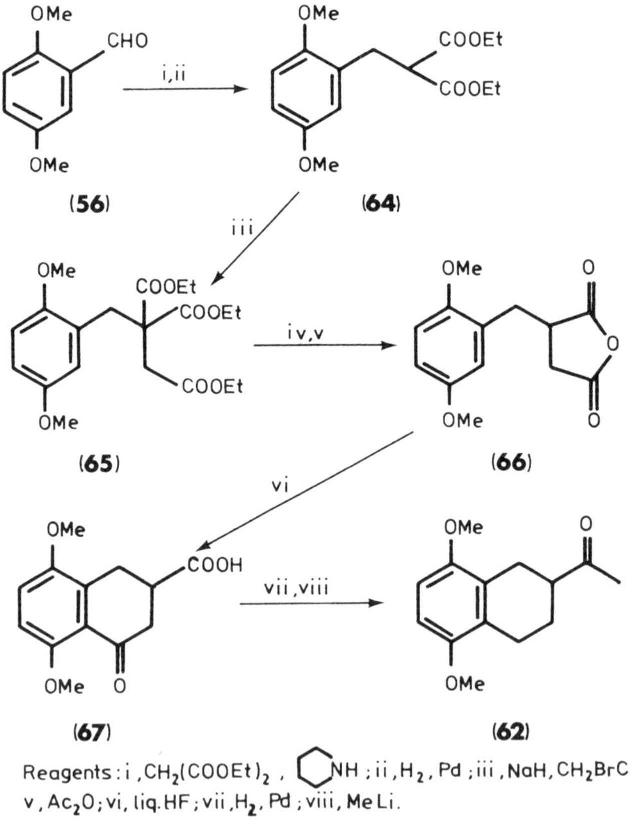

OMe, CHO, OMe **(56)** —i,ii→ OMe, COOEt, COOEt, OMe **(64)**

**(64)** —iii→ OMe, COOEt, COOEt, COOEt, OMe **(65)** —iv,v→ OMe, O, O, O, OMe **(66)**

**(66)** —vi→ OMe, COOH, OMe, O **(67)** —vii,viii→ OMe, O, OMe **(62)**

Reagents: i, $CH_2(COOEt)_2$, (piperidine) NH; ii, $H_2$, Pd; iii, NaH, $CH_2BrCOOEt$; iv, $OH^-$; v, $Ac_2O$; vi, liq. HF; vii, $H_2$, Pd; viii, MeLi.

SCHEME 4.4

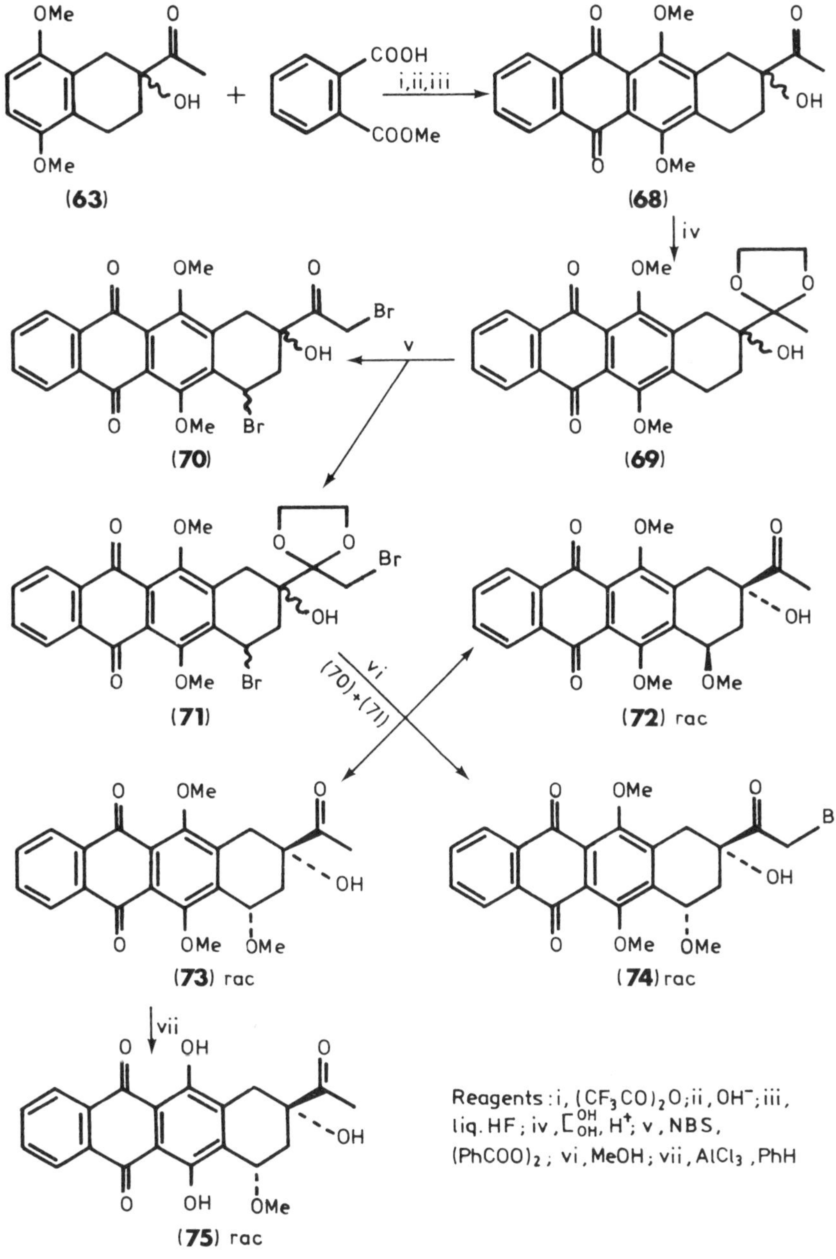

(63) (68) (70) (69) (71) (72) rac (73) rac (74) rac (75) rac

Reagents: i, $(CF_3CO)_2O$; ii, $OH^-$; iii, liq. HF; iv, $\left[^{OH}_{OH}\right.$, $H^+$; v, NBS, $(PhCOO)_2$; vi, MeOH; vii, $AlCl_3$, PhH

The synthesis of racemic 4-demethoxy-7-O-methyldaunomycinone is presented in Scheme 4.4. Acylation of **(63)** with phthalic acid monomethylester in trifluoroacetic anhydride solution and at reflux temperature, followed by saponification and treatment with hydrogen fluoride, gave **(68)**. This compound

SCHEME 4.5

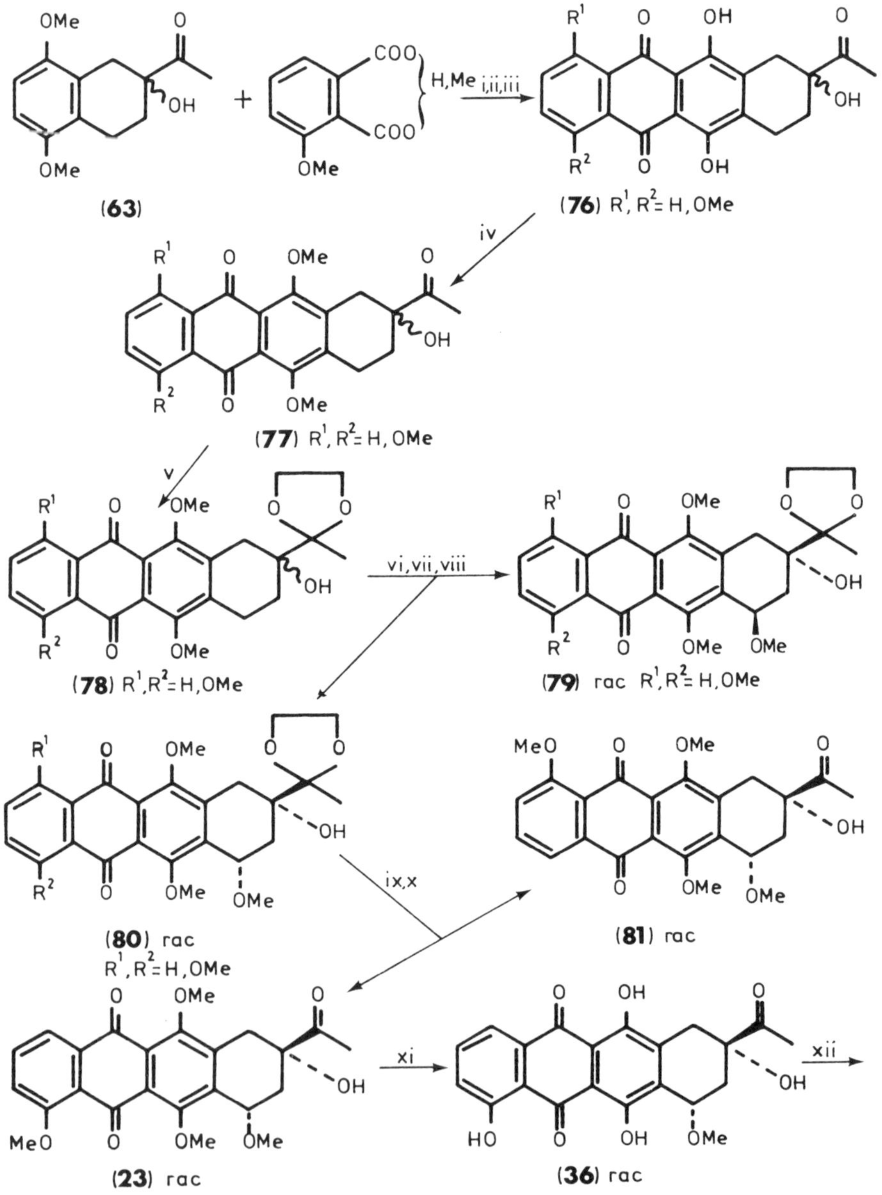
(63)
H,Me i,ii,iii
(76) R¹, R² = H, OMe
iv
(77) R¹, R² = H, OMe
v
(78) R¹,R² = H,OMe
vi,vii,viii
(79) rac R¹,R² = H,OMe
(80) rac R¹,R² = H,OMe
ix,x
(81) rac
(23) rac
xi
(36) rac
xii

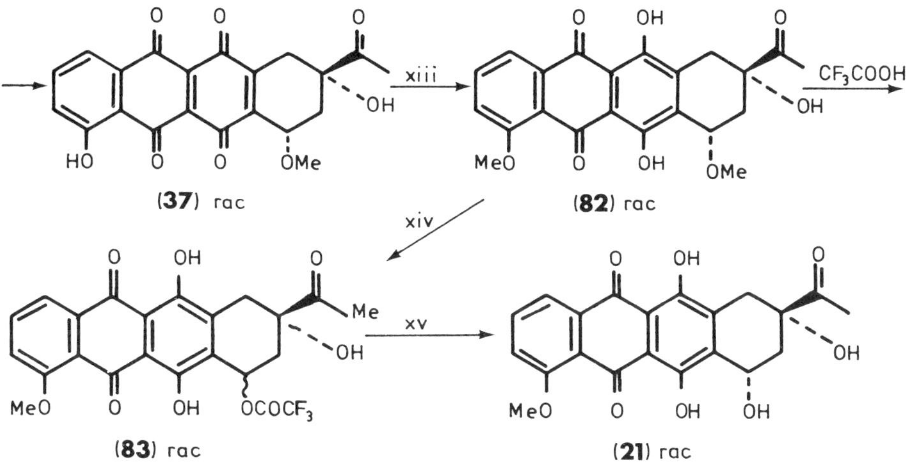

(37) rac → xiii → (82) rac → $CF_3COOH$

xiv → (83) rac → xv → (21) rac

Reagents: i, $(CF_3COO)_2$; ii, $OH^-$; iii, liq. HF; iv, $Me_2SO_4$, $K_2CO_3$; v, $\left[\begin{smallmatrix}OH\\OH\end{smallmatrix}\right.$, $H^+$; vi, NBS; vii, MeOH; viii, TLC; ix, $H^+$; x, TLC; xi, $AlCl_3$; xii, $Pb(OAc)_4$; xiii, $Me_2SO_4$, $K_2CO_3$; $Me_2CO$; xiv, $CF_3COOH$; xv, $NH_4OH$.

was converted to **(69)** which was selectively brominated in the less hindered of the two benzylic positions. The mixture of **(70)** and **(71)** was refluxed with anhydrous methanol to give 4-demethoxydaunomycinone trimethyl ether **(73)** as the main product together with the diastereoisomer **(72)** and the bromoketone **(74)**. The last step was accomplished by the O-demethylation of **(73)**, affording racemic 4-demethoxy-7-O-methyldaunomycinone **(75)**.

The total synthesis of racemic daunomycinone was performed by Wong and his co-workers [39] as outlined in Scheme 4.5. Reaction of **(63)** with 3-methoxyphthalic acid monomethyl ester in trifluoroacetic anhydride solution followed by saponification and ring closure afforded a mixture of quinones with the general formula **(76)**. Methylation of the mixture quantitatively gave the mixture **(77)** which was converted into **(78)**. Benzylic bromination of **(78)**, followed by methanolysis and chromatographic separation of ring A isomers, afforded the *trans*- and *cis*-isomeric mixtures **(79)** and **(80)**. Ring D isomers **(81)** and **(23)** could be separated by chromatography after deblocking of the methylketone side chain in **(80)** by an acid treatment. The synthetic sequence was continued with the demethylation of racemic daunomycinone trimethylether to give racemic 4-O-demethyl-7-O-methyldaunomycinone **(36)** which was oxidized to the unstable anthradiquinone **(37)**, allowing remethylation to **(82)** in 10% yield. Replacement of the benzylic methoxyl group with the trifluoroacetoxy group and hydrolysis of resulting **(83)** gave racemic daunomycinone. In a similar way the 1-methoxy-4-demethoxy analogue of daunomycinone was obtained from **(81)**.

The preparative usefulness of Wong's synthetic sequence for the synthesis of daunomycinone analogues with symmetrical substitution on ring D has been demonstrated in the Author's laboratory. A modification affording the preparation of optically active compounds instead of racemates was developed [40]. This synthetic development, which opened a route to a number of different daunomycinone analogues obtained in optically pure form, is based on the resolution of racemic **(63)** into its enantiomers and on other modifications aimed at preserving the optical homogeneity of the various intermediates. Following this method both enantiomeric forms of 4-demethoxydaunomycinone were prepared [40]. A recently improved procedure is presented in Scheme 4.6, where it is exemplified for the 7(S), 9(S) stereoisomers. (S),(-)-1,4-Dimethoxy-6-hydroxy-6-acetyltetralin **(63)** was heated with phthalic anhydride or a substituted derivative thereof, **(84)**a-f, in the presence of aluminium chloride to give 7-deoxy-4-demethoxy daunomycinone derivatives **(85)**a-f. Ketalization of the

SCHEME 4.6

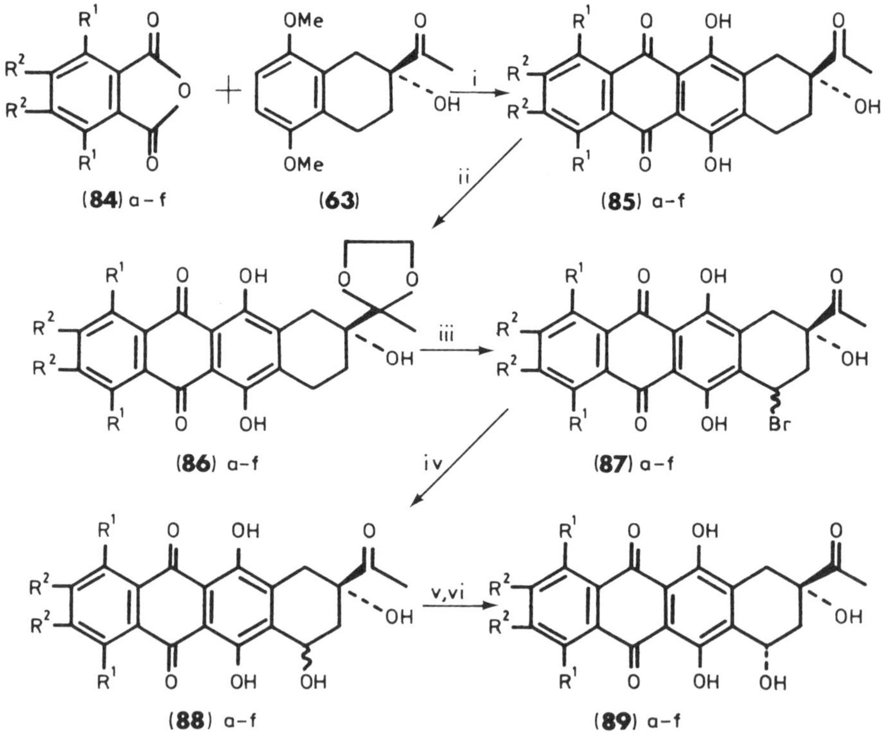

(**84**) a–f (**63**) (**85**) a–f

(**86**) a–f (**87**) a–f

(**88**) a–f (**89**) a–f

a, $R^1 = R^2 = H$; b; $R^1 = H$, $R^2 = CH_3$; c, $R^1 = CH_3$, $R^2 = H$; d, $R^1 = H$, $R^2 = Cl$; e, $R^1 = Cl$, $R^2 = H$; f, $R^1 = H$, $R^2 + R^2 = CH{=}CH{-}CH{=}CH$.

Reagents: i, $AlCl_3$; ii, $\left[{}^{OH}_{OH}\right.$, TsOH; iii, $Br_2$, AIBN; iv, $H_2O$; v, $CF_3COOH$; vi, $NH_4OH$

latter gave (**86**)a-f which was brominated with homosuccinimide and 2,2′-azo-bis-isobutyronitrile to afford the desired selective substitution at C-7 as in (**87**) a-f. Working up of the reaction product gave (**88**)a-f, a mixture of *cis*- and *trans*-isomers with the latter predominating. Subsequent treatment with trifluoroacetic acid followed by saponification with ammonia afforded the daunomycinone analogues (**89**)a-f. This procedure has been used, as shown in Scheme 4.6 for the synthesis of 4-demethoxydaunomycinone (**89**)a, 4-demethoxy-2,3-dimethyldaunomycinone (**89**)b, 4-demethoxy-1,4-dimethyldaunomycinone (**89**)c, 4-demethoxy-2,3-dichlorodaunomycinone (**89**)d, 4-demethoxy-1,4-dichlorodaunomycinone (**89**)e, and the benzo-analogue (**89**)f [41].

A completely different variant of the scheme DC + BA → DCBA for the synthesis of 1-methoxy-6,11-dihydroxy-7,8,9,10-tetrahydronaphthacene-5,12-dione (**93**), allowing enough regioselectivity to deserve further investigations for its application to the synthesis of adriamycinone, has been reported [42]. As shown in Scheme 4.7, the reaction of the dilithiophenolate of 1.4-dihydroxy-5,8-dihydronaphthalene, obtained upon treatment of (**90**) with two equivalents of lithium hydride, with 3-methoxyphthalic anhydride, followed by methylation with diazomethane, gave 4′-hydroxy-5′,8′-dihydronaphthyl-2-methoxy-6-carbomethoxybenzoate (**91**) as the main product. Compound (**91**) origi-

SCHEME 4.7

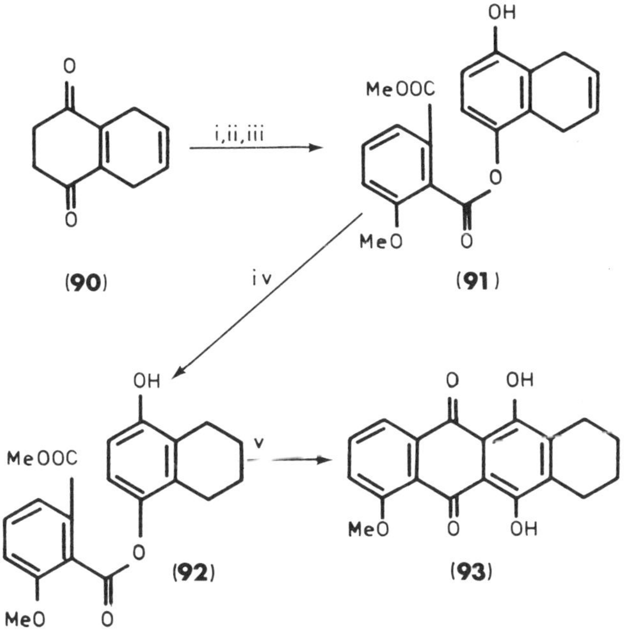

(**90**) (**91**) (**92**) (**93**)

Reagents: i, LiH, THF; ii, 3-methoxyphthalic anhydride; iii, $CH_2N_2$; iv, $H_2$, Pd; v, $BF_3-Et_2O$.

nated from the predominant attack of the phenolate ion to the more hindered carbonyl of 3-methoxy-phthalic anyhdride and its structure was established by its preparation from 2-methoxy-6-carbomethoxybenzoic acid according to a known procedure [43]. Hydrogenation of **(91)** afforded **(92)** which was cyclized

SCHEME 4.8

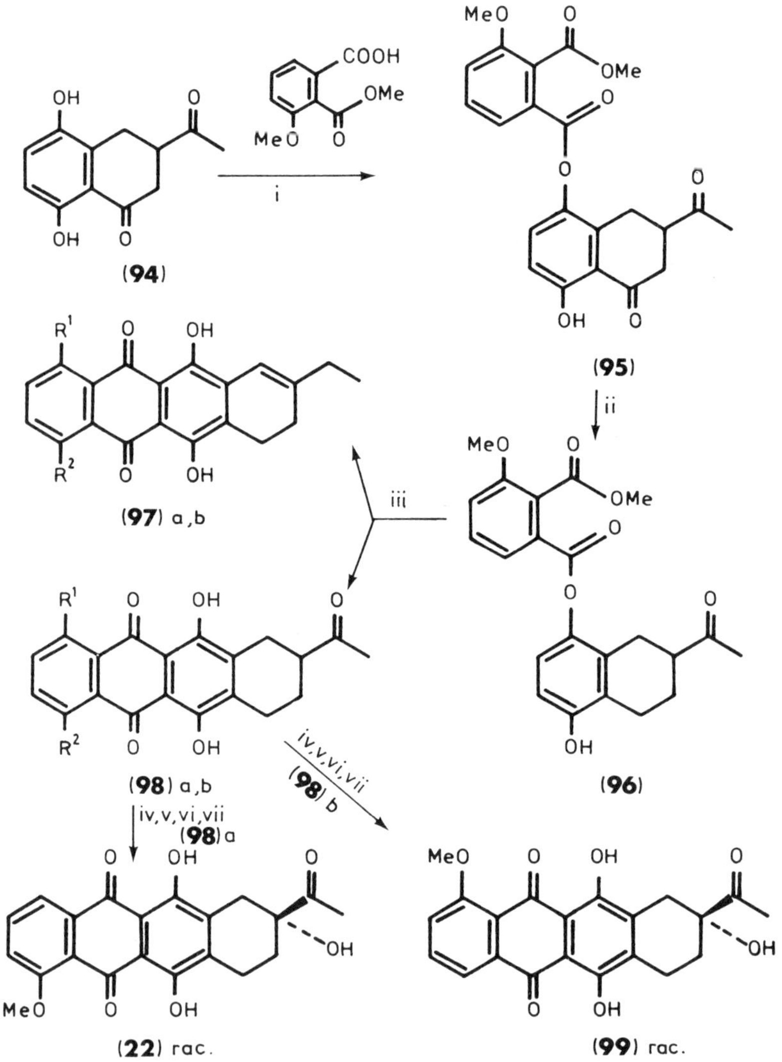
(94)
(95)
(96)
(97) a,b
(98) a,b
(22) rac.
(99) rac.
i
ii
iii
iv,v,vi,vii (98) a
iv,v,vi,vii (98) b

a: $R^1$=H, $R^2$=OMe; b: $R^1$=OMe, $R^2$=H

Reagents: i, TsCl, pyr; ii, $H_2$, Pd–C; iii, $BF_3-Et_2O$, heat; iv, $Ac_2O$, TsOH, heat; v, m-$ClC_6H_4CO_3H$; vi, $OH^-$; vii, $H^+$.

with boron trifluoride etherate at 90° to give (**93**). The latter reaction was considered to proceed *via* a Fries rearrangement and subsequent dehydrative cyclization [42].

The difficulties encountered in this approach to the regiospecific synthesis of daunomycinone are however revealed in a following paper by the same workers of the University of Wisconsin [44]. As indicated in Scheme 4.8, compound (**95**) was obtained by acylation [43] of 2-acetyl-5,8-dihydroxy-4-tetralone (**94**). Attempts to cyclize (**94**) or the corresponding 4-hydroxy compound with the boron-trifluoride-etherate reagent led to very low yields of tetracyclic products. Compound (**95**) was therefore converted into (**96**) and the latter, when treated with the above mentioned reagent, gave, after silicagel chromatography, the mixture (**97**)a, (**97**)b and two regioisomers (**98**)a and (**98**)b. Low yields of tetracyclic compounds were obtained starting from the 5-O-methyl- or 5-O-carboisobutoxy derivatives of (**96**). However the sequence represented by enol acylation, followed by epoxidation, alkaline treatment, and finally acid hydrolysis, afforded the conversion of (**98**)a to (±)-7-deoxy-daunomycinone in 50% overall yield and, similarly, of (**98**)b to (±)-7-deoxy-isodaunomycinone (**99**).

In a recently published paper the regiospecific synthesis of a daunomycinone analogue through selective attack at one of the carbonyl groups of 3-methoxyphthalate was carried out as outlined in Scheme 4.9 [45]. Tetralin derivative (**100**), itself obtained starting from the readily available 3-bromo-2,5-dimethoxybenzaldehyde, was converted to (**101**) and the latter, in three steps, to (**102**).

Protection of the side chain ketone by ketalization and oxidation of the protected intermediate at a platinum anode in 1% methanolic potassium hydroxide afforded (**103**), which, *via* the corresponding lithium derivative, was coupled to dimethyl 3-methoxyphthalate to give the tricyclic derivative (**104**) in 70% yield after silicagel chromatography. Conversion of (**104**) to (**98**)a was carried out without isolation of intermediates by reductive hydrolysis followed by saponification and hydrogen fluoride cyclization in overall reasonable yield. Since ketone (**98**)a, as it was already shown, has been converted to 7-deoxy-daunomycinone, this route represents a regiospecific synthesis of this aglycone.

The DCB + A → DCBA scheme for the synthesis of the dihydroxytetrahydronaphthacenedionc ring system has been approached by making use of the Diels-Alder reaction of quinizarinquinone with suitable butadienes, a reaction already reported in the literature [46]. The problems related to this approach are well documented in the study carried out at the Stanford Research Institute [47], and some reactions investigated by these authors are presented in Scheme 4.10. Although the reaction of (**105**) with 1,3-butadiene and, under optimum conditions, with 1-acetyoxy-1,3-butadiene, afforded the desired adduct (**106**) as the main product, and the internal adduct (**107**) as a minor product, a similar result was not obtained with 2-methoxybutadiene. The latter

SCHEME 4.9

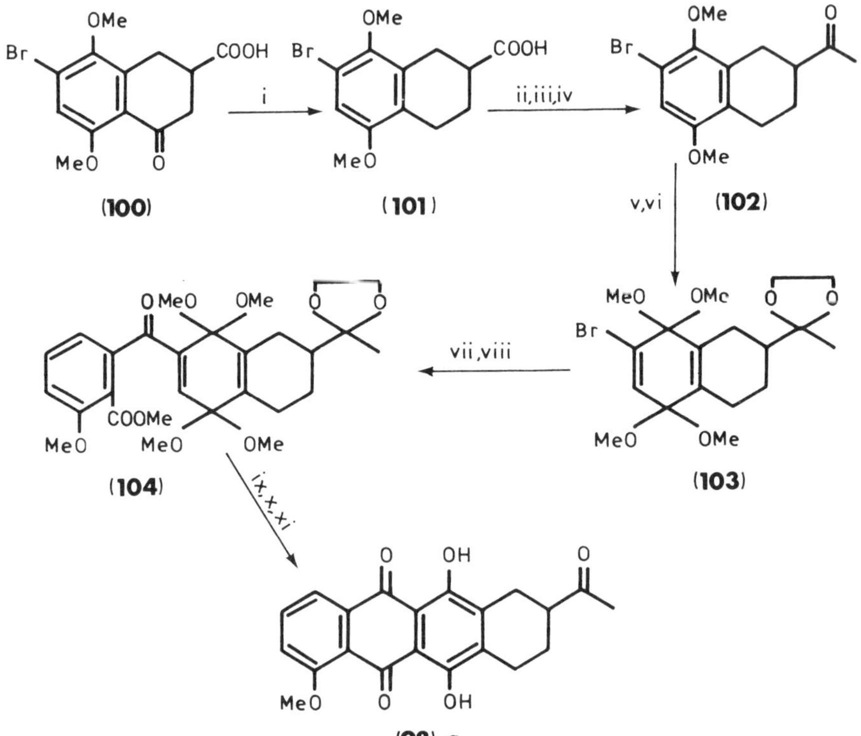

**(100)** —i→ **(101)** —ii,iii,iv→ **(102)** —v,vi→ **(103)** —vii,viii→ **(104)** —ix,x,xi→ **(98)** a

Reagents: i, $Et_3SiH$, $CF_3COOH$; ii, $CH_2N_2$; iii, $CH_3SOCH_2Li$; iv, Al–Hg; v, $HOCH_2CH_2OH$, $H^+$; vi, *e*, $OH^-$, MeOH; vii, BuLi; viii, 3-methoxyphthalic acid dimethyl ester (COOMe, COOMe, OMe); ix, $CF_3COOH$, $H_2O$, $SnCl_2$; x, $OH^-$; xi, HF.

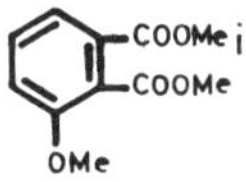

reaction would have given a more direct method to the desired compounds **(113)** and **(115)**. The adducts of general formula **(106)** could be converted into the anthraquinones **(108)**, but these appeared to be unsuitable for further modification because of their insolubility and instability. The compounds of structure **(109)**, obtained from **(106)** by a reduction step, were instead used for a variety of transformations which included further reduction to **(110)**, reoxidation to **(112)**, and conversion of the latter to the simple anthracyclinone analogue **(55)**, as well as synthesis of ketones **(113)** and **(115)**. This synthesis consisted of the methylation of leuco **(109)** (R = H) to **(111)** and conversion of the latter compound, *via* a boronation reaction followed by treatment with hydrogen to **(114)**. Oxidation of **(114)** by the Pfitzner and Moffat procedure [48] afforded **(113)**, while demethylation with aluminium trichloride and subsequent oxidation gave **(115)**.

SCHEME 4.10

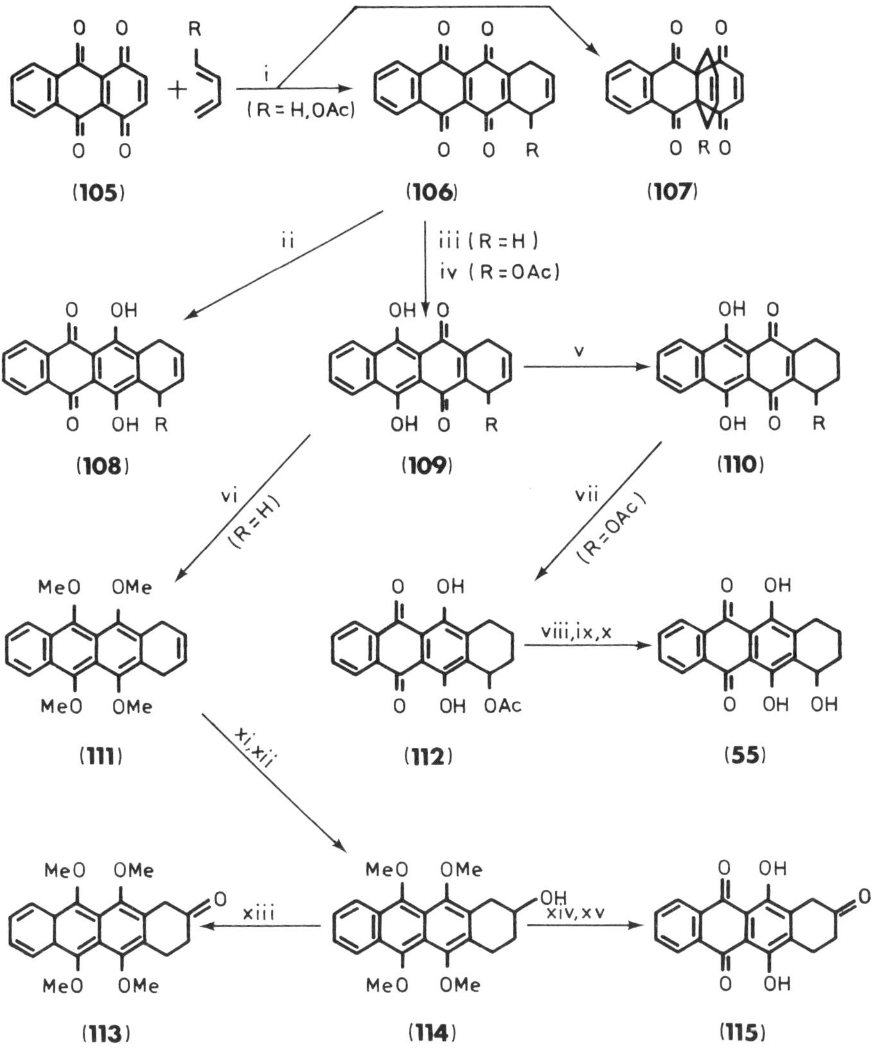

Reagents : i,ii,heat;iii,Zn,AcOH;iv,$H_2$,Pd–$BaSO_4$ ; v,$H_2$,Pd; vi,$Me_2SO_4$,BaO; vii,$Ag_2O$; viii, $CF_3COOH$; ix,MeONa,MeOH; x,AcOH; xi $B_2H_6$; xii, $H_2O_2$,$OH^-$; xiii,DCC,DMSO; xiv, $AlCl_3$; xv,DCC,DMSO.

Functionalization of ring A in the 4-methoxylated analogue (**116**) of tetracyclic ketone (**115**) has been carried out as shown in Scheme 4.11 [49]. Compound (**116**), prepared by periodate oxidation of 7-deoxy-13-dihydrodaunomycinone (**22**), was converted into the cyanohydrin (**117**) and the latter to the tetrahydropyranyl derivative (**118**). Treatment of (**118**) with methylmagnesium iodide and then with hot aqueous acetic acid gave (±)-7-deoxydaunomycinone (**22**). The overall yield of racemic (**22**) from (**116**) was approximately 27%. The following conversion of racemic (**22**) into racemic daunomycinone (**21**) and to its 7-epiderivative (**119**) was performed in three steps, without isolation of the intermediaries: first a benzylic bromination in carbon tetrachloride (the role played by the solvent in the regioselectivity of the bromination was found exceptionally important), then substitution of the halogen with the trifluoroacetate anion and finally methanolysis of the intermediate trifluoroacetate to give the mixture of the racemic *cis*- (**21**) and *trans*- (**119**) daunomycinone. The greater yield of (**119**) (35%) in comparison with that of (**21**) (9%) from (**22**) was explained by attributing a $S_N1$ mechanism to the substitution of bromine with the trifluoroacetate and considering the approach of the nucleophilic reagent should more favourably take place from the side of the molecule which is *trans* to the axial hydroxyl at C-9. In the same paper the conversion of (**21**) to adriamycin was also described [49].

SCHEME 4.11

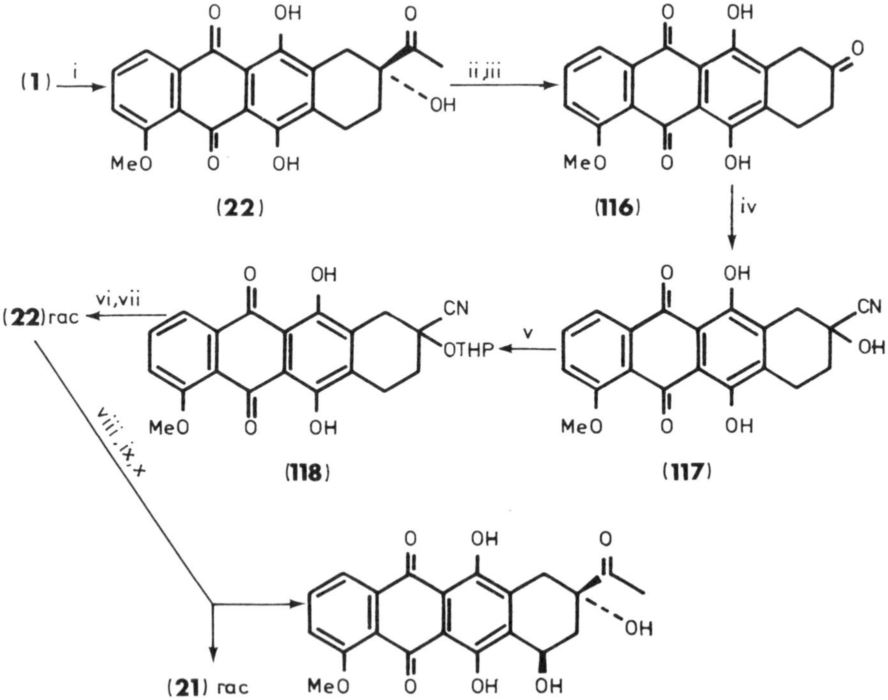

(**1**) →(i) (**22**) →(ii,iii) (**116**) →(iv) (**117**) →(v) (**118**) →(vi,vii) (**22**) rac →(viii,ix,x) (**21**) rac + (**119**) rac

Reagents: i, 2equiv. $Na_2S_2O_4$; ii $LiAlH(O-{}^tBu)_3$; iii, $NaIO_4$; iv, HCN; v, dihydropyran, $H^+$; vi, MeMgI; vii, 60% AcOH; viii, $Br_2$, AIBN; ix, $CF_3COONa$; x, MeOH.

More successfully, Kende and his coworkers [50], in a concurrent study, treated 5-methoxyl-1,4,9,10-anthradiquinone (**121**), which was available in practically quantitative yield from 1,4,5-trimethoxyanthraquinone (**120**), with 2-acetoxybutadiene to give the 1:1 regioisomeric adduct mixture (**122**) in 71% yield (Scheme 4.12). This result was in agreement with deductions based on analysis and on MO calculations suggesting that internal addition was favoured for electron rich dienes (such as 2-ethoxybutadiene), while terminal addition appeared more likely for slightly electron-deficient or unsubstituted dienes (such as 1,3-butadiene and 2-acetoxybutadiene).

SCHEME 4.12

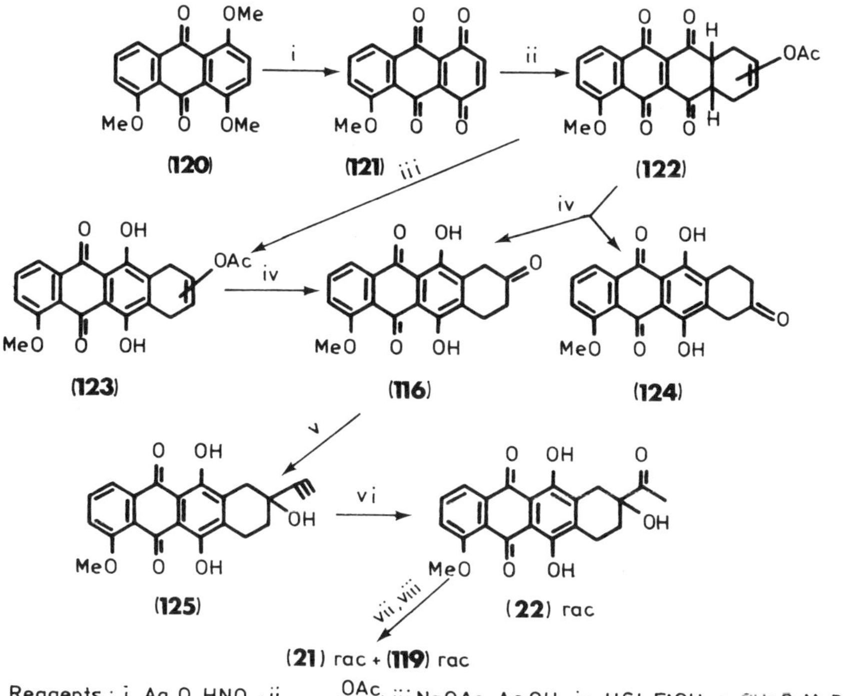

Reagents : i, $Ag_2O$, $HNO_3$; ii, [2-acetoxybutadiene, OAc]; iii NaOAc, AcOH; iv, HCl, EtOH; v, CH≡C-MgBr; vi, HgO, $H_2SO_4$; vii, $Br_2$, hν; viii, $SiO_2$, $H_2O$.

The mixture (**122**) was converted, either directly or *via* the anthraquinone derivative (**123**), to the mixture of ketones (**116**) and (**124**), the former being isolated by means of its lower solubility in solvents like ethanol and pyridine. Ketone (**116**), a key intermediate in the synthesis of the anthracyclinones, was converted into daunomycinone following a procedure different from the one presented in Scheme 4.11. The desired side chain was built up by a Grignard reaction followed by oxidation of the ethynl derivative (**125**) to (±)-7-deoxy-duanomycinone (**22**). Selective radical bromination of (**22**) at C-7, followed by hydrolysis during chromatography on moist silica gel plates, afforded (±)-daunomycinone (**21**) and (±)-7-epidaunomycinone (**119**), the latter being epimerized *via* the 7-O-trifluoroacetate to the desired natural aglycone in 76% yield. The synthetic sequence reported in Scheme 4.12 for the preparation of racemic daunomycinone from (**120**) involves eight steps and an overall yield of approximately 4%.

In a study dealing with the Diels-Alder reaction of anthradiquinones with a variety of dienes, Ross Kelly and his group at Boston College [51] expressed some doubts that the regioselectivity of the reaction could be easily rationalized, their deductions being based on the experimental results obtained with twentyone different dienes. The same authors, therefore, were led to explore an alternative DCB + A → DCBA approach to the functionalized anthradiquinone tetracyclic system [52]. This approach was based on previous work of Spanish authors [53], who had obtained adduct (**128**) by treating (**126**) with butadiene at 150° (Scheme 4.13), the reaction being considered to involve the less stable

SCHEME 4.13

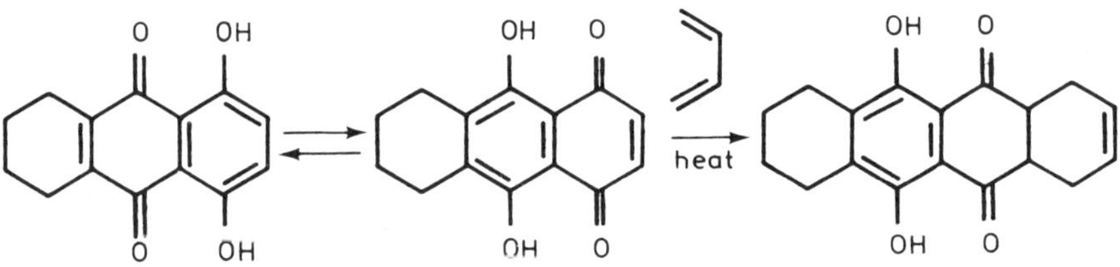

(**126**) (**127**) (**128**)

tautomer (**127**). A similar reaction did not however take place with quinizarine (**129**), apparently because of the presence of the additional aromatic ring. The reaction sequence (**130**) → (**134**) was eventually developed (Scheme 4.14), affording an almost 50% overall yield of the mixture of (**134**)a and (**134**)b starting from naphthazarin (**130**). The structure of the final products was established *via* their conversion to the mixture of (**135**)a and (**135**)b, and comparison of the infrared spectrum of the latter product with the spectra of

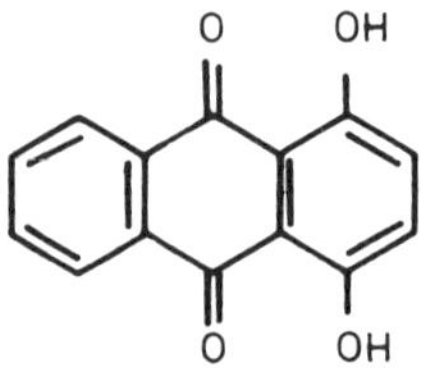

(**129**)

authentic material. Because isomer (**135**)b was the major component, it was concluded that the Diels-Alder reaction between (**133**) and 1-methoxy-3-ethylbutadiene proceeds, primarily, in the regiochemically unfavourable direction. The high yield of the adducts suggested, however, a high potential for this approach to the synthesis of anthracyclinone analogues.

SCHEME 4.14

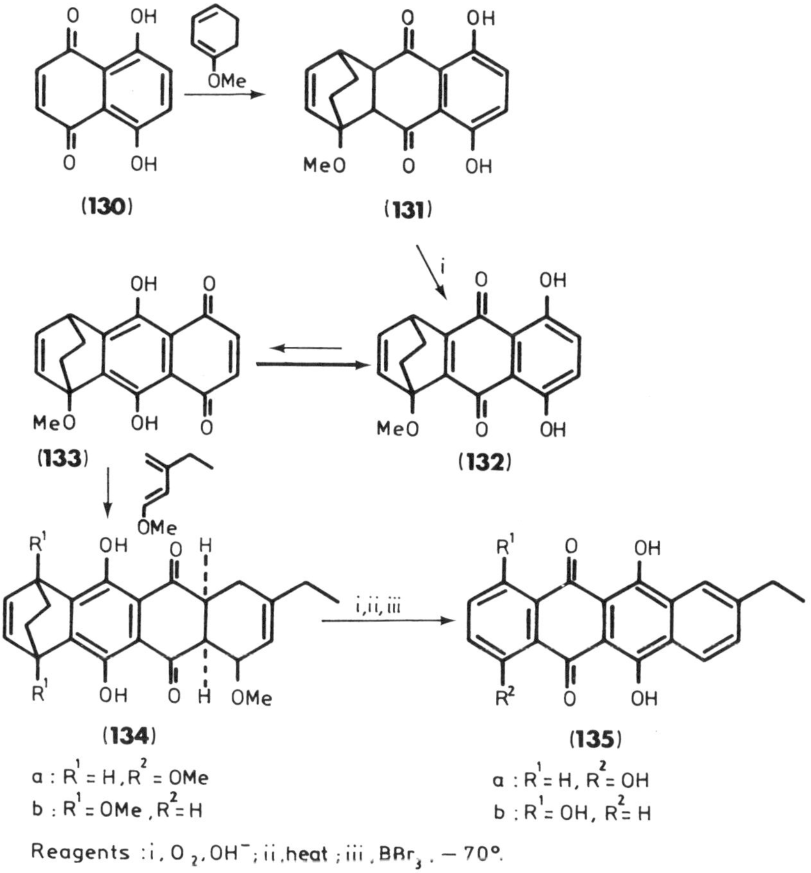

(**130**) (**131**) (**133**) (**132**) (**134**) (**135**)

(**134**) a : $R^1$ = H, $R^2$ = OMe
b : $R^1$ = OMe, $R^2$ = H

(**135**) a : $R^1$ = H, $R^2$ = OH
b : $R^1$ = OH, $R^2$ = H

Reagents : i, $O_2$, $OH^-$; ii, heat ; iii, $BBr_3$, − 70°.

The problem of regioselectivity in the Diel-Alder reaction of substituted naphthaquinones has been further investigated by Ross Kelly and coworkers [54]. An experimental solution has been provided on the basis of a rationale which involved the resonance effects of the *peri* substituent in the 1,4-naphthoquinone derivatives on the C-2, C-3 double bond, and their consequences towards the addition of the substituted diene. Taking account of the above mentioned unfavourable course of the reaction of 1-methoxy-3-ethylbutadiene with (**133**), and of the results of the reaction of juglone (5-hydroxy-1,4-naphthoquinone) and of its acetate with substituted dienes reported in the literature [55, 56, 57, 58], the latter being explained by the increased electron withdrawing character of the C-4 carbonyl in juglone which determines the regiochemical course of the reaction [57, 58], or by the electron feeding properties of the *peri*-acetoxy group, American workers have investigated the reaction sequence presented in Scheme 4.15. The reaction of naphthazarin monopivalate (**136**) with 1-methoxy-3-ethylbutadiene gave the adduct (**137**), in reported

SCHEME 4.15

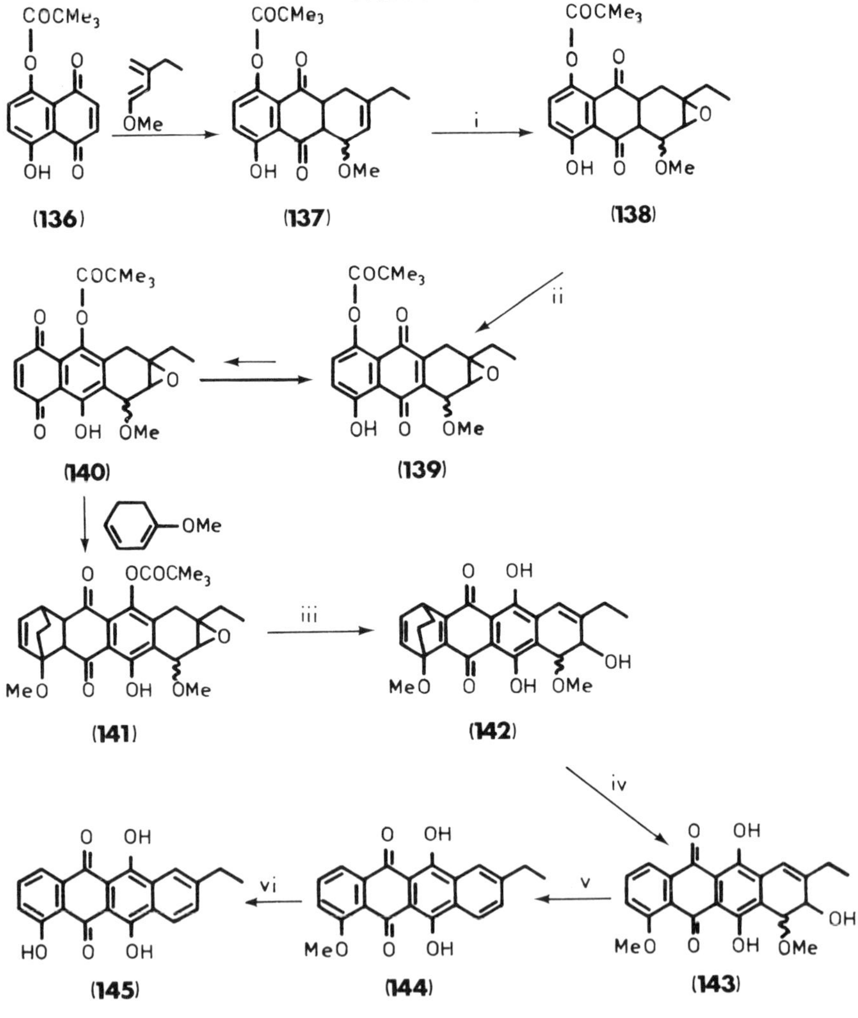

Reagents: i, m-ClPhCOOOH; ii, $PbO_2$; iii, $OH^-$, $O_2$; iv, heat; v, $H_2$, Pd–C; vi, $BBr_3$.

yields of 92-99%, a very regioselective result. Conversion of **(137)** into the epoxide **(138)** and oxidation of the latter gave **(139)** in reasonable yields. Reaction of **(139)** with 1-methoxycyclohexa-1,3-diene afforded **(141)**, the less stable isomer **(140)** from **(139)** being the reactive dienophile.

The structure of **(141)** was proven by its conversion into **(142)** with dilute aqueous alkalis in the presence of oxygen, followed by pyrolysis of **(142)** to

SCHEME 4.16

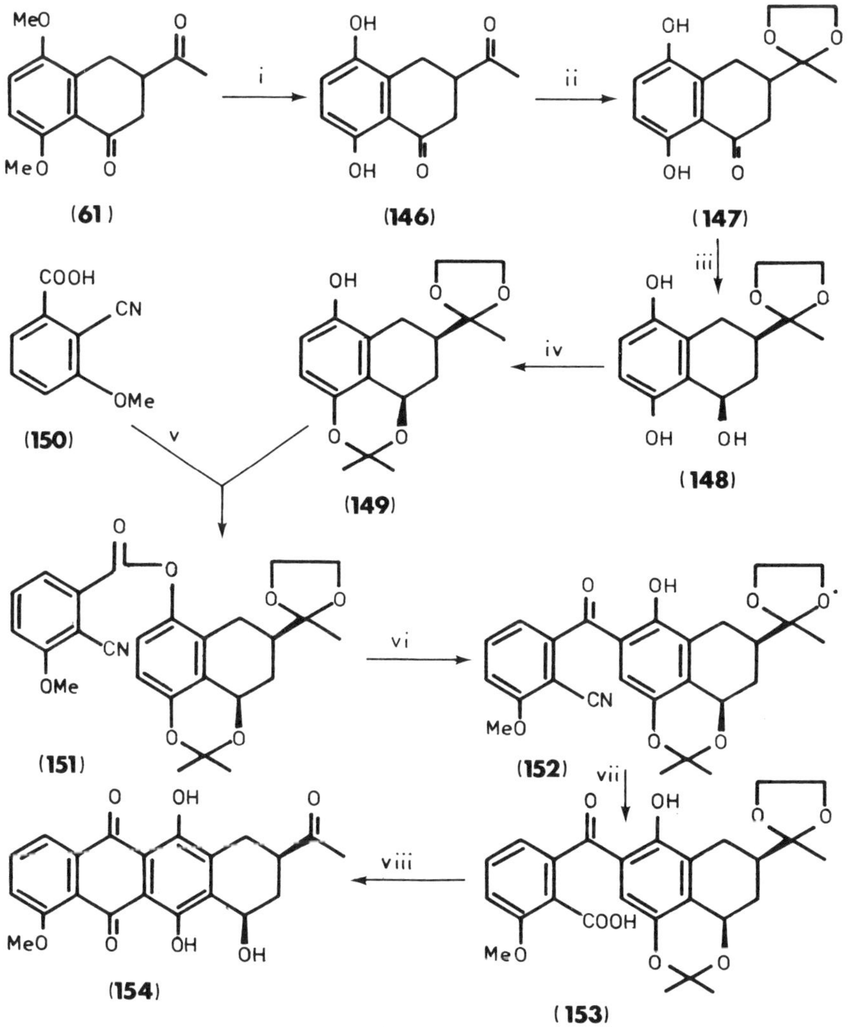

**(61)** **(146)** **(147)** **(150)** **(149)** **(148)** **(151)** **(152)** **(154)** **(153)**

Reagents: i, $BBr_3$, −78° to −10°; ii, (ethylene glycol: $HOCH_2CH_2OH$), TsOH; iii, $NaBH_4$; iv, $(CH_3)_2C(OMe)_2$, TsOH; v, TsCl, pyr; vi, $h\nu$; vii, $OH^-$; viii, liq. HF.

(**143**) and hydrogenation of the latter to (**144**), whose demethylation with boron tribromide gave the known bisanhydro-anthracyclinone (**145**).

A regiospecific synthesis of (±)-9-deoxydaunomycinone has been reported by Kende and coworkers [59] and the corresponding reaction sequence is presented in Scheme 4.16. This synthesis is centred on the photochemical Fries rearrangement of the o-cyanobenzoate ester (**151**). This compound was obtained in a five step procedure starting from Wong's tetralone (**61**), which was demethylated to (**146**) in 76% yield. The latter compound was converted into the key intermediate (**151**) in approximately 50% overall yield. This conversion involved the protection of the side chain ketone by ketalization as in (**147**), the subsequent reduction of the benzylic carbonyl group to give the alcohol (**148**), and, finally, the acylation of the acetonide (**149**) with 2-cyano-3-methoxybenzoic acid (**150**). Irradiation of (**151**) afforded, after a chromatographic isolation step, the ketone (**152**) in 48% yield. The conversion of (**152**) into the acid (**153**), followed by cyclization in liquid hydrogen fluoride, afforded (±)-deoxydaunomycinone (**154**), in 23% yield after chromatographic purification.

SCHEME 4.17

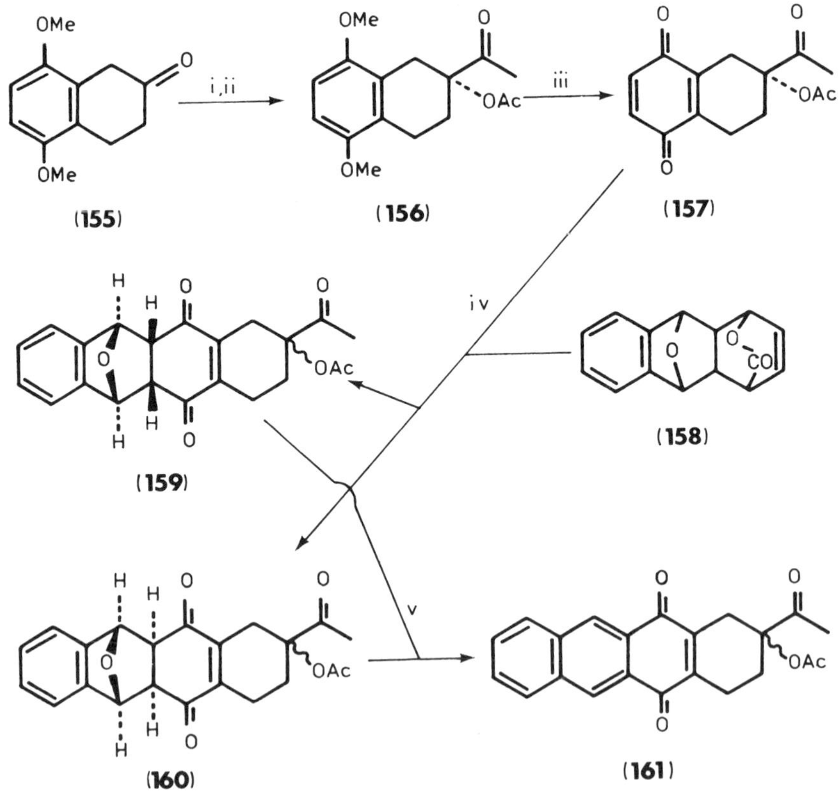

(**163**) (**162**)

(**164**) (**89**) a rac (R = H)

(**165**) rac

Reagents: i, $CH{\equiv}CMgBr$; ii, $Hg(OAc)_2$; iii, AgO; $HNO_3$; iv, heat; v, AcONa, AcOH, heat, vi, Zn, $Ac_2O$, vii, $CrO_3$; viii, HCl; AcOH; ix, $Br_2$, AIBN; x, $CF_3COOAg$; xi, $H_2O$; xii, $CF_3COOH$; xiii, MeOH.

An alternative route to racemic anthracyclinones has been recently reported by Kende and his coworkers as the third different synthesis of daunomycinone derivatives published by the Rochester group during three years [60]. The key step is the Diels-Alder reaction of an isobenzofuran derivative arising by thermolysis of a suitable intermediate, such as compound (**158**) in Scheme 4.17, with a functionalized tetralone, for example (**157**), which represents rings A and B in the final tetracyclic aglycone. The tetralone derivative (**157**) was prepared in good yield starting from 1,4-dimethoxy-6-tetralone (**155**) by ethynylation and conversion into the acetoxyketone (**156**), followed by oxidative demethylation.

Heating (**157**) and (**158**) in diglyme at 140° afforded the mixture of (**159**) and (**160**) which was aromatized to (**161**). The latter compound was reduced and acetylated and the resulting triacetate (**162**) was oxidized to (**163**). Racemic 4-demethoxy-7-deoxy-daunomycinone (**164**) was obtained upon mild acid hydrolysis of (**163**). Conversion of (**164**) to racemic 4-demethoxydaunomycinone (**89**)a (R = H) was carried out in a five step procedure involving homolytic benzylic bromination at C-7, displacement of the halogen atom with the trifluoroacetate anion, equilibration of the C-7 epimeric mixture with trifluoroacetic acid and finally methanolysis to give racemic (**89**)a in 45% yield from (**162**). Introduction of the C-14 hydroxyl group by bromination followed by nucleophilic displacement by a mild alkaline treatment afforded the new aglycone 4-demethoxyadriamycinone (**89**)a (R = H).

Application of this procedure in the daunomycinone series necessitated the use of methoxylated intermediates. To this end (Scheme 4.18) the 3-methoxybenzyne-furan adduct (**166**) was treated with α-pyrone to give (**167**)a and b. This mixture was heated with the tetralone derivative (**157**) to give, after aromatization of the regio- and stereoisomeric mixture of (**168**)a and (**168**)b, the quinones (**169**)a and b. Treatment of the latter compounds, as described above for the 4-demethoxy analogues, afforded the two regioisomeric compounds (**170**)a and (**170**)b. Overall yield of racemic 7-deoxydaunomycinone (**170**)a from (**155**) was indicated to be approximately 10%.

SCHEME 4.18

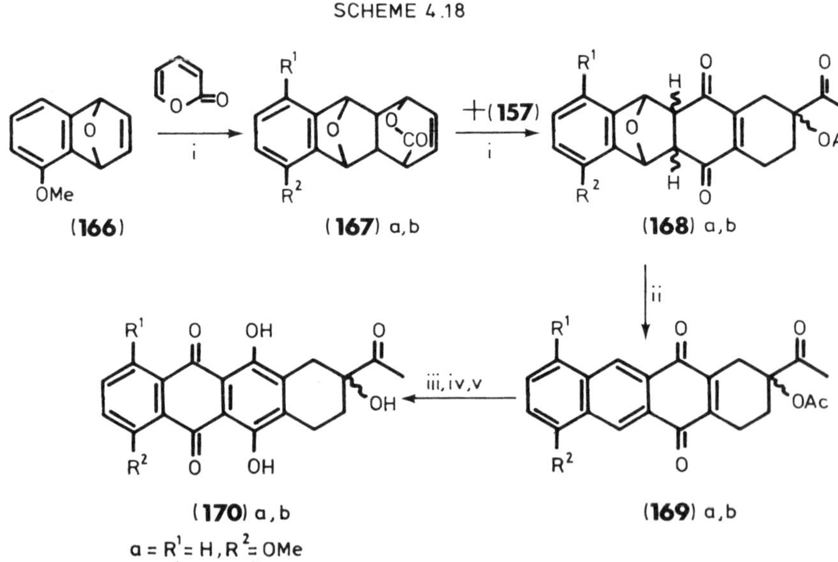


a = $R^1$ = H, $R^2$ = OMe
b = $R^1$ = Me, $R^2$ = H

Reagents: i, heat; ii, AcOH, AcONa, heat; iii, Zn, $Ac_2O$, heat; iv, $CrO_3$, aq. $H_2SO_4$, heat; v, $H^+$

## 5 SYNTHESIS OF DAUNOSAMINE AND RELATED COMPOUNDS

The synthesis of the aminosugar moiety of the antitumour anthracycline antibiotics has been studied in several laboratories since the structure and stereochemistry of daunosamine **(39)** were reported in 1964 [11]. The earlier studies were concerned with the synthesis of derivatives of 3-amino-2,3,6-trideoxy-D-*lyxo*-hexose **(174)**, which are enantiomorphically related to the corresponding derivatives of daunosamine. This preference was clearly related to the more ready availability of the D-sugar intermediates which could be prepared by well established procedures from D-glucose. The results of such studies were also of interest because they afforded confirmation of conclusions drawn from the degradation and physico-chemical investigations originally reported. The synthesis of L-daunosamine has been achieved starting from L-rhamnose and, more recently, from D-mannose. DL-Triacetyldaunosamine has been obtained from non-sugar precursors.

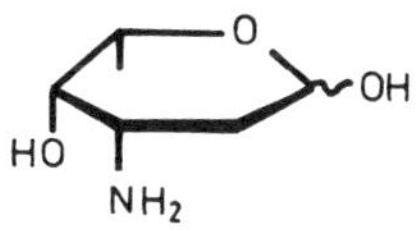

**(39)** 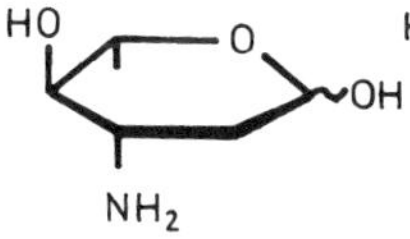 **(171)** 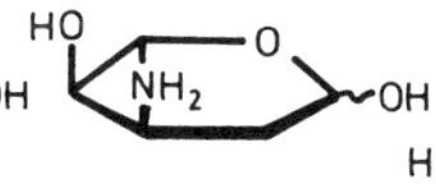 **(172)** 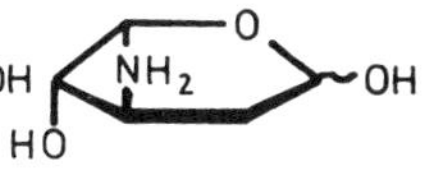 **(173)**

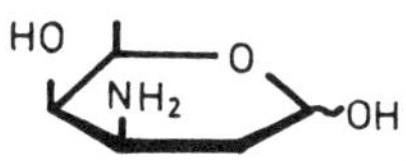

**(174)** 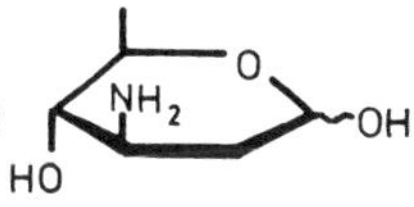 **(175)** 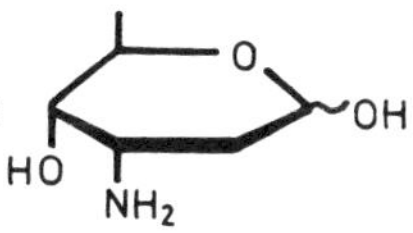 **(176)** 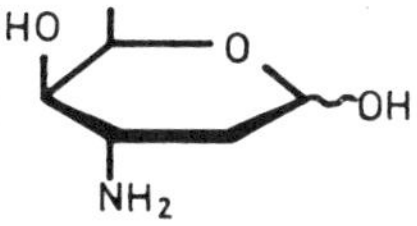 **(177)**

The other configurationally related 3-amino-2,3,6-trideoxyhexoses are **(171)**, **(172)** and **(173)**, which possess, respectively, the L-*arabino*, L-*ribo* and L-*xylo* configurations. Compounds **(171)**, acosamine, and **(172)**, ristosamine, are also important because they have been found as components of other antibiotics, which are actinoidin for acosamine [61], and ristomycin for ristosamine [62]. These aminosugars are of interest because of their close relationship with daunosamine, which renders them likely substitutes for the natural aminosugar in new semi-synthetic or totally synthetic antitumour glycosides. The D-isomers of sugars **(171)**-**(173)** are represented by structures **(175)**-**(177)** respectively.

## 5.1 Synthesis of D-and L-Daunosamine

The first synthetic study aimed at a daunosamine analogue was reported by Richardson [63] and was concerned with the synthesis of N-benzoyl-D-daunosamine (Scheme 5.1). The starting material was methyl 4,6-O-benzylidene-3-deoxy-α-D-*ribo*-hexopyranoside, an intermediate easily accessible from D-glucose, which was converted into the 3-O-methanesulphonate (**178**). This compound gave a facile replacement reaction with inversion of configuration upon treatment with sodium azide, resulting in the 3-azido D-*arabino* derivative (**179**). Catalytic hydrogenation of the latter, followed by N-acetylation of the resulting amine, afforded (**180**), a compound also obtained by another route [64]. Removal of the benzylidene substituent with methanolic hydrogen chloride without a concomitant anomerization of the glycosidic group was possible and afforded methyl 3-acetamido-2,4-dideoxy-α-D-*arabino*-hexopyranoside (**181**). Selective monotosylation of (**181**) gave (**182**). The selectivity of the tosylation reaction was ascribed to the steric hindrance acting

SCHEME 5.1

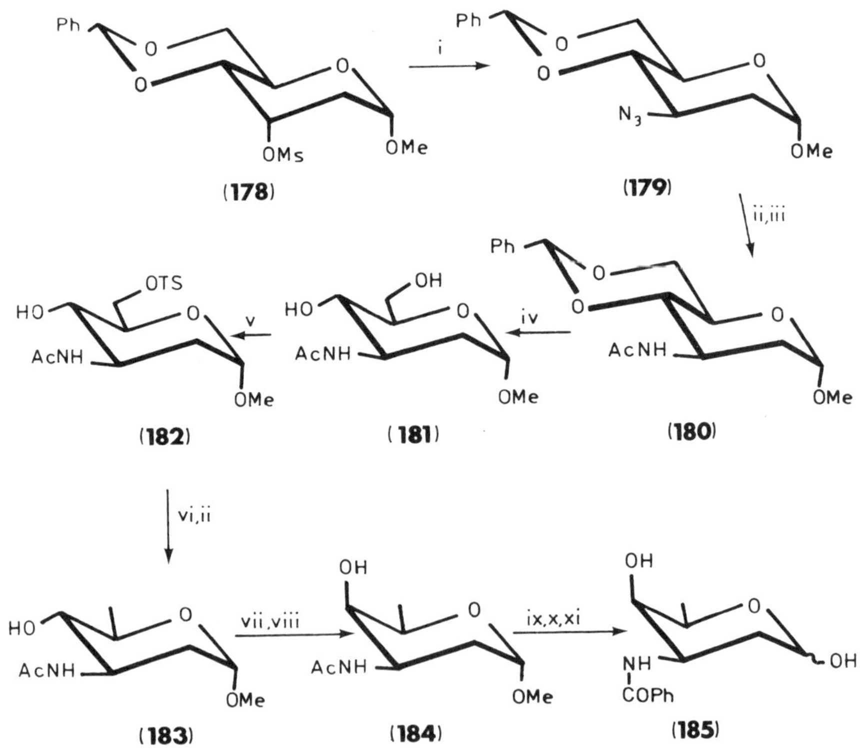

(**178**) (**179**) (**180**) (**181**) (**182**) (**183**) (**184**) (**185**)

Reagents: i, $NaN_3$, DMF, heat; ii, $H_2$, Raney Ni; iii, $Ac_2O$; iv, HCl, MeOH; v, TsCl, pyr; vi, NaI; vii, MsCl, pyr; viii, NaOAc, $NaHCO_3$; ix, $OH^-$; x, $(PhCO)_2O$; xi, aq. AcOH.

on the 4-hydroxyl group. Displacement of the 6-tosyl-group in **(182)** with iodide in acetone followed by reductive dehalogenation gave methyl 3-acetamido-2,3,6-trideoxy-α-D-*arabino*-hexopyranoside **(183)**. This compound was subjected to inversion of configuration at C-4 by solvolysis of the corresponding 4-methanesulphonate. The resulting **(184)**, which possessed the desired D-*lyxo* stereochemistry, was deacetylated, N-benzoylated, and hydrolyzed to the free sugar **(185)**. This compound was enantiomorphic with N-benzoyldaunosamine as deduced by direct comparison with the corresponding derivative of the natural aminosugar.

A study concerning the synthesis of D-daunosamine has been carried out by Baer [65]. This study (Scheme 5.2) involves the use of intermediate compounds in which the nitrogenous function at C-3 came from the oxidation of methyl β-D-glucopyranoside with periodate, to give a dialdehyde, followed by reaction of the latter with nitromethane, a general procedure developed by this author [66, 67]. The major products of the above mentioned reactions are methyl 3-nitro-β-D-glucopyranoside and methyl 3-nitro-β-D-galactopyranoside, both compounds being useful as precursors of the, otherwise scarce, 3-aminohexoses [68, 69]. The 4,6-benzylidene derivatives of the said precursors are presented as starting intermediates in Scheme 5.2. Another feature of Baer's synthesis is the use of β-glycosides, whereas Richardson's approach made use of methyl α-glycosides as intermediates.

Methyl 4,6-O-benzylidene-3-nitro-3-deoxy-β-D-glucopyranoside **(186)** was acetylated and converted, by the Schmidt-Rutz reaction, into a nitroolefin which was hydrogenated with remarkable stereoselectivity to methyl 4,6-O-benzylidene-2,3-dideoxy-3-nitro-β-D-*arabino*-hexopyranoside **(187)**. Hydrolytic removal of the benzylidene group followed by catalytic reduction and N-acetylation of the resulting amine gave methyl 3-acetamido-2,3-dideoxy-β-D-*arabino*-hexopyranoside **(188)**. Conversion of **(188)** into the 6-deoxy-derivative **(190)** involved monotosylation of the primary hydroxyl and O-acetylation to **(189)**, followed by treatment of the latter with sodium iodide to afford the corresponding 6-iodo derivative, which gave **(190)** by reductive dehalogenation. Compound **(190)**, possessing the D-*arabino* configuration, was converted into the stereoisomer with the D-*lyxo* configuration **(192)** *via* the 4-O-mesyl derivative **(191)** which was subjected to inversion of configuration at C-4 by solvolysis with neighbouring group participation.

Methyl N-acetyl-β-D-daunosaminide **(192)** was also obtained starting from methyl 4,6-O-benzylidene-3-nitro-β-D-galactopyranoside **(193)** and following a similar procedure in which, however, the entry into the D-*lyxo* series was more straightforward because no inversion of configuration was necessary once the 2-deoxy and 6-deoxy groups were introduced (Scheme 5.2).

The first synthesis of L-daunosamine was carried out at the Stanford Research Institute (Cal.) [70], and is presented in Scheme 5.3. This synthesis started from L-rhamnose (6-deoxy-L-mannose) **(197)** which was converted into

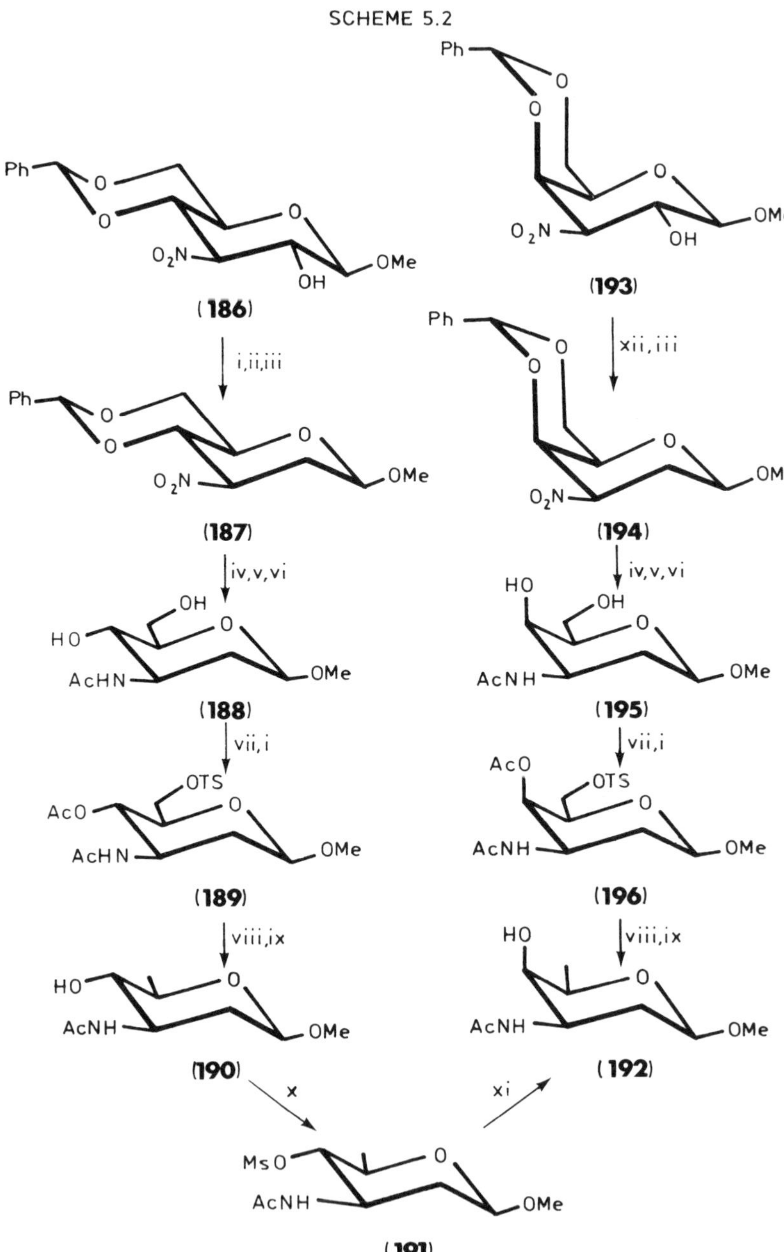


Reagents : i, $Ac_2O$, pyr ; ii, $NaHO_3$, PhH, heat ; iii, $H_2$, Pd–C ; iv, $H^+$ ; v, $H_2$, Pt ; vi, $Ac_2O$, Dowex 1($CO_3^{--}$) ; vii, TsCl, pyr ; viii, NaI ; ix, $H_2$, Ra–Ni ; x MsCl, pyr ; xi, NaOAc, aq. $MeOCH_2CH_2OH$, heat ; xii, $Ac_2O$, AcONa.

L-rhamnal (**200**) according to a known procedure [71]. Methoxymercuration of (**200**) and reduction of (**201**) afforded the 2,6-dideoxy methylglycoside (**202**). Tosylation of the latter gave, after a chromatographic isolation step, mainly (**203**), which was used to give the epoxide (**204**). Nucleophilic opening of the oxirane ring in (**204**) with azide afforded the 3-azido compound (**205**) as the major product. Mesylation of the latter to (**206**), followed by inversion at C-4 by a displacement reaction, afforded the benzoate (**207**) with the L-*lyxo* configuration. L-Daunosamine was obtained from (**207**) upon saponification of the ester group, catalytic hydrogenation, and, finally, hydrolysis of the glycosidic linkage. Alternatively compound (**206**) was hydrogenated to the corres-

SCHEME 5.3

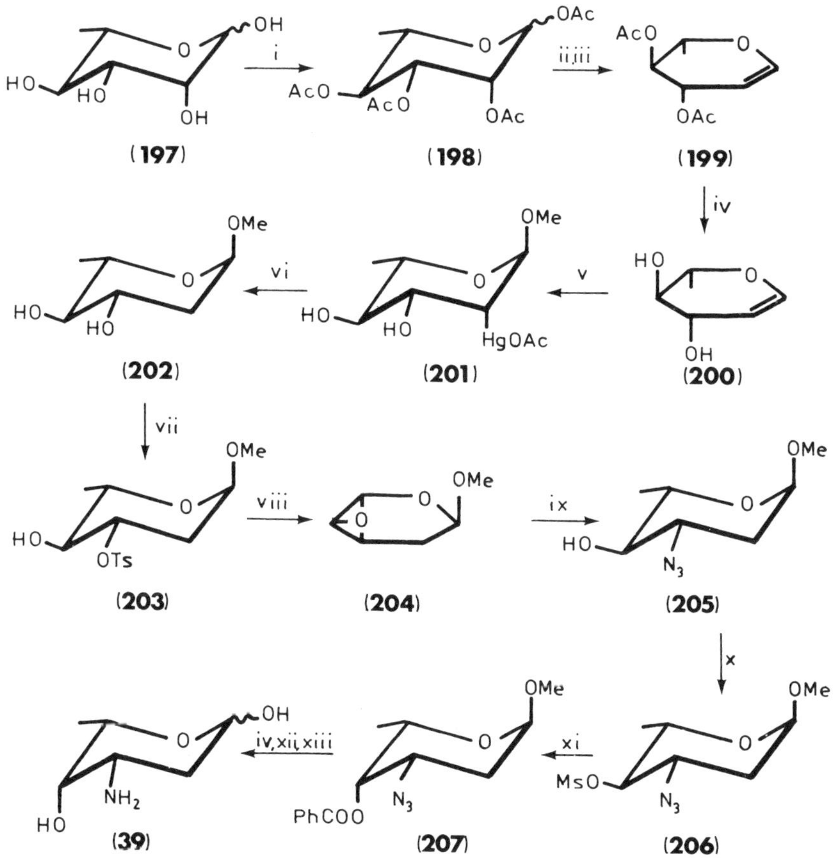

Reagents: i, $Ac_2O$, pyr; ii HBr.AcOH; iii, Zn, AcOH; iv, $OH^-$; v, $Hg(OAc)_2$, MeOH; vi, $KBH_4$; vii, TsCl, pyr; viii, MeONa, MeOH; ix, $NaN_3$; x, MsCl, pyr; xi, PhCOONa, DMF, heat; xii, $H_2$, cat.; xiii, $H^+$.

ponding 3-amino-4-O-mesyl derivative which was N-acetylated and submitted to neighbouring group-assisted displacement of the methansulphonate group with sodium acetate. Obvious steps allowed the conversion of methyl N-acetyl-α-L-daunosaminide to the desired final product.

In view of the high cost of L-rhamnose as a starting material for the preparation of daunosamine and the number of steps required for its synthesis from this sugar, Horton and Weckerle [72] have developed a new synthesis which started from D-mannose (Scheme 5.4). This synthesis required nine steps and afforded L-daunosamine in 40% overall yield from methyl-α-D-mannopyranoside **(208)**. Benzylidenation of **(208)** gave **(209)** which was converted to methyl 4,6-O-benzylidene-2-deoxy-α-D-erythro-hexopyranosid-3-ulose **(210)** by a modification of the Klemer and Rodemeyer reaction [73]. The conversion of **(209)** to **(210)** was carried out with 20g of **(209)** and a yield of 91% was reported for this important step. The reaction sequence followed with the preparation of oxime **(211)** whose reduction and subsequent acetylation gave **(212)** as the major product, the stereoisomer with D-*arabino* configuration being formed in relatively small amount. The conversion of **(212)** to **(213)** following the Hanessian procedure [74] allowed the preparation of the 5,6-unsaturated

SCHEME 5.4

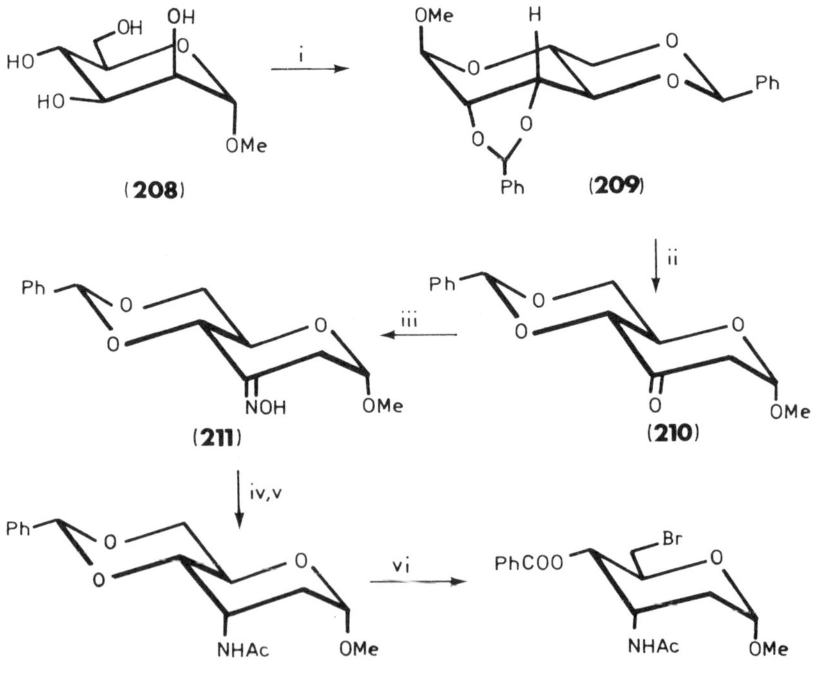

**(208)** →(i) **(209)** →(ii) **(210)** →(iii) **(211)** →(iv,v) **(212)** →(vi) **(213)**

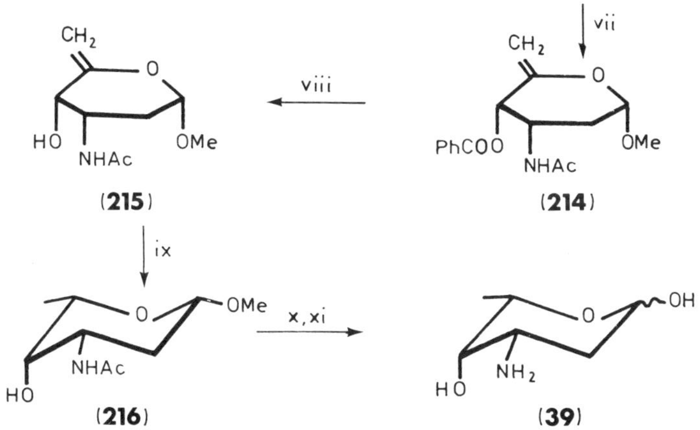

Reagents : i, $PhCH(OMe)_2$, TsOH; ii, BuLi, −30°; iii, $NH_2OH$; iv, $LiAlH_4$; v, $Ac_2O$, pyr.; vi, NBS, $BaCO_3$; vii, AgF, pyr.; viii, MeONa, MeOH; ix, $H_2$, Pd−$BaSO_4$; x, $Ba(OH)_2$; xi, HCl.

derivative (**214**) upon dehydrobromination with silver fluoride. The corresponding O-deacylated compound (**215**) was hydrogenated catalytically with addition of the hydrogen from the less hindered side of the molecule to give, with complete stereoselectivity, the L-*lyxo* derivative (**216**). The latter gave L-daunosamine by N-deacylation and hydrolysis of the methylglycoside.

The third reported synthesis of daunosamine is that of Wong [75] and was carried out starting from non-sugar precursors. The final product reported in this synthesis was DL-triacetyldaunosamine. Wong's daunosamine synthesis started from the oxazole derivative (**217**), the preparation of which was carried out by treatment of 2,4-pentanedione enamine with benzoyl peroxide followed by heating in acetic acid of the thus formed benzoyloxy derivative [76]. Bromination of (**217**) to (**218**), followed by displacement of the halogen with cyanide, gave (**219**) which was converted into (**220**). Ring closure afforded the oxazolo-*α*-pyrone (**221**), the desired intermediate for daunosamine synthesis. Selective hydrogenation of (**221**) gave (**222**), which could be converted into (**223**) in three steps (Scheme 5.5). Removal of the benzylidene group and reacetylation afforded the racemic form of (**42**).

SCHEME 5.5

(217) (218) (219) (220) (221) (222) rac. (223) rac. (42) rac.

Reagents : i, NBS; ii, KCN, liq.HCN; iii; HCl, MeOH, iv, $H_3O^+$; v, $SOCl_2$; vi, $H_2$, Rh–$Al_2O_3$; vii, $NaAl(OCH_2CH_2OMe)_2H_2$; viii; $Ac_2O$, pyr.

## 5.2 Synthesis of Daunosamine analogues

The synthesis of aminosugars related to daunosamine has been carried out starting from daunosamine itself, from L-rhamnose, from L-glucose or L-arabinose, from D-mannose, and from D-glucose.

### 5.2.1 *Synthesis from daunosamine*

Methyl α-daunosaminide (**40**) has been used as starting material for the preparation of daunosamine analogues modified at C-4, as in the derivatives of 4-epidaunosamine (acosamine) and of 4-deoxydaunosamine (Scheme 5.6).

Synthesis of 2,3,6-trideoxy-3-trifluoroacetamido-L-*arabino*-hexose or N-trifluoroacetylacosamine **(227)** was achieved [77] by converting **(40)** into the N-trifluoroacetyl derivative **(224)** by methanolysis of an intermediate N,O-ditrifluoroacetylderivative, followed by oxidation of **(224)** to the keto derivative (225) and stereoselective reduction of the latter to give the equatorial alcohol (226). Acid hydrolysis of (226) afforded acosamine as the N-trifluoroacetyl derivative (227). For the synthesis of 2,3,4,6-tetradeoxy-3-trifluoroacetamido-L-threo-hexose **(231)** compound **(224)** was converted into the 4-p-bromo-benzenesulphonyl derivative **(228)** which was submitted to a nucleophilic displacement reaction with iodide. The resulting iodo derivative (229) gave **(230)** by reductive dehalogenation. Acid hydrolysis of **(230)** afforded the desired N-trifluoroacetyl-daunosamine (231) [78].

SCHEME 5.6

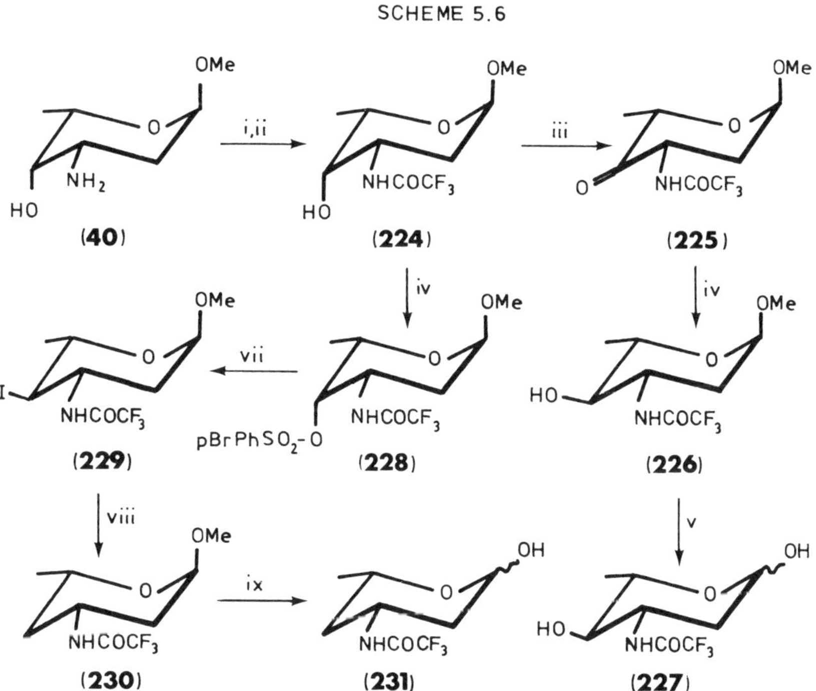


Reagents : i, $(CF_3CO)_2O$ ; ii, MeOH ; iii, $RuO_4$ ; iv, $NaBH_4$ ; v, $H_3O^+$ ; vi, p-$BrC_6H_4SO_2Cl$, pyr. ; vii, NaI, heat ; viii, $H_2$, Pt ; ix, aq. AcOH.

5.2.2 *Synthesis from L-rhamnose*

Entry into the 3-amino-2,3,6-trideoxy-L-*arabino*-hexose series of derivatives was afforded by the availability of the intermediates of daunosamine synthesis from L-rhamnal reported above. Catalytic hydrogenation of **(205)** afforded methyl α-acosaminide **(232)** [79, 80]. As shown in Scheme 5.7 illustrating the synthesis of acosamine and ristosamine derivatives, compound **(232)** was converted into acosamine by acid hydrolysis. In the same study [80], **(232)** was converted into the acetylated derivatives **(233)** and **(234)**, which appeared identical with the same derivatives derived from biosynthetic material. Compound **(233)** was also O-methylated to **(235)**, the N-acetyl derivative of methyl actinosaminide, another compound derived from the antibiotic actinoidin [81, 61]. Intermediate **(203)** was instead used for the synthesis of ristosamine **(172)**, which differs from daunosamine in the absolute configuration at C-3 and C-4 [82]. Displacement of the tosyloxy group in **(203)** with azide afforded **(236)**, displaying the desired L-*ribo* configuration. Catalytic reduction of **(236)** followed by acid hydrolysis of the intermediate aminoglycoside gave ristosamine.

SCHEME 5.7

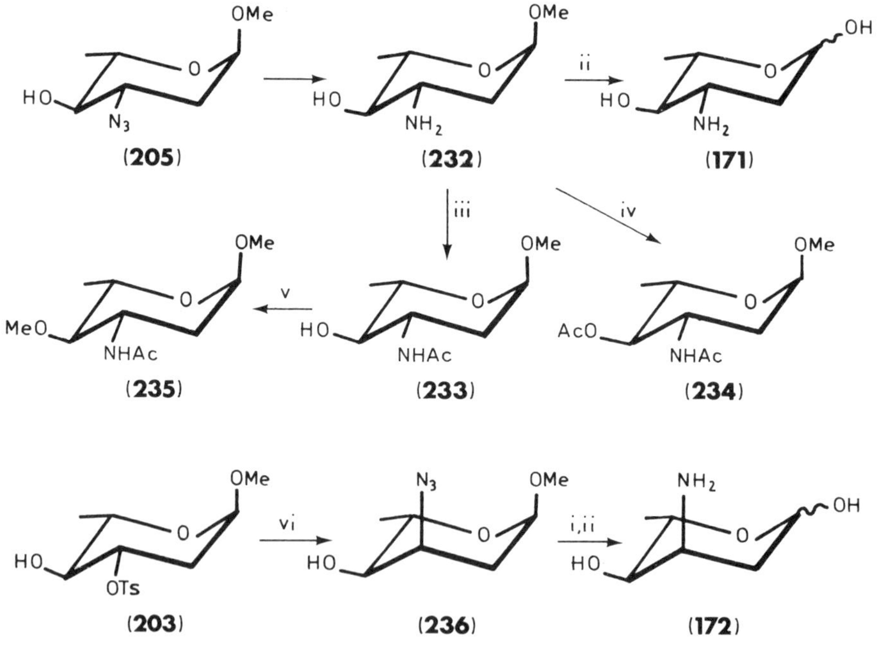

(**205**) → (**232**) →[ii] (**171**)

(**232**) →[iii] (**233**); (**232**) →[iv] (**234**); (**233**) →[v] (**235**)

(**203**) →[vi] (**236**) →[i,ii] (**172**)

Reagents : i, $H_2$, Pd–C ; ii, $H_3O^+$ ; iii, $Ac_2O$, MeOH ; iv, $Ac_2O$, pyr. ; v, $Me_2SO_4$ ; vi, $NaN_3$, DMF, heat.

The 4-O-mesyl derivative of (**205**) was also used for the synthesis of the 4-amino analogues of daunosamine [83]. In this study (Scheme 5.8) compound (**237**) was treated with sodium benzylsulphinate and thiobenzyl alcohol to give (**238**). This reaction is considered to occur through the intermediate formation of an aziridine. This would derive from intramolecular nucleophilic attack at C-4 by the amino nitrogen resulting from the reduction of the azide. Compound (**238**) would then originate as a consequence of the nucleophilic displacement at C-3 due to a benzylsulphide anion. Identification of compound (**238**) was carried out by $^1$H n.m.r. and mass spectrometry on the aminoglycoside itself, as well as on its N-trifluoroacetyl derivative. Desulpherization of (**228**) afforded (**239**).

SCHEME 5.8

MsO, $N_3$, OMe (**237**) —i→ $PhCH_2S$, OMe, $NH_2$ (**238**) —ii→ OMe, $NH_2$ (**239**)

Reagents : i, $PhCH_2SO_2Na$, $PhCH_2SH$; ii, Raney Ni.

The synthesis of N-benzylristosamine from L-rhamnal following a procedure essentially similar to that described in schemes 5.3 and 5.7 has been reported by Hungarian chemists [84].

L-Rhamnal has been used by German authors [85] as starting material in a new reaction sequence leading to both acosamine and ristosamine (Scheme 5.9). According to this procedure di-O-acetyl-L-rhamnal (**199**) was submitted to an allylic displacement with boron trifluoride etherate as catalyst. The nucleophilic reagent, in this case represented by the azide anion, enters in the C-1 position as in (**240**), which, however, readily equilibrates with the more stable 3-azido compound (**241**). Although substantial quantities of a dimeric product were also formed, the reaction is of considerable practical interest because compound (**241**) is clearly an outstanding intermediate for the synthesis of 3-amino-2,3,6-trideoxy-L-hexoses. Iodomethylation of the equilibrium mixture of (**240**) and (**241**) followed by catalytic hydrogenation and acetylation afforded (**242**) and (**243**), the former (methyl-N,O-diacetyl-α-acosaminide) being formed in greater amount than the latter (methyl N,O-diacetyl-α-ristosaminide).

SCHEME 5.9

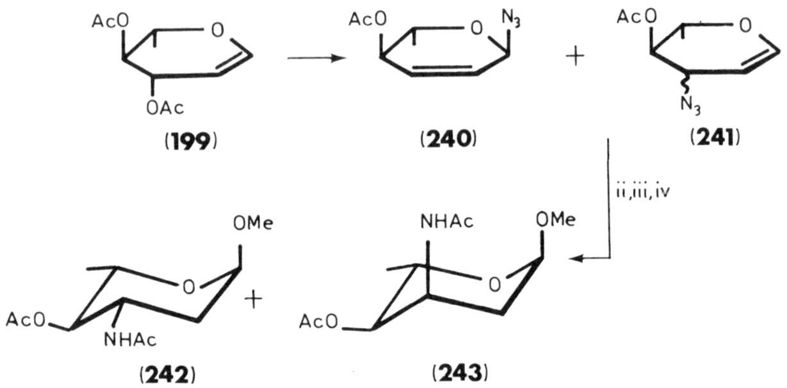

(199) → (240) + (241)

ii,iii,iv

(242) + (243)

Reagents: i, $NaN_3$, $BF_3$–$Et_2O$; ii TlOAc, $I_2$, MeOH; iii, $H_2$, Pd; iv, $Ac_2O$, pyr.

Horton and his coworkers have also used L-rhamnose as starting material in a study aimed at the evaluation of the Klemer and Rodemeyer reaction [73] for the development of new synthetic procedures affording analogues [86]. In this study (Scheme 5.10) methyl-α-L-rhamnopyranoside **(244)** was converted to the 2,3-benzylidene acetal **(245)**. This compound gave a mixture of different products when treated with butyl lithium, because of the interference of the 4-oxyanion formed in these conditions. Benzylation of **(245)** gave **(246)** which could be resolved into the two epimeric forms a and b differing in the configuration at C-2′. Compound **(246)** also failed to give a straightforward reaction with butyllithium, probably because of the formation of a carbanion as a consequence of the abstraction of the benzylic proton. On the contrary the 4-O-methyl derivative **(247)** gave the desired methyl 2,6-dideoxy-4-O-methyl-α-L-*erythro*-hexopyranosid-3-ulose **(248)** in 40% yield. Hydroxylamine converted **(248)** into the corresponding oxime **(249)**, a potential precursor of the 4-O-methyl derivatives of ristosamine, of acosamine, and of the other derivatives in the L-ribo and L-arabino series.

SCHEME 5.10

(244) (245) (247) (246) (249) (248)

(246)
a : $R^1$ = Ph, $R^2$ = H
b : $R^1$ = H, $R^2$ = Ph

Reagents : i $PhCH(OMe)_2$, TsOH; ii, $PhCH_2Br$, NaI, DMF; iii, MeI, NaH, DMF; iv, BuLi, hexane, − 30°; v, $NH_2OH$.

5.2.3 *Synthesis from L-arabinose and L-glucose*

As part of a programme aimed at the synthesis of new semisynthetic anthracycline glycosides related to daunomycin and adriamycin and at the pharmacological evaluation of the new compounds in order to establish structure-activity relationships and possibly develop more efficient drugs possessing a broader spectrum of activity and decreased toxicity, the synthesis of amino-sugars related to L-daunosamine from commercially available L-arabinose was studied in the author's laboratory. This sugar can be converted into 2-deoxy-L-*arabino*-hexose (2-deoxy-L-glucose) by the procedure of Sowden and Fischer [87]. Standard procedures [88, 89] were also available for the conversion of 2-deoxy-L-glucose to methyl 4,6-O-benzylidene-2-deoxy-α-L-*arabino*-hexopyranoside (**250**). This protected intermediate (Scheme 5.11) displayed the free 3-hydroxyl group, suitable for the introduction of a nitrogenous function, thus representing a suitable intermediate for the fulfilment of the programme.

SCHEME 5.11

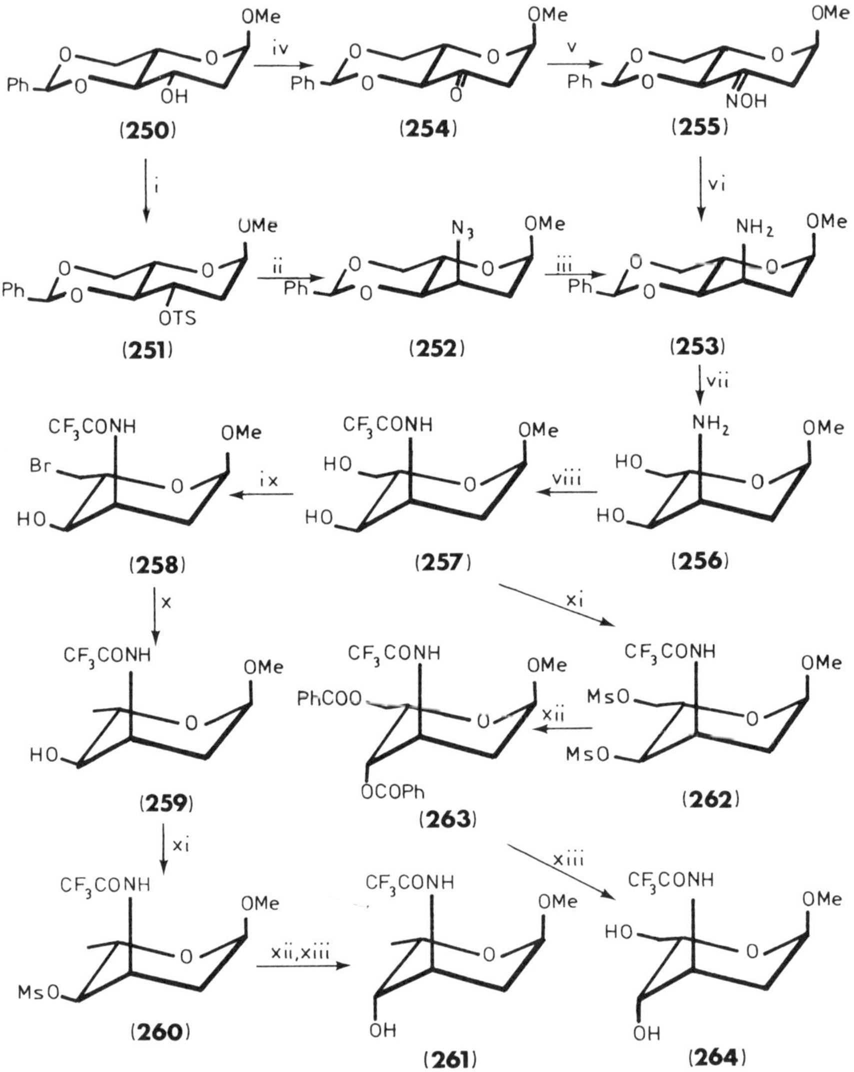

Reagents : i, TsCl, pyr ; ii, $NaN_3$, DMF, heat ; iii, $H_2$, Pd–C ; iv, $RuO_4$ ; v, $NH_2OH$ ; vi, $LiAlH_4$ ; vii, HCl, MeOH ; viii, $(CF_3CO)_2O$ ; ix, NBS, $PPh_3$, DMF ; x, $H_2$, Pd–C, $BaCO_3$ ; xi, MsCl, pyr ; xii, PhCOONa, DMF, heat ; xiii, MeONa, MeOH.

Access into the series possesing an axial amino group at C-3 (L-*ribo* and also L-*xylo*) was ensured by the high yield conversion of **(250)** to methyl 3-amino-4,5-O-benzylidene-2-deoxy-α-L-*ribo*-hexopyranoside **(253)** *via* the tosyl derivative **(251)**, nucleophilic displacement of the tosyloxy group with azide, and final catalytic hydrogenation of **(252)** to give **(253)**, in 86% overall yield from **(250)** [90]. A similar conversion had been reported for the D-series, but the recorded yields were considerably lower [91, 92]. An alternative synthesis of **(253)** from **(250)** was represented by the oxidation of **(250)** to the known [93] methyl 4,6-O-benzylidene-2-deoxy-α-L-*erythro*-hexopyranosid-3-ulose **(254)** and conversion of the latter to the oxime **(255)** which was then reduced with lithium aluminium hydride to give a mixture containing 85% of the L-*ribo* amine **(253)** and 10% of the corresponding L-*arabino* isomer. The overall yield of the alternative route was 65% [90, 94]. Removal of the benzylidene group in **(255)** afforded methyl 3-amino-2,3-dideoxy-α-L-*ribo*-hexopyranoside, **(256)** a compound whose D-enantiomorphy was already known [92, 95]. The corresponding N-trifluoroacetyl derivative **(257)** was a key intermediate for both the preparation of compounds belonging to the 6-deoxy-L-*ribo*-series and of L-*xylo* analogues.

Conversion of **(257)** into the 6-bromo derivative **(258)** according to a literature procedure [96], followed by reductive dehalogenation, afforded methyl 2,3,6-trideoxy-3-fluoroacetamido-α-L-*ribo*-hexopyranoside (methyl N-trifluoroacetyl-α-ristosaminide) **(259)** [94].

Conversion of **(259)** to the corresponding L-*xylo* analogue **(261)**, which is the α-methylglycoside of the previously unknown (L and D-series) 3′-epidaunosamine, was achieved by treatment with methanesulphonyl chloride in pyridine and by nucleophilic displacement followed by sodium methoxide catalyzed methanolysis of the intermediate crystalline **(260)** [97]. On the other hand mesylation of **(257)** afforded the 4,6-di-O-mesyl derivative **(262)** which was subjected to nucleophilic displacement in order to carry out the inversion of configuration at C-4 and the entry in the L-*xylo* series. O-Debenzoylation of **(263)** afforded methyl 2,3-dideoxy-3-trifluoroacetamido-α-L-*xylo*-hexopyranoside **(264)** [90]. This appears to be the first synthesis of derivatives of 3-amino-2,3-dideoxy-L-*xylo*-hexose, but the corresponding D-series had already been explored by Overend and his coworkers, who prepared methyl 2,3-dideoxy-3-formamido-α-D-*xylo*-hexopyranoside and its L-*lyxo* analogue by reduction and N-formylation of the mixture of methyl 4,6-O-benzylidene-2-deoxy-α-*threo*hexopyranoside-3-ulose *syn* and *anti* oximes [92].

For access to the series possessing an equatorial amino group at C-3 (L-*arabino* and also L-*lyxo*), the L-*ribo* analogue **(265)** of **(250)** was a suitable intermediate. Compound **(265)** and was made available according to two procedures reported in the literature for the D-series. The first was based on the already mentioned oxidation of **(250)** to **(254)** [98 followed by a stereoselective

SCHEME 5.12

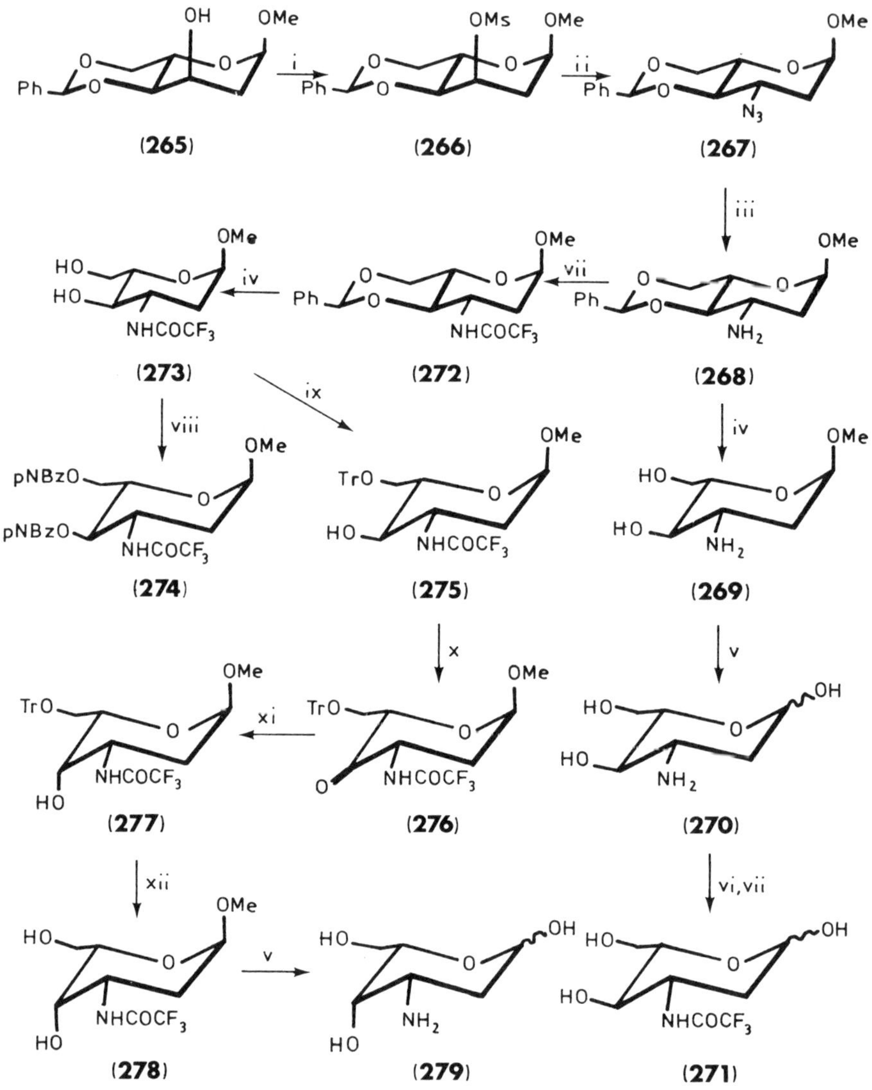

Reagents : i, MsCl, pyr; ii, $NaN_3$ DMF; iii, $H_2$, Raney Ni; iv, HCl, MeOH; v, $H_3O^+$, heat; vi $(CF_3CO)_2O$; vii, MeOH; viii, p-$NO_2C_6H_4COCl$ (pNBzCl), pyr; ix; TrCl, pyr; x, $RuO_4$, $K_2CO_3$; xi, LiBH(sec. Bu$)_3$H, THF, −78°; xii, aq. AcOH.

reduction with lithium aluminium hydride [97], and resulted in a 82% conversion of **(250)** to methyl 4,6-O-benzylidene-2-deoxy-α-L-*ribo*-hexopyranoside **(265)** [90]. The second consisted in the known procedure available for the preparation of the D-enantiomer of **(265)** starting from D-glucose *via* methyl 2,3-anhydro-4,6-O-benzylidene-α-L-*allo*-pyranoside [99, 100, 63]. In the application of this procedure to the synthesis of **(265)** from L-glucose an overall yield of 30% was recorded [90].

The conversion of **(265)** to methyl 3-amino-4,6-di-benzylidene-2,3-dideoxy-α-L-*arabino*-hexopyranoside **(268)** was essentially based on work done in the D-series [92, 63]. Mesylation of **(265)** followed the displacement with azide and catalytic hydrogenation of **(267)** afforded **(268)** in 59% overall yield. Compound **(268)** was a pivotal intermediate in that it represented the entry into the L-*arabino* series of 3-amino-2,3-dideoxy hexoses and also the precursor of the new derivatives possessing the L-*lyxo* configuration (Scheme 5.12).

Debenzylidenation of **(268)** gave methyl 3-amino-2,3-dideoxy-α-L-*arabino*-hexopyranoside **(269)** which was hydrolyzed to the free aminosugar **(270)**. The latter compound had already been reported in the D-series, together with the corresponding methyl β-glycoside, but obtained by a different route [68]. N-Trifluoroacetylation of **(268)** afforded **(272)** which was converted into methyl 2,3-dideoxy-3-trifluoroacetamido-α-L-*arabino*-hexopyranoside **(273)**, also characterized as the 4,6-di-O-*p*-nitrobenzoate **(274)**. Compound **(273)** was tritylated and the resulting 6-O-trityl derivative **(275)** was oxidized to methyl 2,3,-dideoxy-3-trifluoroacetamido-6-O-triphenylmethyl-α-L-*threo*-hexopyranosid-4-ulose **(276)**. Reduction of **(276)** with lithium selectride afforded a stereoselective hydride attack from the upper side of the molecule owing to the presence of the two equatorial substituents at C-3 and C-5. The resulting axial alcohol **(277)** was stepwise hydrolyzed to methyl 2,3-dideoxy-3-trifluoroacetamido-α-L-*lyxo*-hexopyranoside **(278)** and then to 3-amino-2,3-L-*lyxo*-hexopyranose (6-hydroxydaunosamine) **(279)** [90]. A synthesis of methyl 3-amino-2,3-dideoxy-β-D-*lyxo*-hexopyranoside had been reported by Baer and Kinzle starting from methyl 3-deoxy-3-nitro-β-D-galactopyranoside [69].

### 5.2.4 *Synthesis from D-mannose*

A synthesis of 3-amino-2,3,6-trideoxy-D-*ribo*-hexose, the C-5 epimer of daunosamine and enantiomorph of ristosamine, from methyl 3-acetamido-4-O-benzoyl-6-bromo-2,3,6-trideoxy-α-D-*ribo*-hexopyranoside **(213)** has been reported [101]. As shown in Scheme 5.13, catalytic hydrogenation of **(213)** removed the bromine atom and O-debenzoylation of **(280)** by Zemplén transesterification with catalytic sodium methoxide in methanol afforded methyl N-acetyl-α-D-ristosaminide **(281)**. The latter compound was subjected to different transformations, including N-deacetylation followed by N-benzoylation to **(282)**, a highly acid-labile compound which underwent easy conversion

SCHEME 5.13

Reagents: i, $H_2$, Ni; ii, MeONa; iii, $Ba(OH)_2$; iv, PhCOCl; v, $H_3O^+$; vi, HCl.

into the benzamido sugar (**283**). On the other hand N-deacetylation of (**281**) followed by acid hydrolysis gave D-ristosamine (**284**), which was obtained in 38% overall yield from D-mannose, the original precursor of (**213**) (see Scheme 5.4).

### 5.2.5 *Synthesis from D-glucose*

Two syntheses of D-ristosamine (**176**) (the already above mentioned 5-epimer of daunosamine) starting from tri-O-acetyl-D-glucal have been published recently.

The first one is presented in Scheme 5.14[102]. According to this procedure (**285**) was converted into methyl 2-deoxy-$\beta$-D-*arabino*-hexopyranoside (**286**) by addition of hydrogen chloride and subsequent glycosidation followed by Zemplén deacetylation. Mesylation of the 4,6-O-benzylidene derivative (**287**) and treatment with azide gave (**289**). The Hanessian reaction allowed the conversion of (**289**) to (**290**), which was hydrogenated in order to remove the bromine atom. Reduction was, however, accompanied by a partial migration of the benzoyl residue to the amino group. Benzoylation of the resulting mixture gave (**291**). O-Deacetylation of (**291**) to methyl N-benzoyl-$\beta$-ristosaminide and subsequent mild acid hydrolysis of the latter gave N-benzoyl-D-ristosamine (**283**).

In the second synthesis, part of which is presented in Scheme 5.15, the 3-O-tosyl analogue (**292**) of (**288**) was similarly converted into (**289**) with sodium azide and then to (**290**), this compound affording D-ristosamine (**176**) upon O-debenzoylation, catalytic hydrogenation and acid hydrolysis [103].

SCHEME 5.14

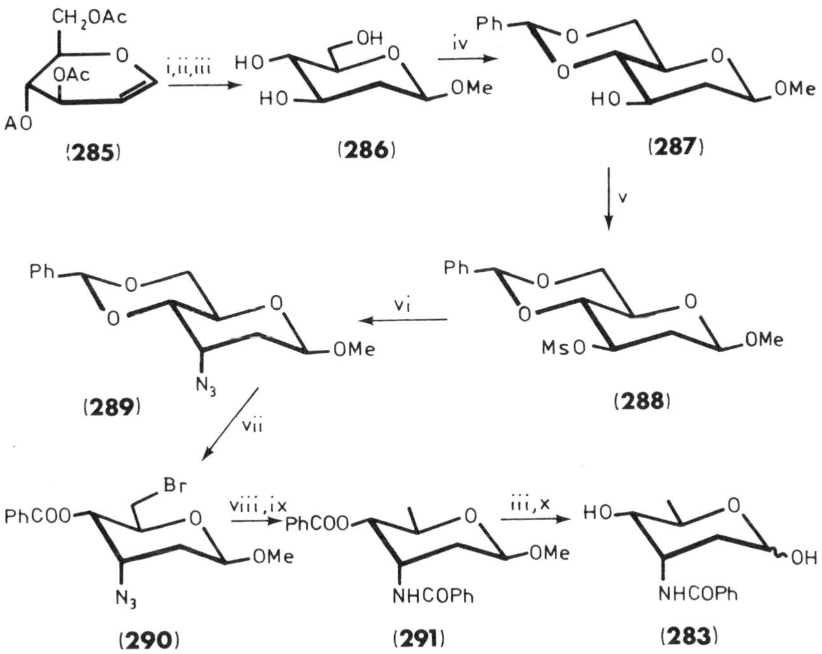

Reagents : i, HCl ; ii, MeOH, $Ag_2CO_3$ ; iii, MeONa ; iv, PhCHO, $ZnCl_2$ ; v, MsCl, pyr. ; vi, $NaN_3$, HMP, 100° ; vii, NBS ; viii, $H_2$, Ni ; ix, PhCOCl, pyr. ; x, aq. AcOH.

SCHEME 5.15

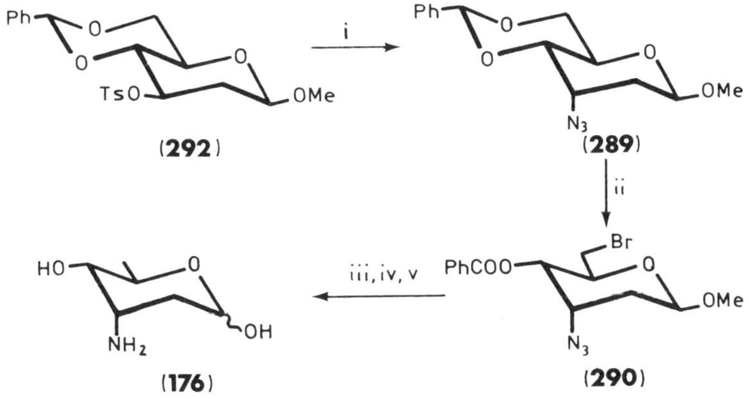

Reagents : i, $NaN_3$ ; ii, NBS ; iii, MeONa ; iv, H , Pd ; v, HCl.

## 6 GLYCOSIDE SYNTHESIS

The synthesis of anthracycline and anthracycline-like glycosides has recently received considerable attention. The development of suitable methods for the synthesis of the glycoside bond between the aglycone and the aminosugar was a prerequisite for any attempt at the preparation of daunomycin and adriamycin by total synthesis. Total synthesis could provide an alternative method, possibly competitive with the biosynthetic process, for the preparation of clinically useful antibiotics. Although this possibility seems remote at the present time, the synthesis of the glycosidic linkage remains an essential step in the preparation of new potential antitumour agents related to the anthracycline antibiotics but not accessible by direct chemical modification of the biosynthetically available glycosides. It allows, for instance, the coupling of the new, modified aminosugars to daunomycinone and adriamycinone or that of daunosamine to new aglycones obtained by total synthesis or by chemical modification of daunomycinone. When adequate information concerning the relationship between the aglycone and aminosugar structures with biological activity becomes available,† new glycosides will be synthesized starting from unnatural aglycones and aminosugars, thus combining different structural modifications in order to increase selectivity of action. In any case a high yield, stereoselective reaction for glycoside synthesis is required. In fact, although data presently available do not allow definite conclusions to be made for the limited pharmacological action of $\beta$-glycosides, it should be noted that the natural configuration present in the $\alpha$-glycosides renders these the best candidates for optimal biological activity. In the following we shall describe the different, successful approaches to the synthesis of the glycosidic linkage in the anthracycline glycosides and the variety of new structural and stereochemical analogues thus obtained, so witnessing both the contribution of organic chemists to cancer research, and the potentiality of these recently developed methods for the preparation of new antitumour agents.

### 6.1 The Koenigs Knorr and related reactions

The most frequently used reactions for glycoside synthesis are the Koenigs-Knorr and related condensations of a suitably protected sugar halide with an alcohol in the presence of an insoluble silver or mercuric salt. The reaction is, in principle, a nucleophilic displacement but its features, such as the rate and the steric course, are, in the absence of a participating group at C-2, dependent on a number of factors operating on a complex mechanism which is presently not completely understood. These factors include the nature of the halide and of the alcohol, the excess of the alcohol, the solvent, the silver or mercuric salt, and the temperature [104]. A push-pull mechanism has been proposed in which the 'pull' is represented by the silver complexing the halogen and the 'push' by the

†See Part D for current ideas on mode of action of these antibiotics.

entering nucleophile. Such a type of mechanism could involve a varying degree of $S_N1$ and $S_N2$ character depending on whether the 'pull' or the 'push' is predominant. The complete inversion of configuration at the anomeric centre, which often takes place when a large excess of the alcohol is used, is not generally the case when the amounts of the reagents are stoichiometric [105].

The first synthesis of a daunomycinone glycoside was carried out by Penco [106] who treated daunomycinone (**21**) with 2,3,4,6-tetraacetyl-α-D-glucosyl bromide (**293**) or with 2-deoxy-3,4,6-triacetyl-2-trifluoro-acetamido-α-D-glucosyl bromide (**294**) in 1,2-dichloroethane and in the presence of silver carbonate (Scheme 6.1). Upon hydrolysis with dilute alkali the condensation products (**295**) and (**296**) afforded, respectively, 7-O-(β-D-glycopyranosyl)-daunomycinone (**297**) and 7-O-(2-amino-2-deoxy-β-D-glucopyranosyl)-daunomycinone (**298**). The structure of the two semisynthetic glycosides was

SCHEME 6.1

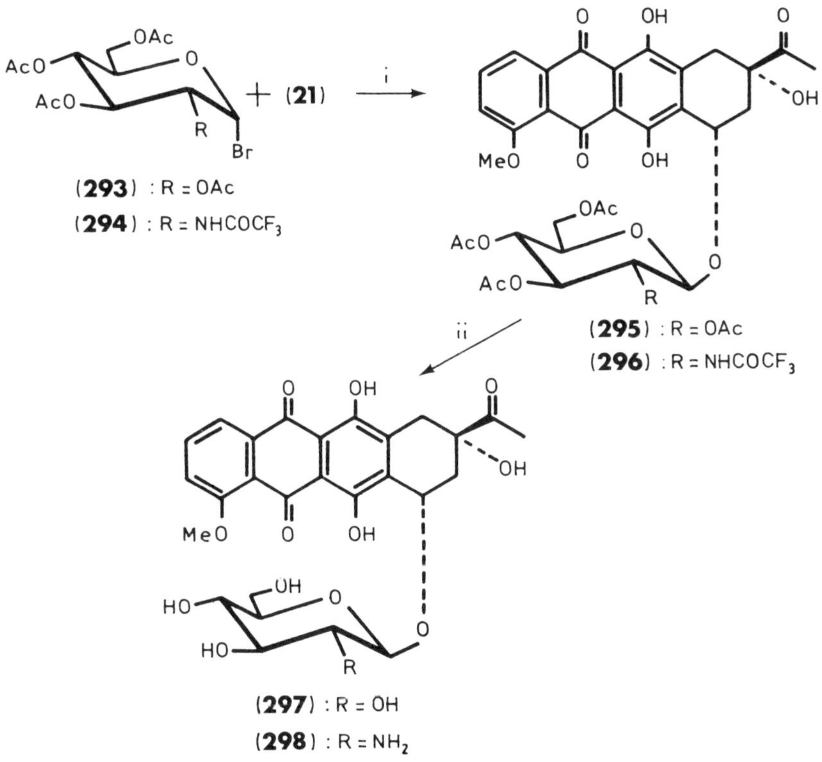

(**293**) : R = OAc
(**294**) : R = $NHCOCF_3$

(**295**) : R = OAc
(**296**) : R = $NHCOCF_3$

(**297**) : R = OH
(**298**) : R = $NH_2$

Reagents : i, $Ag_2CO_3$, ii, $OH^-$.

proved by their conversion into 7-deoxy-daunomycinone and the free sugars upon catalytic hydrogenolysis. The β-configuration was assigned to the glycosidic linkage on the basis of the known effect of participating groups at C-2 in the glucosyl halide [107, 108].

In the same year (1968) glycoside **(300)** was synthesized starting from acetobromoglucose **(293)** which was coupled with the tetracyclic daunomycinone analogue **(55)** in the presence of mercuric cyanide to give **(299)** which was then converted to glycoside **(300)**, as shown in Scheme 6.2 [37].

SCHEME 6.2

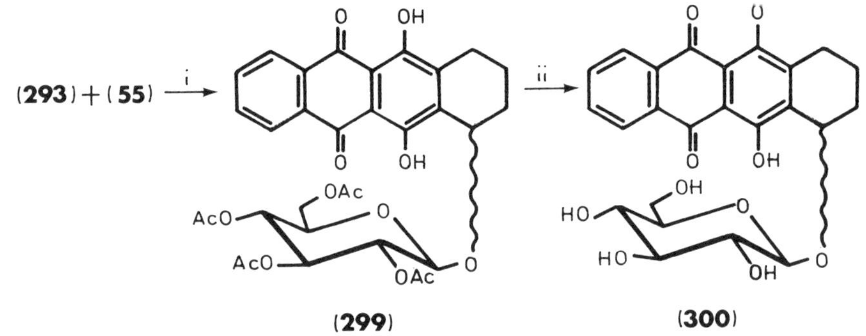

**(293)** + **(55)** $\xrightarrow{i}$ **(299)** $\xrightarrow{ii}$ **(300)**

Reagents : i, $Hg(CN)_2$ ; ii, MeONa, MeOH.

A synthesis of daunomycin starting from aglycone and O-p-nitrobenzoyl-N-trifluoroacetyldaunosaminyl bromide **(302)** was published by Acton *et al.* [109]. As shown in Scheme 6.3, **(302)** was prepared from 1,4-bis(O-p-nitrobenzoate) **(301)**, which was treated in dichloromethane and at 0° with anhydrous hydrogen bromide. The coupling of **(302)** and **(21)** was carried out with mercuric cyanide, mercuric bromide and powdered molecular sieve in boiling anhydrous tetrahydrofuran. A threefold molar excess of **(302)** was used to give a 50% yield of **(303)**. Deblocking of **(303)** gave daunomycin. This coupling took place with unexpected stereoselectivity, because only the α-anomer was isolated.

The synthesis of the daunomycin glycosidic linkage was also investigated as a model study in the author's laboratory where the synthetic procedure reported in Scheme 6.4 was developed [110]. In this study N,O-ditrifluoroacetyl-α-daunosaminyl chloride **(306)** was used as the glycosylating agent in a modified Koenigs-Knorr reaction, in which mercuric oxide, mercuric bromide, and mole-

SCHEME 6.3

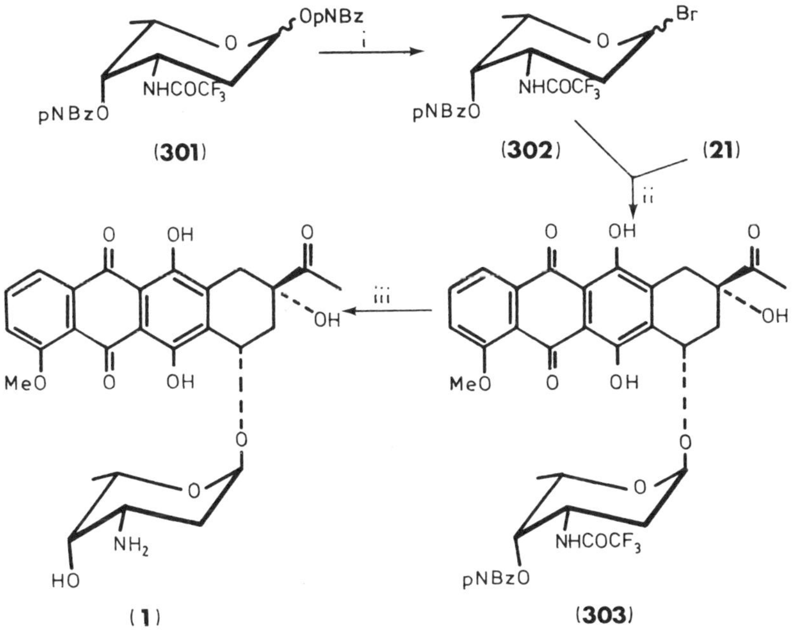

(301) (302) (21) (1) (303)

Reagents : i, HBr ; ii, $Hg(CN)_2$, $HgBr_2$, molecular sieve ; iii, $OH^-$ ; pNBzO = *p*-nitrobenzoate.

cular sieve were the reagents and dichloromethane was the solvent. Recovery of the reaction products followed by hydrolysis of the O-trifluoroacetate grouping upon treatment with methanol afforded the α and β-N-trifluoroacetyl glycosides **(308)** and **(310)** in the approximate ratio of 7:3. Chromatographic separation followed by mild alkaline treatment gave the two aminoglycosides, daunomycin **(1)** and β-daunosaminyl-daunomycinone **(313)**. The same reaction sequence was carried out for the synthesis of 4′-epidaunomycin and of its β-anomer, but starting from N,O-ditrifluoroacetyl-α-acosaminyl chloride **(307)**. The latter was obtained from N-trifluoroacetyl-acosamine **(232)**, which was converted into **(305)** and then treated with hydrogen chloride to afford **(307)**. Coupling of **(307)** and **(21)**, according to the procedures outlined above, gave **(309)**, **(311)** and, finally, the 4′-epianalogues **(312)** and **(314)**.

SCHEME 6.4



(304), (306) $R^1 = OCOCF_3$, $R^2 = H$

(305), (307) $R^1 = H$, $R^2 = OCOCF_3$

(308), (310), (1), (313): $R^1 = OH$, $R^2 = H$

(309), (311), (312), (314): $R^1 = H$, $R^2 = OH$

Reagents: i, HCl; ii, HgO, $HgBr_2$, molecular sieve; iii, MeOH; iv, $SiO_2$; v, $OH^-$.

SCHEME 6.5

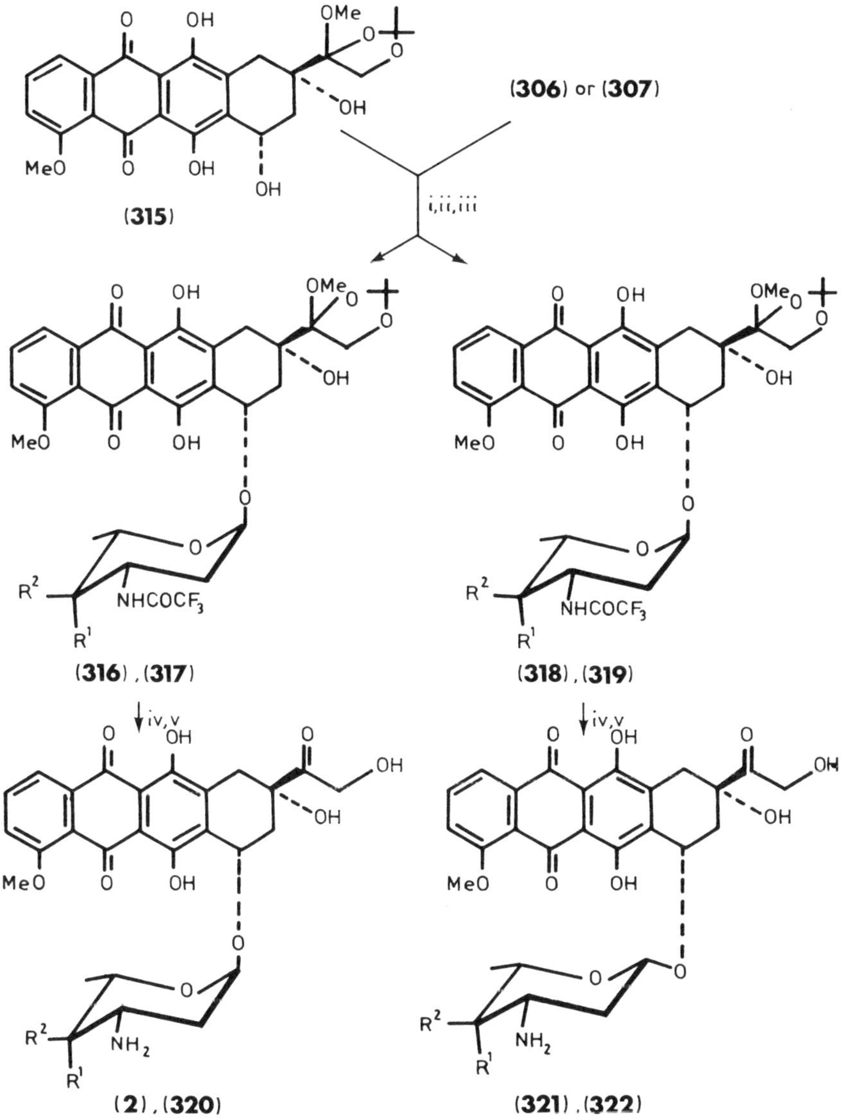

(**315**)

(**306**) or (**307**)

i,ii,iii

(**316**), (**317**)

(**318**), (**319**)

iv,v

(**2**), (**320**)

(**321**), (**322**)

(**316**), (**318**), (**2**), (**321**) : $R^1 = OH, R^2 = H$

(**317**), (**319**), (**320**), (**322**): $R^1 = H, R^2 = OH$

Reagents : i, $HgO.HgBr_2$, molecular sieve; ii, MeOH, iii, $SiO_2$; iv, $OH^-$; v, $H^+$.

In order to perform the coupling of daunosamine and adriamycinone, the hydroxymethylketone function of the latter was protected as in **(315)** (Scheme 6.5). This compound was obtained by treatment of adriamycinone with 2,2-dimethoxypropane under anhydrous acid conditions. Its structure was established, *inter alia,* by analysis of its mass spectrum [110]. Condensation of **(315)** with **(306)** under the above mentioned conditions and removal of the O-trifluoroacetyl grouping with methanol afforded the two anomeric glycosides **(316)** and **(318)** which were separated by chromatography. Removal of the protecting groups, first using a mild alkaline treatment and then deblocking the side chain with dilute acid, afforded adriamycin **(2)** and its β-anomer **(321)**. This reaction sequence (Scheme 6.5) was also used for the synthesis of 4′-epiadriamycin **(320)**, a new analogue which has shown interesting pharmacological properties and which is presently under clinical trial, together with 1′,4′-

SCHEME 6.6

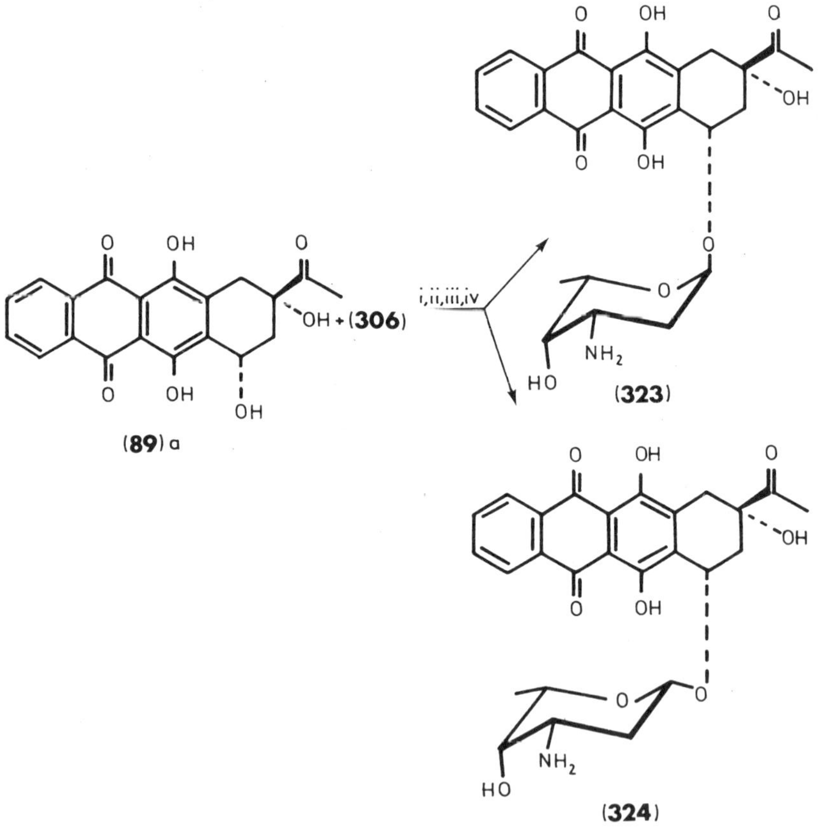

**(89)** a + **(306)** → (i, ii, iii, iv) → **(323)** + **(324)**

Reagents: i, HgO, $HgBr_2$, molecular sieve; ii, MeOH; iii, $SiO_2$; iv, $OH^-$.

diepiadriamycin (**322**). In this case (**315**) was condensed with (**307**) to give the protected derivatives (**317**) and (**319**), these compounds affording, after removal of the protecting groups, the new adriamycin analogues in which the aminosugar moiety exhibits the L-*arabino* configuration [110].

Another example of the procedure described above is represented by the synthesis of the $\alpha$ and $\beta$ anomers of 7-O-daunosaminyl-4-demethoxydaunomycinone (Scheme 6.6). The starting material was 4-demethoxydaunomycinone obtained by total synthesis, as already shown in Scheme 4.12. The two anomeric N-trifluoroacetyl derivatives arising from the condensation of (**89**)a with N,O-ditrifluoroacetyl-$\alpha$-daunosaminyl chloride (**306**) followed by methanolysis of the O-trifluoroacetate were separated by chromatography and converted to (**323**) and (**324**) with dilute sodium hydroxide. Similarly, starting from the 7(R), 9(R) stereoisomer (**325**) of 4-demethoxy-daunomycinone (Scheme 6.7), the two glycosides (**326**) and (**327**) were obtained [40].

SCHEME 6.7

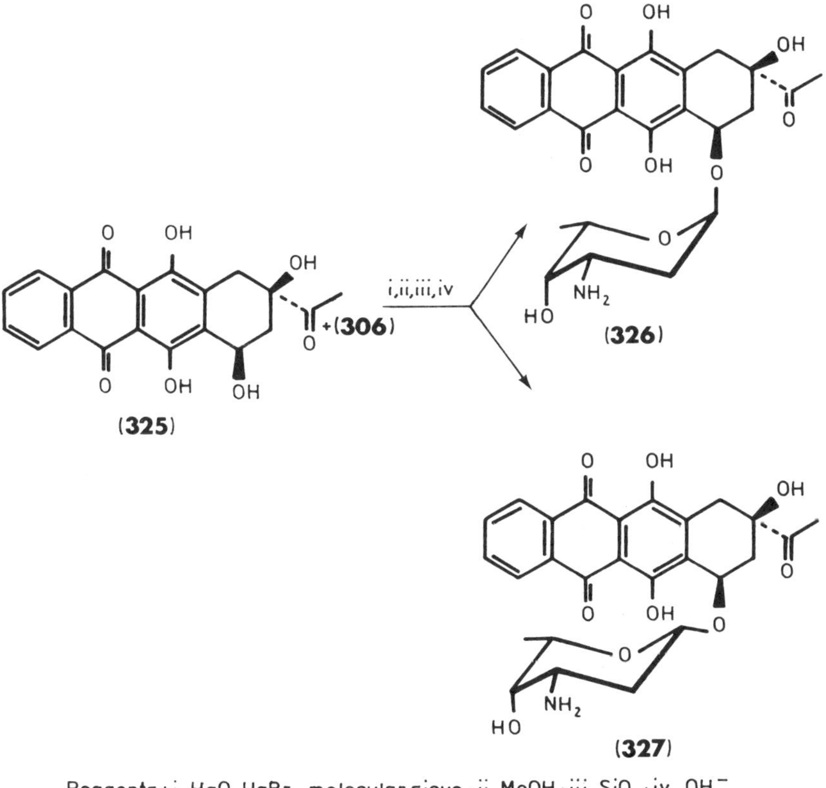

(**325**) + (**306**) —i,ii,iii,iv→ (**326**) + (**327**)

Reagents: i, HgO, $HgBr_2$, molecular sieve; ii, MeOH; iii, $SiO_2$; iv, $OH^-$.

### 6.2 Other reactions

Other methods have also been used for the synthesis of the glycosidic linkage in the semisynthetic anthracyclines, during investigations aimed at improving the yields and at controlling the steric course of the reaction. The following reactions have been reported: the Fischer method of glycoside synthesis, the glycal-alcohol acid-catalyzed reaction, and the glycoside synthesis by the use of soluble silver salts.

#### 6.2.1 *The Fischer method*

The application of the classical Fischer procedure for glycoside synthesis [111] to the coupling of daunomycinone with N,O-ditrifluoroacetyldaunosamine has been reported. The reaction was carried out in anhydrous dioxane and in the presence of dilute hydrogen chloride at room temperature. Conversion of 50% of the aglycone to the N,O-ditrifluoroacetyl glycoside was recorded. The latter was isolated by chromatography on the silicagel column and transformed to daunomycin by an alkaline treatment. Only the α-glycoside was formed [112].

#### 6.2.2 *Acid catalyzed glycosidation of glycals*

The acid catalyzed addition of an alcohol to suitably protected hex-1-enopyranoses is a known method for the synthesis of 2-deoxyglycosides [113]. Its applicability to the anthracycline series was proved by the synthesis of daunomycin N-trifluoroacetate in good yield upon treatment of daunomycinone with 1,2,3,6-tetradeoxy-3-trifluoroacetamido-4-trifluoroacetyl-L-*lyxo*-hex-1-enpyranose (**328**) in anhydrous benzene and in the presence of an acid catalyst, followed by methanolysis of the O-trifluoroacetyl group (Scheme 6.8).

SCHEME 6.8

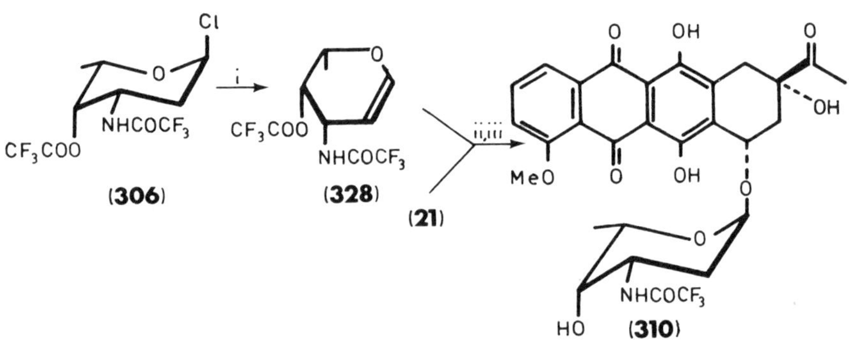

(**306**) (**328**) (**21**) (**310**)

Reagents : i, $Hg(CN)_2$ ; ii, TsOH(cat.) ; iii, MeOH.

Compound **(328)** was obtained from 2,3,6-trideoxy-3-trifluoroacetimido-4-trifluoroacetyl-α-L-*lyxo*-pyranosyl chloride **(306)** upon treatment with mercuric cyanide in a mixture of benzene-dioxane. The method was also used for the synthesis of adriamycin, in which case 9-deacetyl-9-(2′, 2′-dimethyl-4′-methoxy-4′-dioxolanyl)-daunomycinone **(315)** was used instead of daunomycinone in the reaction. The free antibiotics were obtained by deblocking procedures already outlined (Schemes 6.4 and 6.5) [114].

SCHEME 6.9

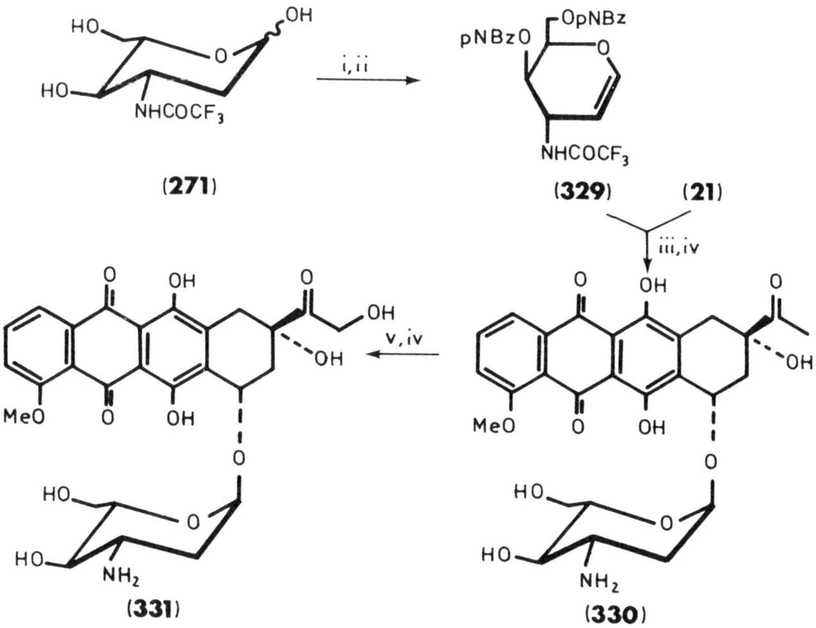

Reagents: i, p−$NO_2C_6H_4$ COCl (pNBzCl), pyr; ii, aq. $NaHCO_3$; iii, TsOH cat., PhH; iv, $OH^-$; v, $Br_2$.

The same reaction has been successfuly applied (Scheme 6.9) for the synthesis of 7-O-(3-amino-2,3-dideoxy-α-L-*arabino*-hexopyranosyl)-daunomycinone, **(330)** the 4′-epi,6′-hydroxy analogue of daunomycin and an intermediate for the preparation of the corresponding adriamycin analogue **(331)** [115]. The key intermediate for the stereocontrolled glycosidation of daunomycinone, 1,2,3-trideoxy-4,6-di-O-nitrobenzoyl-3-trifluoroacetamido-L-*arabino*-hex-1-enopyranose **(329)**, was prepared from 2,3-dideoxy-3-trifluoroacetamido-L-*arabino*-hexopyranose **(271)** which was p-nitro-benzoylated and the resulting 1,4,6-tri-O-p-nitrobenzoate subjected to a mild alkaline treatment to afford

(**329**) in nearly quantitative yield. Condensation of (**329**) with daunomycinone, in the presence of an acid catalyst, gave 7-O-(2,3-dideoxy-4,6-di-O-p-nitro-benzoyl-trifluoroacetamido-α-*arabino*-hexopyranosyl) daunomycinone which afforded 4′-epi-6′-hydroxy-daunomycin (**330**) upon deacetylation with dilute sodium hydroxide. The yield of (**330**) from (**21**) was 56% and no β-anomer was found. The remarkable stereocontrol in the acid catalyzed glycosidation reaction and particularly with a bulky aglycone, is noteworthy although a related reaction in the aminoglycoside series has been described [116]. On the other hand when daunomycinone (Scheme 6.10) was allowed to react in methylene chloride and in the presence of mercuric oxide, mercuric bromide and molecular sieve, with 2,3-dideoxy-4,6-di-O-p-nitrobenzoyl-3-trifluoroacetamido-L-*arabino*-hexopyranosyl bromide (**332**), obtained by reaction of the product of the p-nitrobenzylation of (**271**) with dry hydrogen bromide in methylene chloride, a lower glycosidation yield was obtained and also the β-anomer (**333**) of (**330**) was isolated [115].

SCHEME 6.10

Reagents : i, p-$NO_2C_6H_4COCl$ (pNBzCl), pyr; ii; HBr; iii, HgO, $HgBr_2$, molecular sieve; iv, $OH^-$.

### 6.2.3 *Glycosidation with soluble silver salts*

Silver trifluoromethanesulphonate (silver triflate) was first introduced as a halogen acceptor in the glycosidation of an alcohol with a sugar halide by Krouzer and Schuerch [117] and soon found useful applications (see for instance [118]). This method has been widely used for the synthesis of anthracycline glycosides in the author's laboratory and differs from the various modifications of the Koenigs-Knorr reaction because the reaction takes place in a homogenous medium and is characterized by the low nucleophilicity of the anion. In the case of polar solvents, such as ether, the reaction should conceivably follow a $S_N1$ type mechanism, but a certain degree of $S_N2$ behaviour should be expected in non-polar solvents, such as dichloromethane, because of the formation of ion pairs.

The successful application of the silver triflate assisted glycosidation was reported in the synthesis of 4′-deoxydaunomycin [78]. As shown in Scheme 6.11 the synthesis of the glycosidic linkage was performed by reaction of daunomycinone with 2,3,4,6-tetrahydroxy-3-trifluoroacetamido-L-*threo*-hexopyranosyl chloride **(334)**, prepared from **(231)** by p-nitrobenzylation followed by treatment with dry hydrogen chloride, in methylene chloride and at room temperature in the presence of silver triflate. The reaction was complete in 30 minutes and only the α-anomeric N-trifluoroacetylglucoside was formed. Removal of the N-trifluoroacetyl group afforded 4′-deoxydaunomycin **(335)** whose anomeric configuration was established on the basis of the analysis of the $^{1}$H n.m.r. spectrum. The adriamycin analogue **(336)** was obtained from **(335)** following the already mentioned procedure.

SCHEME 6.11

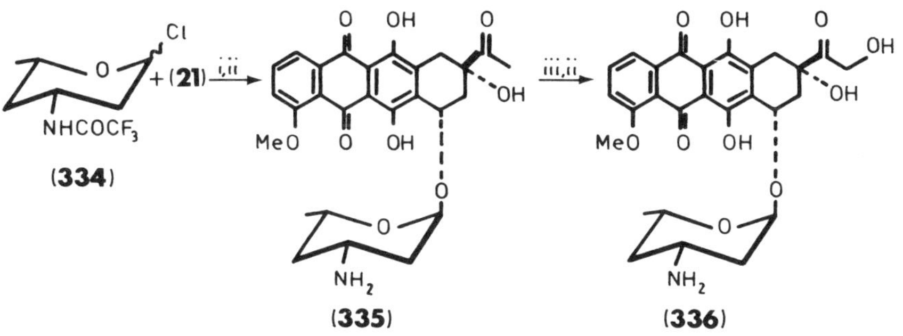

(334) + (21) —i,ii→ (335) —iii,ii→ (336)

Reagents: i, $CF_3SO_3Ag$; ii, $OH^-$; iii, $Br_2$.

Other applications of this procedure were exemplified in the synthesis of 3′,4′-epi-6′-hydroxydaunomycin **(337)**, 3′,4′-epi-daunomycin **(338)**, 4-demethoxy-4′-epi-daunomycin **(339)**, 4′-epidaunomycin **(312)** and of daunomycin itself [119].

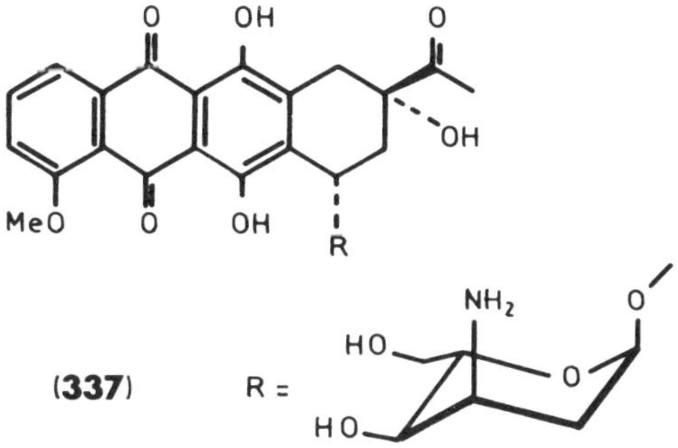

**(337)** R =

(**338**) R =

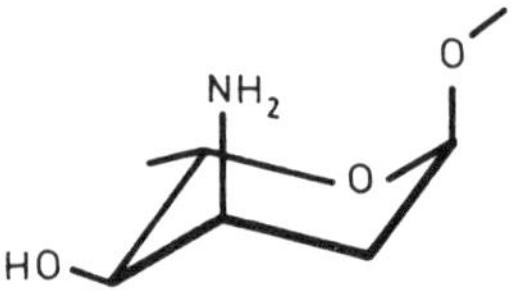
NH2
O
O
HO

(**339**) R =

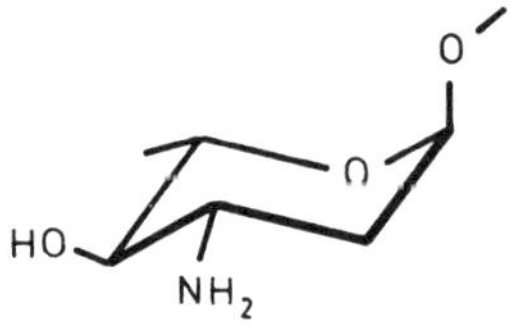
O
O
HO
NH2

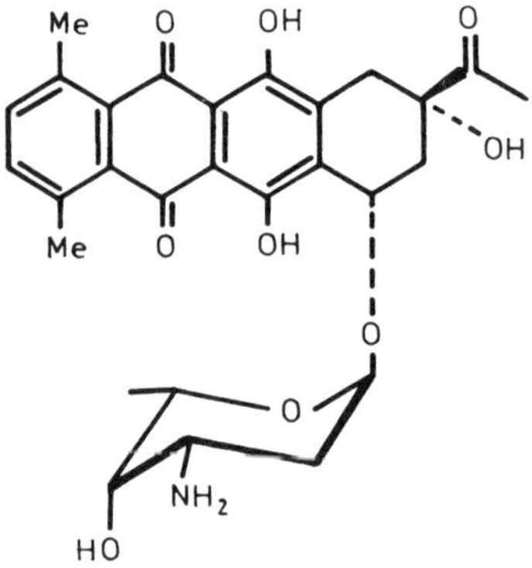
Me
O
OH
O
OH
Me
O
OH
O
O
NH2
HO

(**340**)

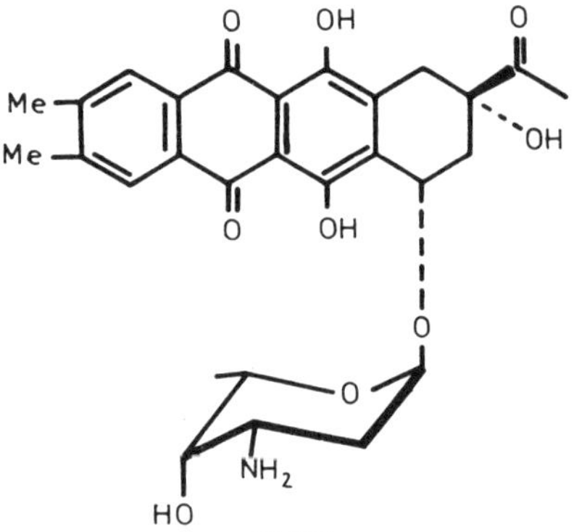
O
OH
O
Me
Me
OH
O
OH
O
O
NH2
HO

(**341**)

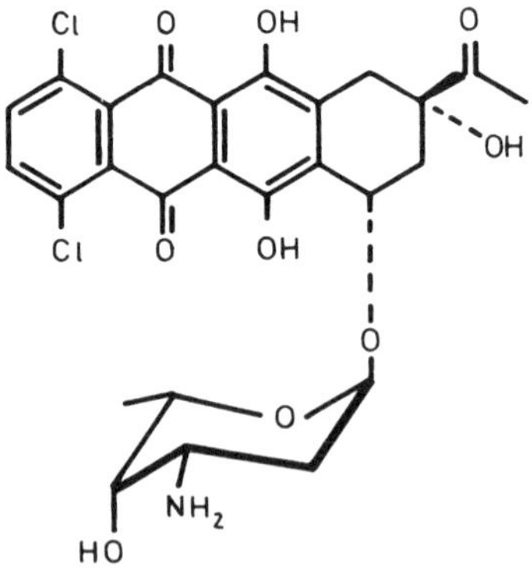
Cl
O
OH
O
OH
Cl
O
OH
O
O
NH2
HO

(**342**)

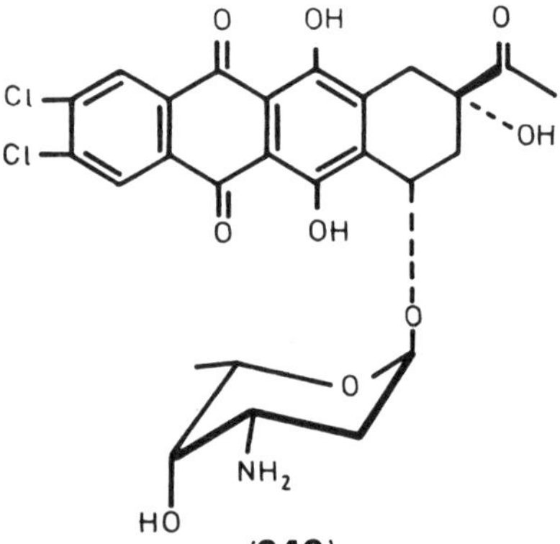
O
OH
O
Cl
Cl
OH
O
OH
O
O
NH2
HO

(**343**)

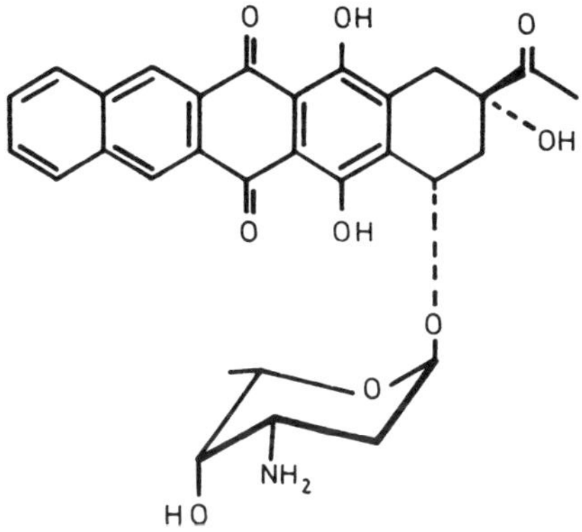

(**344**)

SCHEME 6.12

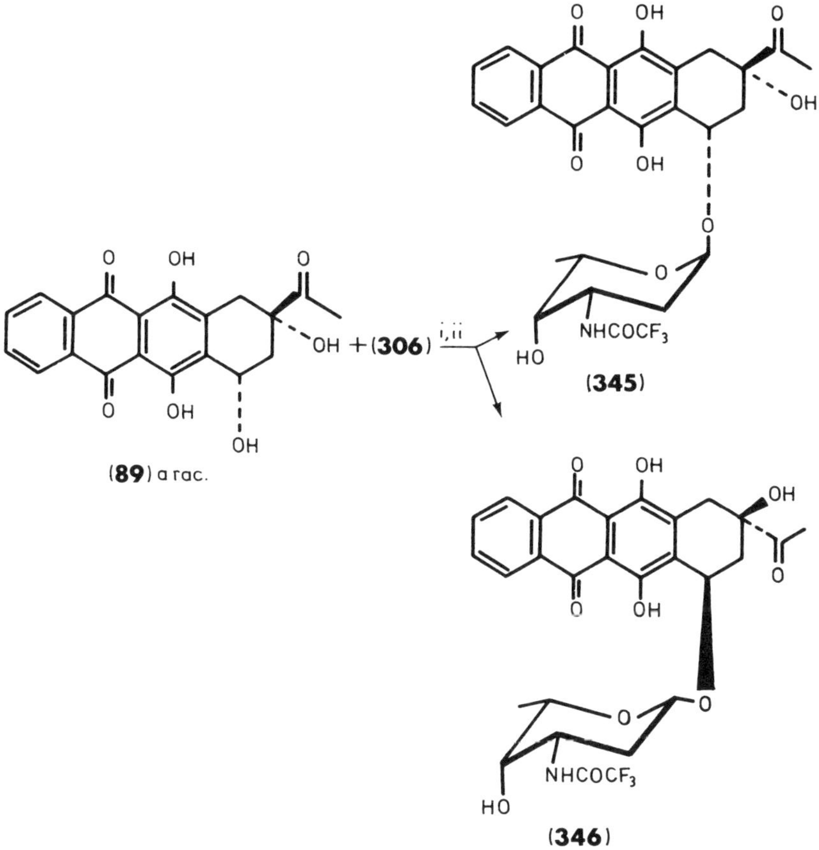

(**89**) a rac. + (**306**) $\xrightarrow{i,ii}$ (**345**) + (**346**)

Reagents: i, $CF_3SO_3Ag$; ii, MeOH.

The silver triflate method was also used successfully for the synthesis of new 7-O-daunosaminylanthracyclinones in which the aglycone moiety was originated by total synthesis. 1,4-Dimethyl-4-demethoxydaunomycin (**340**), 2,3-dimethyl-4-demethoxydaunomycin (**341**), 1,4-dichloro-4-demethoxydaunomycin (**342**), 2,3-dichloro-4-demethoxydaunomycin (**343**), and 2,3-benzo-4-demethoxydaunomycin (**344**) were prepared following this procedure [41]. An interesting finding, which may also have synthetic usefulness, is the clear resolution of the two enantiomorphic forms of racemic 4-demethoxydaunomycinone as a consequence of the coupling with (**306**) using the silver triflate method. As shown in Scheme 6.12 the reaction proceeds with considerable stereoselectivity in that practically only (**345**), the α-glycoside of the 7(S), 9(S), and (**346**), the β-glycoside of the 7(R), 9(R) enantiomer are formed [121].

### 6.2.4 *Synthesis of ϵ-Rhodomycinone glycosides*

The anthracyclinone ϵ-rhodomycinone [122] is a readily available by-product of the anthracycline fermentation [123]. It is understandable, therefore, that attention was paid to glycosidation of this compound as an approach to new biologically active glycosides. The first report concerning the glycosidation of ϵ-rhodomycinone described the stereoselective synthesis of (**348**) upon condensation of (**20**) with 4-O-p-nitrobenzoyl-3-N-trifluoroacetyl-daunosaminyl chloride (Scheme 6.13) followed by removal of the protecting groups in alkaline condition [124]. In a very recent publication El Khadem *et al.* [125] have reported the synthesis of 16 blocked and 10 deblocked none-nitrogen containing glycosides of ϵ-rhodomycinone. The new derivatives included com-

SCHEME 6.13

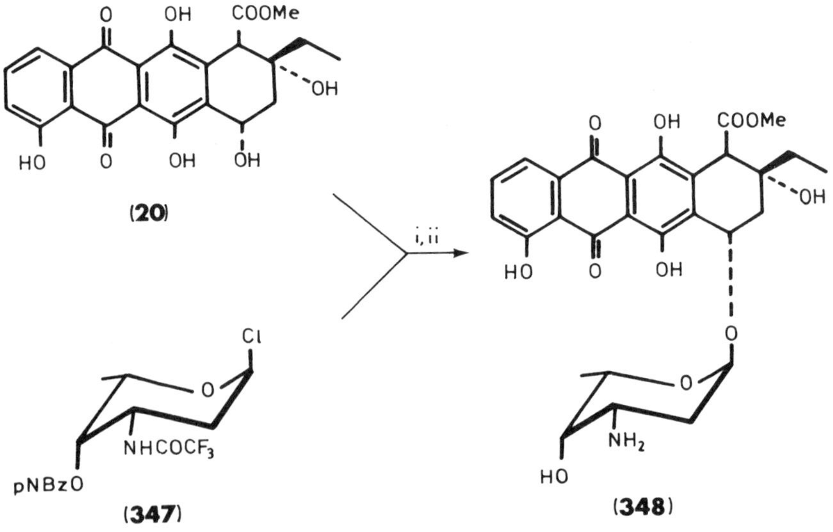

Reagents: i, $Hg(CN)_2$, $HgBr_2$, molecular sieve, THF; ii, $OH^-$.

pounds containing the following moieties: D-glucopyranosyl, 2-deoxy-L-fucopyranosyl, 2-deoxy-L-rhamnopyranosyl, 2-deoxy-D-ribopyranosyl, L-fucopyranosyl as well as other pentosyl derivatives in both the pyranose and furanose forms. The method used was the $Hg(CN)_2$-$HgBr_2$ assisted Koenigs-Knorr type condensation of the aglycone with the required protected glycosyl halides and the yields of the blocked glycosides were highly variable, the best ones being recorded for the 2-deoxysugar derivatives (75 to 83%). Structures of the deblocked glycosides described in this work are **(349)** to **(358)**.

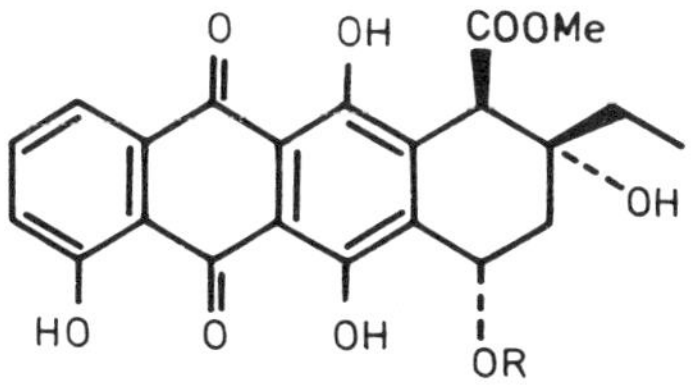

O OH COOMe OH HO O OH OR

**(349)**, R = HO OH O HO OH

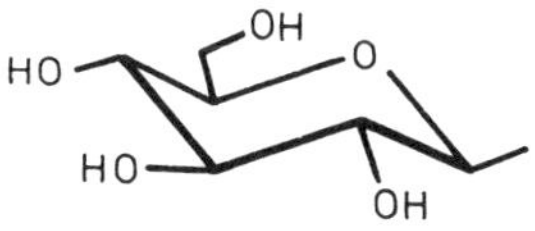

**(354)**, R = 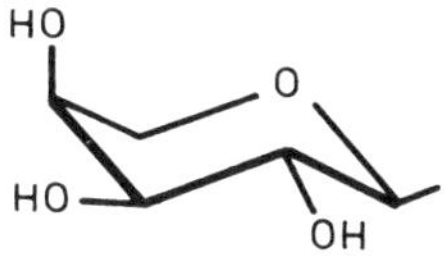 HO O HO OH

**(350)**, R = 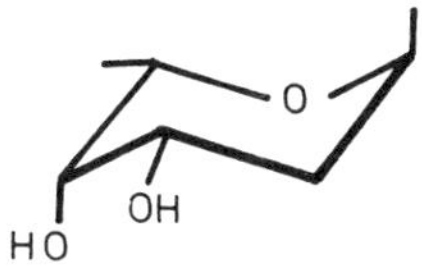 O HO OH

**(355)**, R = 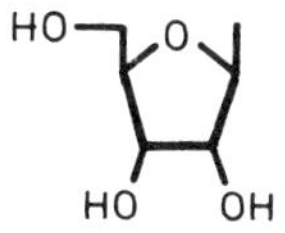 HO O HO OH

**(351)**, R = 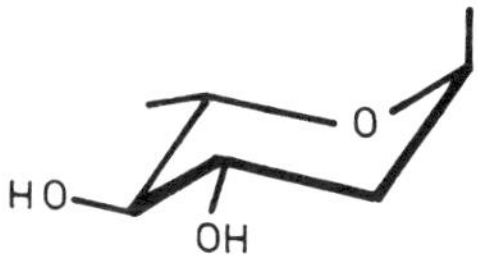 O HO OH

**(356)**, R = 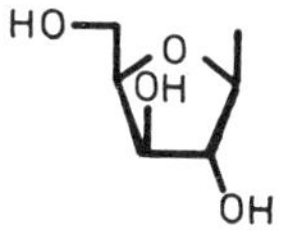 HO O OH OH

**(352)**, R = 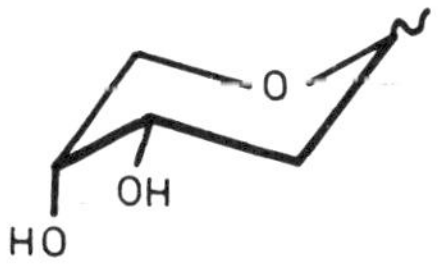 O HO OH

**(357)**, R = 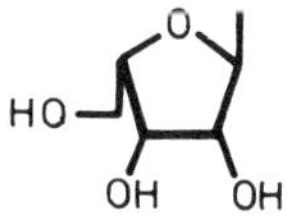 O HO OH OH

**(343)**, R = 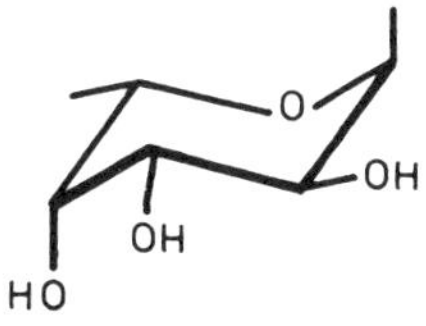 O OH HO OH

**(358)**, R = HO O OH

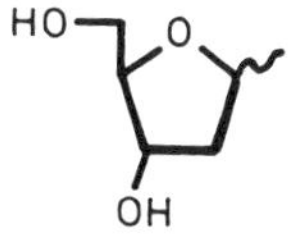

## 7 REACTIONS OF THE ANTITUMOUR ANTHRACYCLINES

Chemical modifications of the natural antitumour anthracyclines have been pursued for several reasons. One was the establishment of chemical correlations amongst the different, related natural products and another for the introduction of radioisotopic labels in the same antibiotics for metabolic and pharmacokinetic investigations. Yet another reason was for the preparation of new derivatives, to be tested as antitumour agents in the laboratory for the optimization of pharmacological activity and for the evaluation of molecular requirements for action.

### 7.1 Chemical correlations and synthesis of radiolabelled compounds

The first prepared interconversion of antitumour anthracyclines was the semisynthesis of adriamycin from daunomycin following the reaction sequence outlined in Scheme 7.1 [126]. Daunomycin (**1**) was converted by trifluoroacetylation, followed by O-acyl exchange, to the N-trifluoroacetylderivative (**310**) which on photohalogenation gave (**359**) after a chromatographic purification. Substitution of iodine with acetate gave (**360**) and the latter was converted into N-trifluoroacetyladriamycin (**361**) upon treatment with a weak base. Because compound (**361**) was also obtained by N-trifluoroacetylation of adriamycin the sequence outlined in Scheme 7.1 established the desired chemical correlation of the two antibiotics. However (**361**) was also converted to (**2**), thus affording a method for the partial synthesis of (**2**) from (**1**). The dihydroxyacetone grouping of (**361**) was protected as the cyclic orthoformate (**362**). This protection was necessary owing to the great instability of the side chain of (**2**) to the alkaline conditions used for the removal of the N-trifluoroacetyl group. Hydrolysis of (**362**) with dilute sodium hydroxide followed by an acid treatment afforded (**2**). A more straightforward synthesis of adriamycin from daunomycin was subsequently carried out [127]. This synthesis involved electrophilic bromination of (**1**) followed by the substitution of bromine with a hydroxyl group in the intermediate 14-bromodaunomycin (**363**) by means of a mild

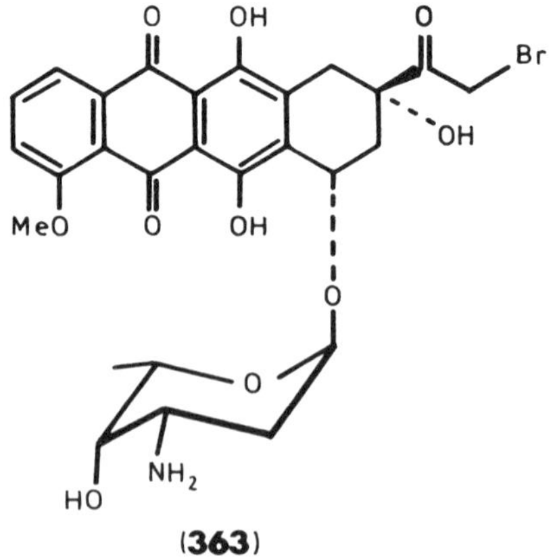

O OH O Br OH MeO O OH O O NH$_2$ HO

(**363**)

SCHEME 7.1

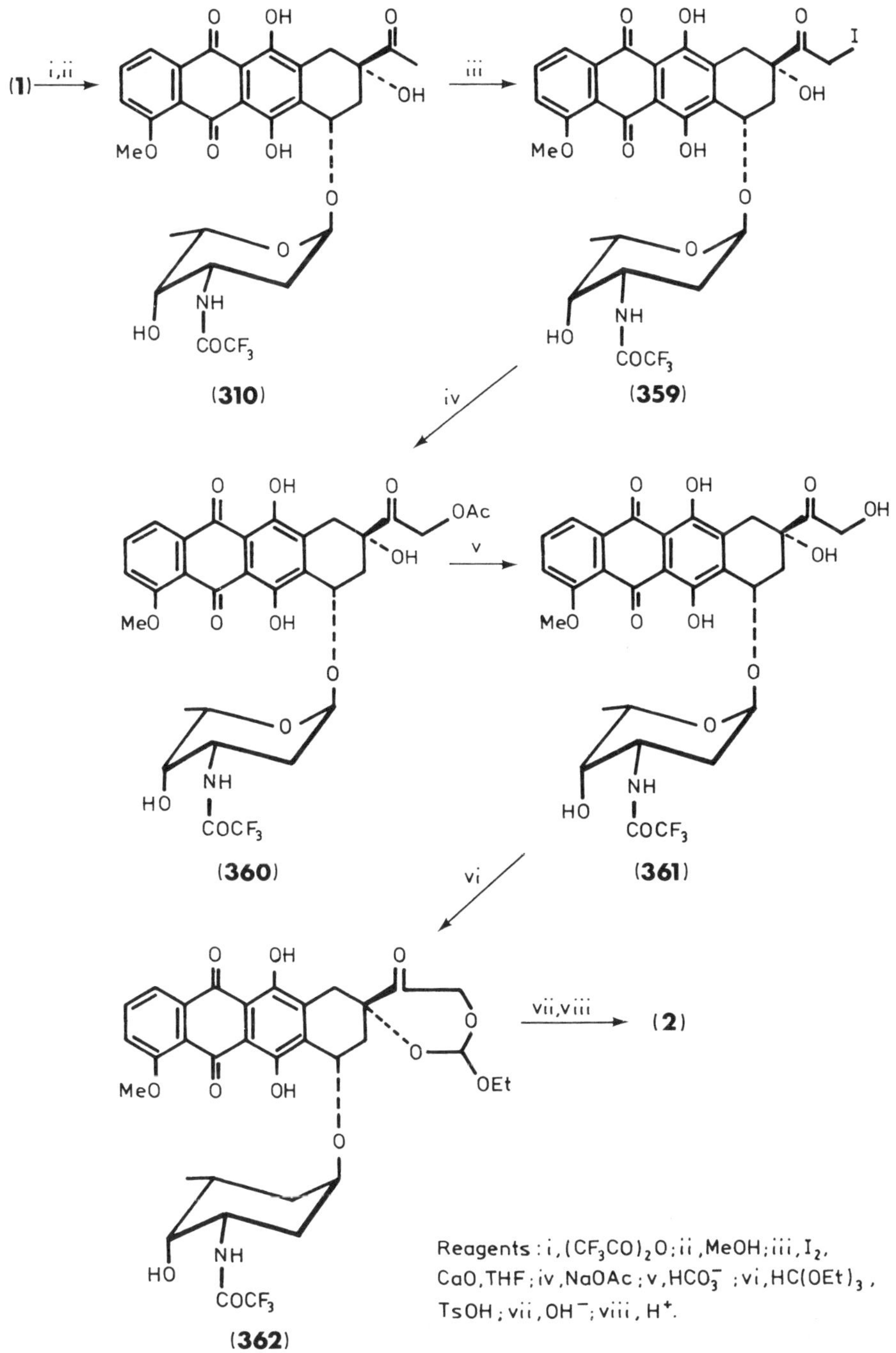

Reagents: i, $(CF_3CO)_2O$; ii, MeOH; iii, $I_2$, CaO, THF; iv, NaOAc; v, $HCO_3^-$; vi, $HC(OEt)_3$, TsOH; vii, $OH^-$; viii, $H^+$.

alkaline treatment. This procedure was also used, for instance, for the preparation of labelled adriamycin from $^{3}H$ or $^{14}C$ labelled daunomycin [128, 129].

The reverse transformation, i.e. the conversion of adriamycin into daunomycin, was used for the synthesis of [14-$^{14}C$]daunomycin. In the author's laboratory N-trifluoroacetyl-13-dihydroadriamycin **(365)**, prepared by N-trifluoroacetylation of 13-dihydroadriamycin [adriamycinol, **(364)**], was oxidized with sodium periodate to give the aldehyde **(366)** in 65% yield (Scheme 7.2). This compound was treated with [$^{14}C$]diazomethane (originating from the labelled N-nitrosourea, via commercially available [$^{14}C$]methylamine) to give a mixture of **(367)** and **(368)**, the former prevailing (60% of total) when the reaction was carried out in dichloromethane and diethyl ether, the latter

SCHEME 7.2

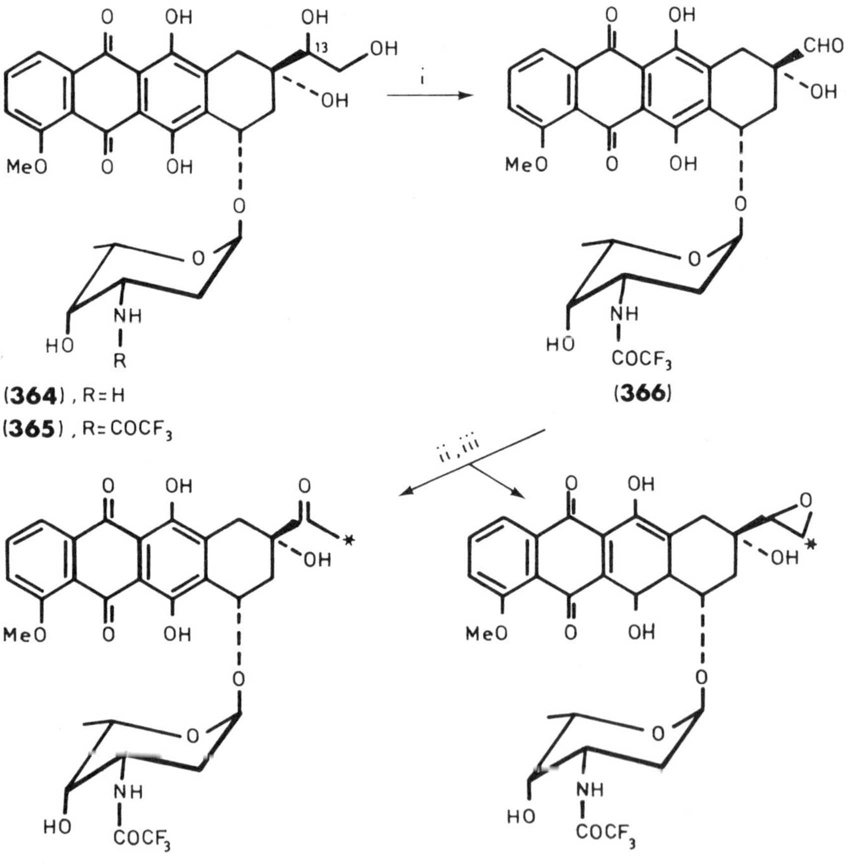

**(364)**, R = H
**(365)**, R = $COCF_3$

**(366)**

**(367)**

**(368)**

**(369)** **(370)**

Reagents : i, $NaIO_4$ ; ii, $^{14}CH_2N_2$ ; iii, $SiO_2$ chrom. ; iv, $OH^-$ ; v, $Br_2$ ; vi, $OH^-$

when protic solvents were used. The two products could be separated chromatographically. [14-$^{14}$C] Daunomycin **(369)** was obtained from **(367)** by mild alkaline treatment, and was converted into [14-$^{14}$C]adriamycin **(370)** via the 14-bromoderivative as already mentioned [129]. This procedure allowed the introduction of radioactive carbon into adriamycin with 9% overall radiochemical yield starting from $NH_2{}^{14}CH_3$. HC1.

Other authors [130] have obtained [14-$^{14}$C]adriamycin following the reaction sequence outlined in Scheme 7.3. The acid **(371)** prepared from N-trifluoroacetyladriamycin **(361)** [131] was converted into the mixed anhydride with t-butylcarbonic acid which, upon treatment with [$^{14}$C]diazomethane afforded **(372)** and **(373)** in 20% yield each. N-trifluoroacetyl-[14-$^{14}$C]adriamycin **(374)** was obtained from **(372)** *via* the 14-bromoderivative. Protection of the 14-hydroxyl of **(374)** as in **(375)** [132], followed by sequential deblocking of the amino group and of the side chain primary hydroxyl group, gave [14-$^{14}$C]-adriamycin **(370)** in 0.17% overall radiochemical yield starting from [$^{14}$C] diazal.

A different synthesis of [$^{14}$C]daunomycin and of [$^{14}$C]adriamycin has been carried out at the Stanford Research Institute [133]. This synthesis (Scheme 7.4) started from adriamycinone **(45)** which was treated with an excess (15 equiv.) of $^{14}$C-labelled Grignard reagent to give the glycol **(376)**. Oxidation of **(376)** resulted in the cleavage of the original $C_{13}$-$C_{14}$ bond to afford [14-$^{14}$C]-daunomycinone **(377)**. Koenigs-Knorr glycosidation of **(377)** with the protected daunosaminyl chloride followed by deacetylation of the resulting $\alpha$-glycoside gave [14-$^{14}$C]daunomycin **(369)**. Bromination of **(377)** and subsequent hydrolysis of the resulting 14-bromoderivative provided [14-$^{14}$C]adriamycinone

SCHEME 7.3

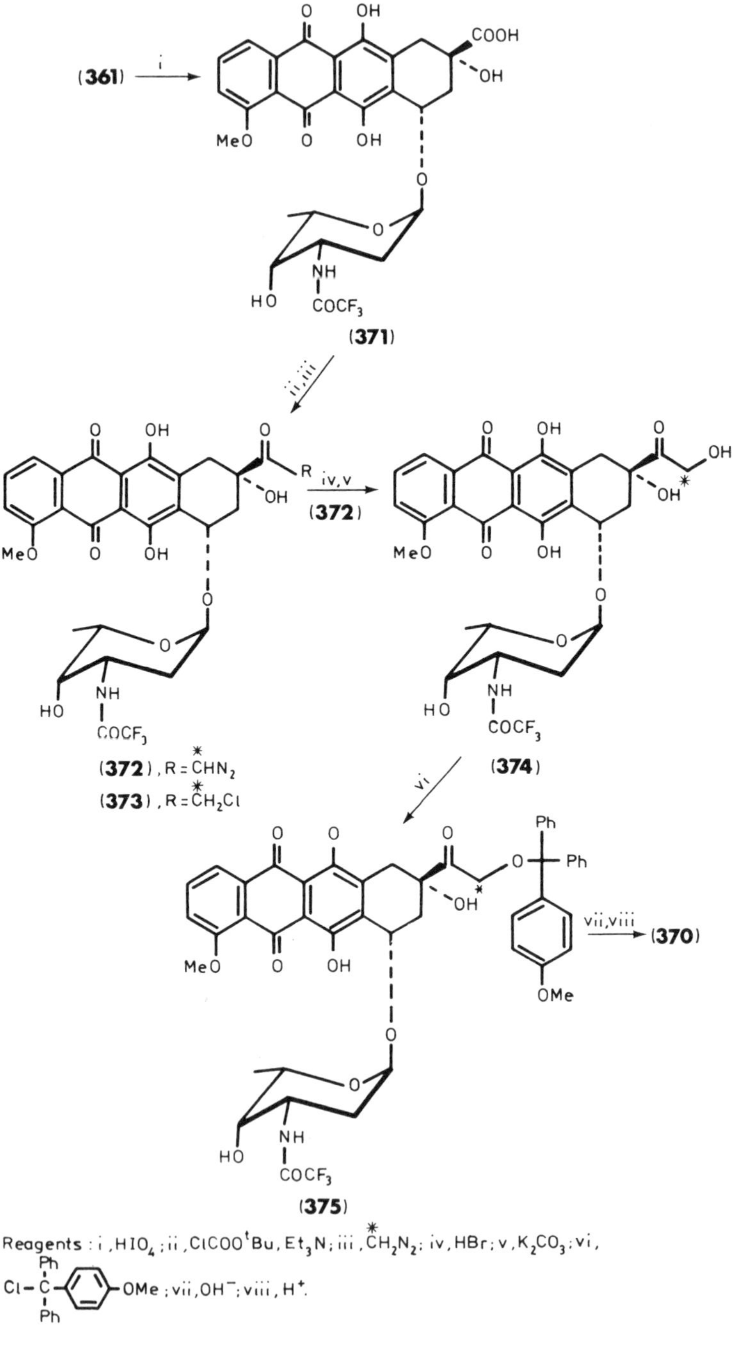

(**361**) $\xrightarrow{\text{i}}$ (**371**)

(**371**) $\xrightarrow{\text{ii, iii}}$ (**372**), R = $\overset{*}{C}HN_2$; (**373**), R = $\overset{*}{C}H_2Cl$

(**372**) $\xrightarrow{\text{iv, v}}$ (**374**)

(**374**) $\xrightarrow{\text{vi}}$ (**375**) $\xrightarrow{\text{vii, viii}}$ (**370**)

Reagents : i, $HIO_4$; ii, $ClCOO^tBu$, $Et_3N$; iii, $\overset{*}{C}H_2N_2$; iv, HBr; v, $K_2CO_3$; vi, $Cl-C(Ph)_2-C_6H_4-OMe$; vii, $OH^-$; viii, $H^+$.

(378). Protection of the 14-OH as in 14-O-p-anisyldiphenylmethyladriamycinone (**379**) followed by glycosidation afforded (**380**). Deblocking of (**380**) afforded [14-$^{14}$C] adriamycin (**370**).

SCHEME 7.4

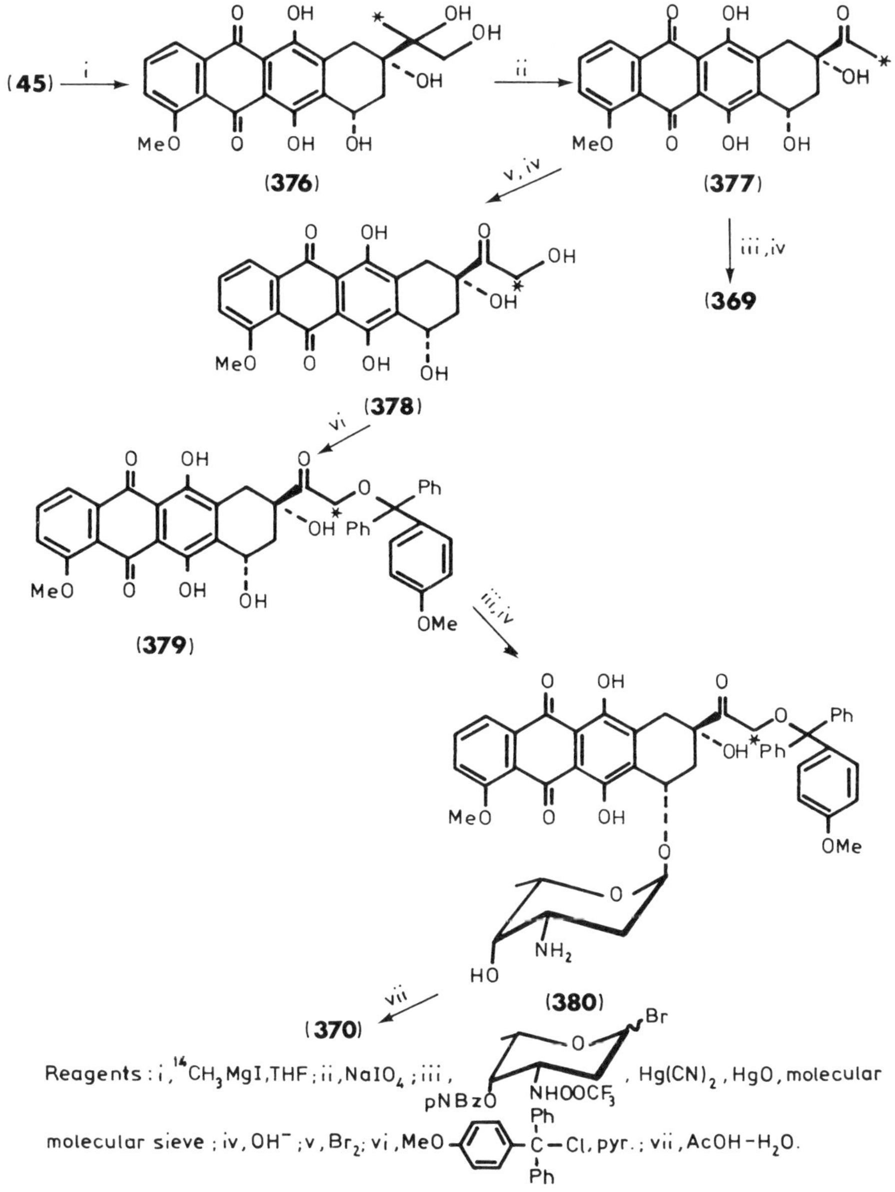

(**45**) → (**376**) → (**377**) → (**369**)

(**377**) → (**378**) → (**379**) → (**380**) → (**370**)

Reagents: i, $^{14}CH_3MgI$, THF; ii, $NaIO_4$; iii, [2,3,6-trideoxy-3-trifluoroacetamido-4-O-p-nitrobenzoyl glycosyl bromide: Br, O, pNBzO, NHOOCF$_3$], $Hg(CN)_2$, HgO, molecular sieve; iv, $OH^-$; v, $Br_2$; vi, MeO–$C_6H_4$–C(Ph)$_2$–Cl, pyr.; vii, AcOH–$H_2O$.

Potassium borohydride reduction of the side-chain carbonyl of daunomycin has been reported [134]. The resulting 13-dihydroderivative was identical, apart from the absolute configuration at the new asymmetric centre (which is not known), to biosynthetic duborimycin **(4)**.

Carminomycin **(3)** was obtained starting from daunomycinone **(21)**, which was O-dimethylated to carminomycinone **(381)**, the latter affording N-trifluoroacetylcarminomycin **(382)** upon condensation with N,O-ditrifluoroacetyldaunosaminyl chloride in the presence of silver trifluoromethane sulphonate and in a mixture of dimethylformamide-dichloromethane, followed by de-O-trifluoroacetylation (Scheme 7.5). De-N-trifluoroacetylation of **(382)** gave **(3)** [135, 136].

SCHEME 7.5

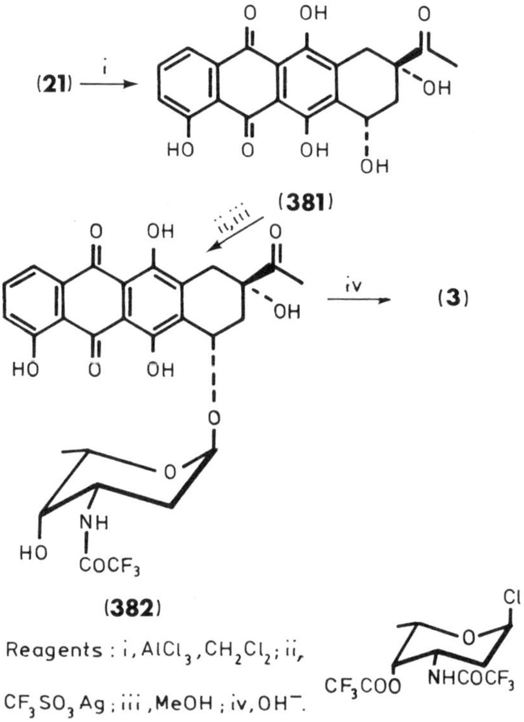

**(21)** → **(381)** → **(382)** → **(3)**

Reagents: i, $AlCl_3$, $CH_2Cl_2$; ii, $CF_3SO_3Ag$; iii, MeOH; iv, $OH^-$.

## 7.2 Other reactions

Chemical modification of daunomycin and adriamycin represents an obvious approach to the development of new antitumour agents. Derivatization was carried out at the ketone and amino functions of the antitumour anthracyclines, as well as at C-14. Other derivatives were obtained by the oxidative breakdown of the C-9 side chain, Daunomycinone has also been used as a substrate for chemical derivatization.

### 7.2.1 *Simple derivatives*

The C-13 ketone function of the antitumour anthracyclines reacts promptly with carbonyl reagents such as hydroxylamine and hydrazine derivatives. Compounds (**383**)a-e have been described [137]. Other similar derivatives including the hydrazone (**383**)f and other substituted hydrazones, have been reported in the patent literature [138, 139]. Reduction of the C-13 ketones (**2**) and (**3**) afforded 13-dihydroadriamycin and 13-dihydrocarminomycin respectively [134, 140].

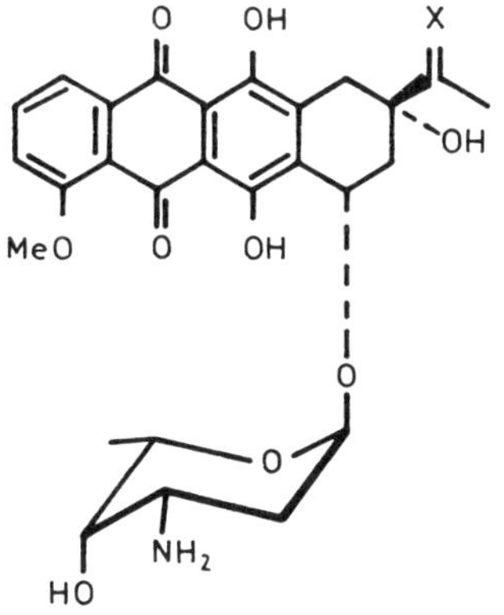

(**383**) a : X = NOH
b : X = NOMe
c : X = $NNHCONH_2$
d : X = NN(piperidino)
e : X = $NNHCOCH_2OH$
f : X = NNHCOPh
g : X = O–CH₂CH₂–O (ethylene ketal)

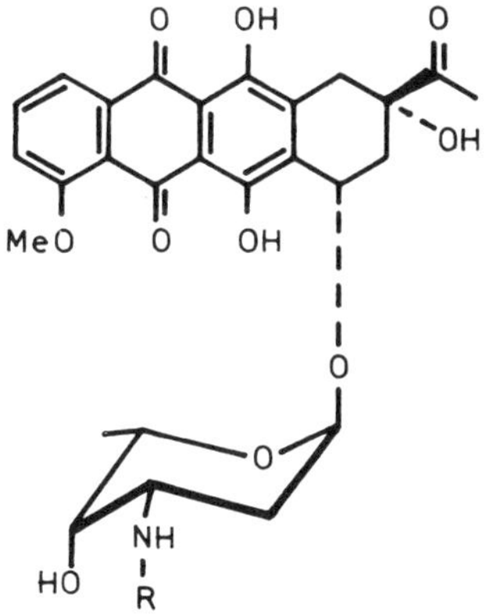

(**384**) a : R = Ac
b : R = COEt
c : R = COPr
d : R = CONHMe
e : R = CONHBu
f : R = CSNHMe
g : R = CSNHBu
h : R = CSNHPh
i : R = COOMe
l : R = $COCH_2NMe_2$
m : R = $COCH_2NHCOCH_2NMe_2$
n : R = $COCH_2NPr_2$
o : R = L-leucyl
p : R = D-leucyl
q : R = L-phenylglycyl

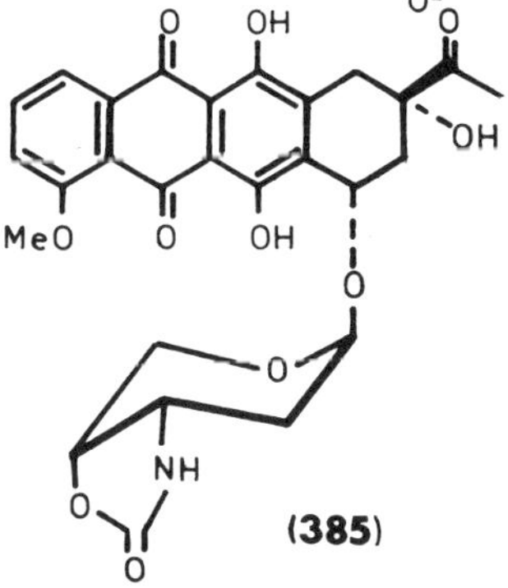

(**385**)

N-Acetyldaunomycin (**384**)a was prepared for $^1$H n.m.r. studies [29], and the N-trifluoroacetyl derivatives of (**1**), (**2**) and (**3**) have already been mentioned above as protected derivatives used for synthetic studies. Compounds (**384**)a-i were prepared in a study concerning the antitumour activity of daunomycin derivatives [137]. Acid anhydrides, alkyl isocyanates, alkyl isothiocyanates, and methyl chloroformate were used as reagents. When daunomycin as the free base was treated in pyridine with phosgene N-carboxydaunomycin γ-lactone (**385**) was obtained [137]. Peptide derivatives (**384**)l-n have been prepared using the mixed anhydride method of peptide synthesis [141]. N-Aminoacyl derivatives of daunomycin have also been reported in a patent [142]. Among others, compounds (**384**)o-q were prepared.

7.2.2 *Synthesis of C-14 substituted analogues*

14-Halogeno-derivatives of daunomycin have been found to be useful intermediates for the derivatization of the side chain with suitable nucleophiles.

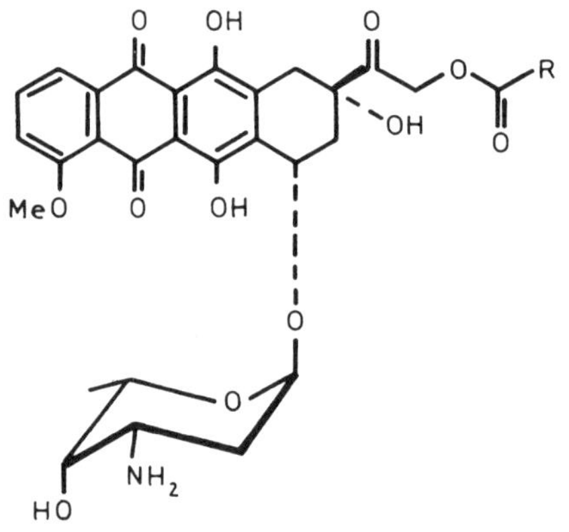

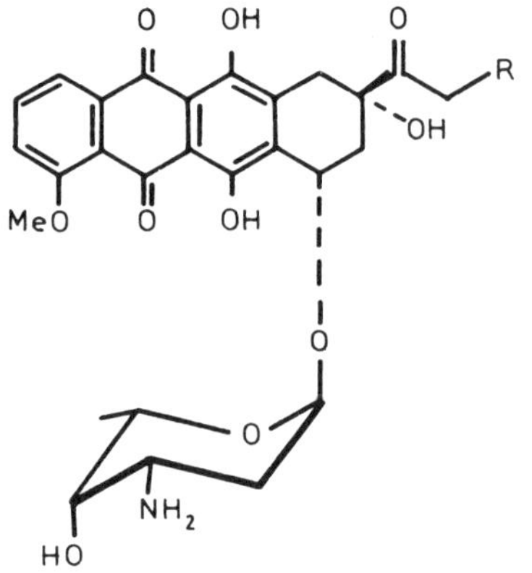

(**386**) a : R = Me
b : R = Et
c : R = $(CH_2)_6Me$
d : R = Ph
e : R = $CH_2Ph$
f : R = 3-pyridyl
g : R = $CH_2OCO(CH_2)_4Me$
h : R = $CH_2OCO(CH_2)_{10}Me$
i : R = $CH_2OCO(CH_2)_{16}Me$
l : R = $CH_2SCO(CH_2)_4Me$

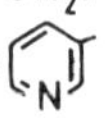

(**387**) a : R = morpholino
b : R = 4-methylpiperazino (N N–Me)
c : R = piperidino
d : R = 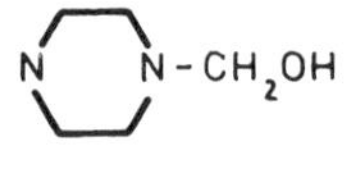 N N–$CH_2OH$
e : R = $N(CH_2CH_2OH)_2$

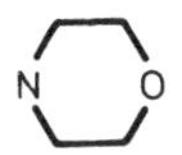

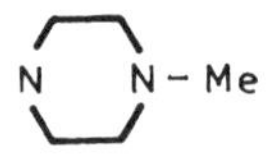

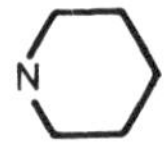

Reaction of 14-bromodaunomycin with the sodium or potassium salts of organic acids afforded the 14-O-acyl derivatives of adriamycin (**386**)a-f [143]. In addition to these, double esters, such as adriamycin 14-O-hexanoglycolate (**386**)g, 14-O-lauroylglycolate (**386**)h, 14-O-stearoylglycolate (**386**)i, and hexanoglycolate (**386**)l have been reported [144]. Reaction of 14-bromodaunomycin with amines gave 14-amino-derivatives (**387**)a-e [145].

SCHEME 7.6

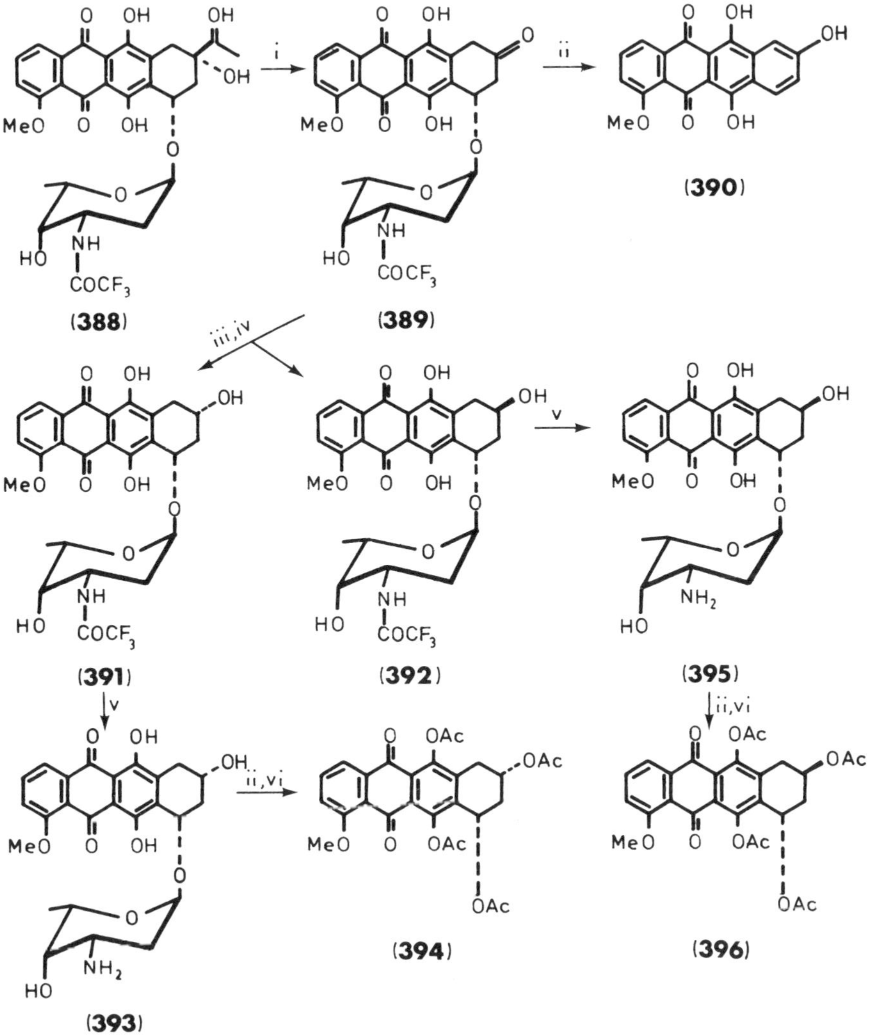

(**388**) (**389**) (**390**)

(**391**) (**392**) (**395**)

(**393**) (**394**) (**396**)

Reagents : i , $NaIO_4$ ; ii , $H^+$ ; iii , $NaCNBH_3$ ; iv , $SiO_2$ chrom. ; v , $OH^-$ ; vi , $Ac_2O$, pyr.

Similar derivatives of N-trifluoroacetyladriamycin have also been prepared, as for instance N-trifluoroacetyladriamycin-14-valerate, which was obtained starting from 14-iodo-N-trifluoroacetyldaunomycin [146].

7.2.3 *Side-chain oxidative degradation*

Starting from 13-dihydro-N-trifluoroacetyldaunomycin (**388**) the ketone (**389**) was obtained upon oxidation with sodium metaperiodate (Scheme 7.6). Compound (**389**), which showed essentially the same ultraviolet and visible spectrum as the starting material, was degraded to (**390**) with acid. The two epimeric alcohols (**391**) and (**392**) were obtained when (**389**) was reduced with sodium cyanoborohydride, and the *cis*-compound (**391**) was the major product. Removal of the N-trifluoroacetyl group by alkaline treatment afforded the free aminoglycosides (**393**) and (**395**). Assignment of stereochemistry at C-9 was based on the width of the signal corresponding to H-9 in the $^1$H n.m.r. spectrum of the tetraacetates (**394**) and (**396**) [147].

Periodate oxidation of 13-dihydroadriamycin has already been mentioned (Scheme 7.2). Similar treatment of adriamycin itself gave (**397**)a, which was converted into the methyl ester (**397**)b [131].

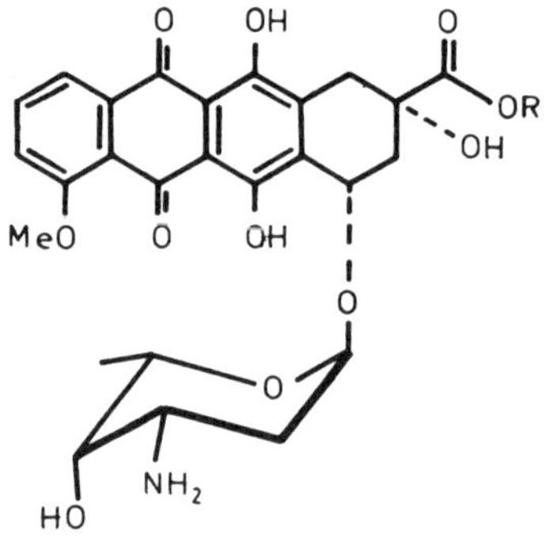

(**397**) a : R = H
b : R = Me

### 7.3 Reactions of Daunomycinone

Chemical modification of daunomycinone **(21)** followed by glycosylation represents an important route for the semisynthesis of new anthracyclines starting from biosynthetic **(1)**. As indicated in Scheme 7.7, 14-bromodaunomycinone **(398)**, easily obtained upon bromination of daunomycinone [127], was converted into the tosylhydrazone **(399)** which afforded the 14-ethers **(400)**a-c upon solvolysis in the presence of silver triflate. Deblocking of the ketone function with acid gave **(401)**a-c which were glycosated to the corresponding daunosaminides **(402)**a-c. The sequence is also of interest because it represents an original procedure of apparently general application for the synthesis of α-alkoxy ketones [148].

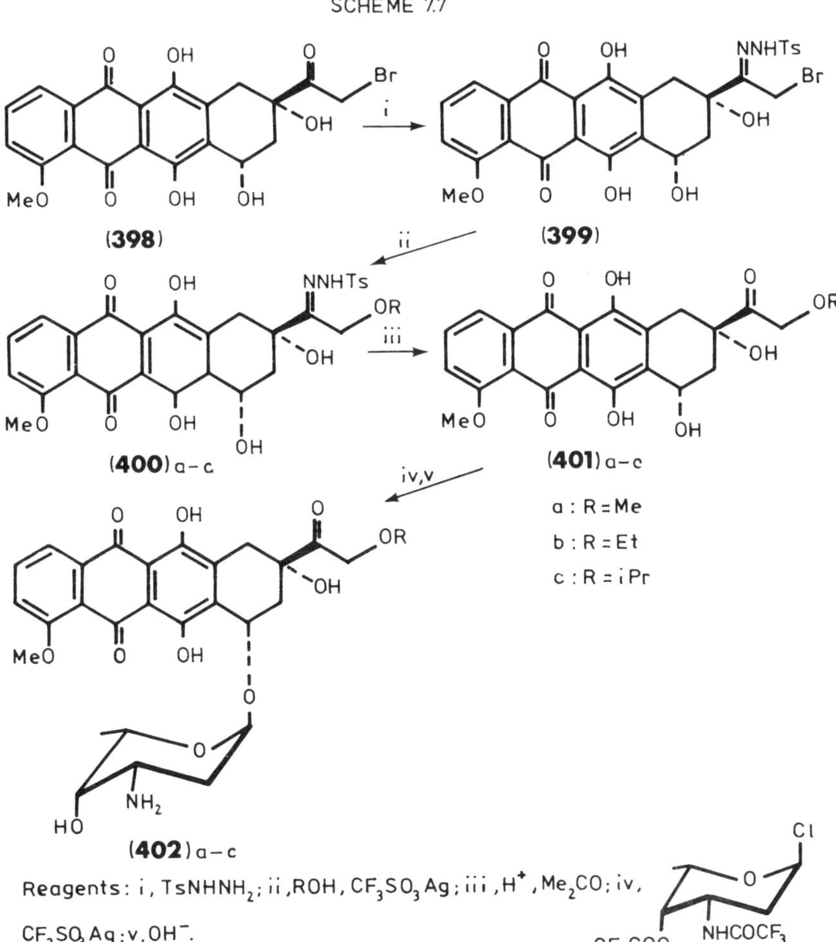

In a different study [149] daunomycinone (**21**) was converted to the triethoxycarbonyl derivative (**403**) which could be dealkylated to give, after a chromatographic separation, (**404**) in approximately 60% yield (Scheme 7.8). Ethoxylation of (**404**) afforded in 85% yield, (**405**)a, which was stepwise hydrolyzed, first to (**406**)a and then to 4-O-demethyl-4-O-ethyldaunomycinone (**407**)a in approximately 50% yield. Glycosidation of (**407**) followed by removal of the protecting groups gave the daunomycin analogue (**408**)a. Similarly compounds (**408**)b-d were obtained.

SCHEME 7.8

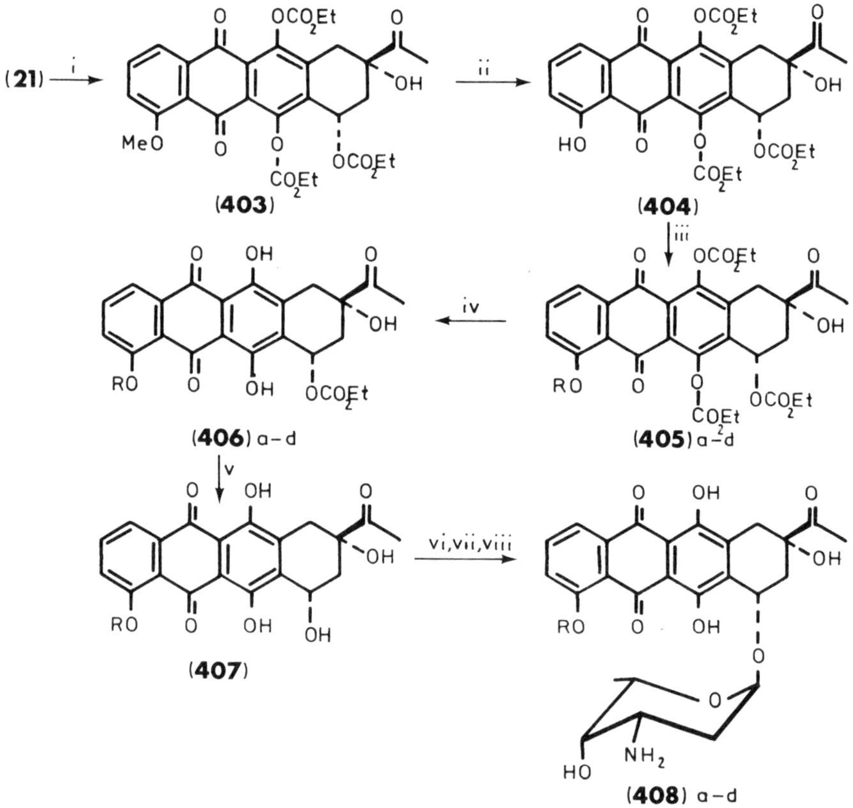

Reagents : i , EtOCOCl , pyridine ; ii , $AlBr_3$ ; iii , RI , $Ag_2O$ ; iv , HN(morpholine)O ; v , $OH^-$ ; vi , (sugar chloride with $CF_3COO$ and $NHCOCF_3$) , $CF_3SO_3Ag$ ; vii , MeOH ; viii , $OH^-$.

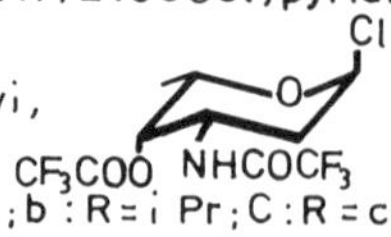

a : R = Et ; b : R = i Pr ; C : R = cyclohexyl ; d : R = $CH_2Ph$.

## 8 PHYSICO-CHEMICAL AND ANALYTICAL STUDIES

Physico-chemical methods and analytical techniques are of paramount importance in the study of natural products and of their derivatives. Structural and configurational investigations of antitumour anthracyclines have involved an extensive use of spectroscopic methods and a summarized account of their applications is presented below. Other examples of the application of these and other refined techniques to the study of the behaviour of anthracycline glycosides in solution and of their complex with small ions or with biological macromolecules will also be shown. Recently $^{13}C$ n.m.r. spectroscopy has been successfully employed for biosynthetic studies. Labelled compounds, fluorescence and polarographic analysis have all been used, together with different separation methods, for the assay of the antitumour anthracyclines in biological fluids.

### 8.1 Structure and conformation studies

Instrumental techniques have been widely used for identification purposes and structure determination of daunomycin and its derivatives or analogues. The usefulness of electronic spectroscopy for the elucidation of the substitution patterns in the chromophoric moiety of the anthracyclines is well documented in the classical works of H. Brockmann [4]. Proton and $^{13}C$ magnetic resonance is a currently used method for the determination of structure and of configurational features in both the natural and synthetically derived compounds of this class. Mass spectra, although not generally obtained from the anthracycline glycosides, have been employed for the study of the aglycone and of the sugar moieties. Circular dichroism has made possible the ready establishment of configurational relationships among the known anthracyclines. Crystallographic X-ray analysis of representative compounds has afforded confirmation of structures and is expected to furnish information of use for the evaluation of molecular requirements for biological activity.

#### 8.1.1 *Ultraviolet, visible and fluorescence spectra*

The electronic spectrum of daunomycinone (maxima at 234, 252, 290, 480, 495, 532 nm), identical to that of daunomycin, is in full agreement with the chromophore substitution in 1,4,5-trihydroxyanthraquinone [29c]. The maxima in the visible region are however less defined and shifted 5-10 nm toward longer wavelengths when compared directly with those exhibited by helminthosporin [150]. The absorption spectrum displays important changes in strong acid or base, owing to the formation of different ionic species. In sulphuric acid daunomycin shows a blue-violet colour with maxima at 257, 303, 545 and 585 nm. In piperidine the colour of the solution is blue and absorption maxima are at 540, 570 and 630 nm [7]. An example of the changes of the visible spectrum in daunomycinone-derived compounds and of the diagnostic usefulness of this method in structural investigations is reported in Table 8.1.

**Table 8.1**
Visible absorption maxima ($\lambda_{max}$ in nm) of daunomycinone and derivatives in different solvents. Absorbance ratios are given in brackets [29c].

| Compounds | Chloroform | Solvent Conc.$H_2SO_2$ | DMF | Piperidine |
|---|---|---|---|---|
| **(21)** | 479,495,530 | 542,582 | 478,495,530 | 566,607 |
| **(24)** | 467,497,521 537 | 542,582 | 480,503,534 | 580,614 |
| **(29)** | 497,518,560 | | | |
| **(30)** | 491,525,566 | 580,626 | 570,625 | 570,612 |
| **(31)** | 486,519,588 (1:2:2.2) | 580,626 (1:1.8) | 571,613 (1:1.3) | 554,596 |
| **(32)** | 482,515,554 (1:2.1:2.5) | 575,620 (1:2) | 566,609 (1:1.1) | 546,590 |
| 5,12-Naphthacenequinone-1,6,7,11 tetrahydroxy [151] | 479,512,560 (1:2.5:3.8) | 552,595 (1:2.2) | 582,626 (1:1.3 | 558,602 |
| 5,12-Naphthacenequinone-1,6,10,11-tetrahydroxy [151] | 482,515,554 (1:2.1:2.5) | 565,618 (1:1.8) | 568,609 (1:1.1) | 546,590 |

Owing to the identity of the chromophore moiety, adriamycin showed essentially the same ultraviolet and visible spectra as daunomycin [128]. The spectra of carminomycin displays differences, as expected because of the different substitution at C-4 [33, 151]. More specifically, carminomycin I shows absorption maxima at 236, 255, 462, 478, 492, 510, 525 nm.

As originally observed by Di Marco and his coworkers [152], daunomycin shows a typical fluorescence spectrum with an emission of 580nm when excited at 485 nm. The same behaviour is shown by derivatives modified in the aminosugar moiety, as for instance N-acetyldaunomycin [152], and by adriamycin [128].

### 8.1.2 *Infrared spectra*

The infrared spectra of anthracyclines and their derivatives were generally determined by the KBr technique and extensively used for identification purposes. Functional analysis has generally been limited to the carbonyl groups typical of this class of compounds.

Because of the chelation of quinone carbonyls of daunomycin and of daunomycinone, the corresponding C=O stretching vibrations exhibit absorptions in the region 1590-1620 $cm^{-1}$. In this range two strong bands are present which are the result of the quinone carbonyl absorptions as well as that of the aromatic C=C band [29]. Substitution of the C-4 methoxyl with a hydroxyl as in carminomycinone is accompanied by the exhibition of a single absorption in the above mentioned range, apparently because of the displacement of the band with higher frequency to 1610 $cm^{-1}$, which can be explained by intensified hydrogen bonds [33]. The quinone absorption shifts near 1670 $cm^{-1}$ when the hydrogen bonds are abolished, for instance upon acetylation of the phenolic hydroxyls. Also, anthracyclinones with non-chelated quinone groupings, as for instance aklavinone, display the non-chelated quinone absorption at approximately 1675 $cm^{-1}$, the other band from the chelated quinone appearing at about 1623 $cm^{-1}$ [4].

The side chain ketone band at 1718 $cm^{-1}$ in daunomycinone (1715 $cm^{-1}$ in daunomycin hydrochloride) is shifted at 1727 $cm^{-1}$ in adriamycinone (1724 $cm^{-1}$ in adriamycin hydrochloride) [153]. In carminomycinone this absorption falls at 1715 $cm^{-1}$ [33]. When the A ring is aromatized following dehydration, the side chain ketone grouping absorbs at 1685 $cm^{-1}$ in bisanhydrodaunomycinone. Classical anthracyclinones, as for instance $\epsilon$-rhodomycinone, show a carbonyl band at about 1740 $cm^{-1}$ resulting from the C-10 carbomethoxy group [4].

### 8.1.3 *Nuclear magnetic resonance*

The $^1H$ n.m.r. spectra of daunomycinone **(21)** and of daunosamine **(39)** together with those of their derivatives and of derivatives of the antibiotic daunomycin **(1)** have been the object of a detailed study [29c]. The spectra were generally determined in different solvents at 60 and 100 MHz, the double resonance was currently used for proton decoupling; The shift values are generally given in $CDCl_3$ and expressed in ppm ($\delta$) from tetramethylsilane. The side chain methyl group was characterized by a signal in the range 2.40-2.45 $\delta$ in daunomycinone and in a number of its derivatives, but the signal appeared at 2.35 $\delta$ in 7-deoxydaunomycinone **(22)** and was shifted at higher field by 0.2 $\delta$ or more in compounds containing a 9-O-acetyl group such as daunomycinone tetracetate and daunomycin pentaacetate. In bisanhydro-daunomycinone dimethyl ether **(26)** the side chain methyl protons appeared at 1.95 $\delta$. Ring A protons of **(21)** and of its derivatives form an ABX system including H-8(A), H-8(B), and H-7, and an A′B′ system corresponding to $CH_2$-10. The benzylic hydrogen at C-7 ($H_x$) was found at 5.35 $\delta$ in **(21)**, at 4.92 $\delta$ in the daunomycinone trimethyl ether **(23)**, and at 5.07 and 5.19 $\delta$ in daunomycin pentaacetyl and N-acetyl **(384)**a derivatives respectively. This proton appeared shifted at 6.42 $\delta$ in daunomycinone pentaacetate and at 6.55 $\delta$ in 7-O-trifluoroacetyl-daunomycinone. In one of the derivatives studied in more detail, daunomycinone trimethylether (**23**), the AB portion of the ABX system was represented by two pairs of doublets at 1.87 and 2.42 δ, the coupling constants being $J_{AB}$= 15,0, $J_{AX}$ = 3.5, and $J_{BX}$ = 2.5 Hz. In pentaacetyl daunomycin H-8(A) appeared at 2.17 and H-8(B) at 2.63 δ, while in (**384**)a the two corresponding signals were found at 2.09 and 2.29 δ. The geminal protons at C-10 appeared in the spectrum of (**23**) as two doublets centred at 3.02 and 3.22 δ (J = 18.5 Hz). In (**384**)a these two signals were found at 2.88 and 3.21 δ.

An interesting feature of the $^{1}H$ n.m.r. spectra of daunomycinone derivatives was the long range coupling between H-$8_{eq}$ and H-$10_{eq}$ [$J_{8e,10e}$ = 1 Hz in (**23**)], also present in (**384**)a. This coupling was stereospecifically restricted between only two of the four hydrogen atoms at C-8 and C-10 (and not averaged among all four), thus indicating the existence of a preferred conformation of the molecule and half-chair conformation of the A ring (Figure 1). This

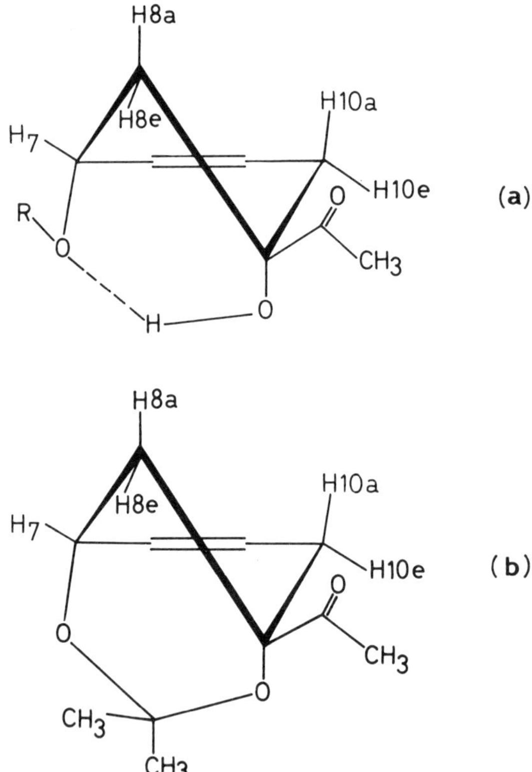


**Figure 1**

Conformation of ring A in daunomycinone derivatives, as deduced by $^{1}H$ n.m.r. spectroscopy in $CDCl_3$ solution; a) Daunomycinone, 7-O-alkyl derivatives and glycosides (N-acetyldaunomycin). b) 7,9-O-Isopropylidenedaunomycinone (35).

finding was in agreement with the deductions based on the values of the coupling constants. The values of $J_{7,8A}$ and of $J_{7,8B}$ were 3.5 and 2.0 Hz respectively in **(384)**a, and were almost identical to those exhibited by **(23)** (3.5 and 2.5 Hz) and by isopropylidenedaunomycinone **(35)** (2,5 and 3.5 Hz), in which the conformation of ring A is fixed, suggesting the same conformation of this ring in the three compounds; The small values of $J_{7,8A}$ and $J_{7,8B}$ indicate a pseudo-equatorial orientation of H-7, the C(7)-H bond nearly bisecting the H-C(8)-H angle. It should be noticed that stabilization of the ring A conformation in daunomycin derivatives possessing the free 9-OH could be the consequence of a hydrogen bond established between 0-9 and 0-7, also suggested by the shift value of OH-9 [4.41 δ for **(384)**a].

As far as the other protons of daunomycinone derivatives are concerned, the C-4 methoxyl group gave the expected singlet in the range from 3.97 to 4.08 δ, while aromatic H-1, H-2 and H-3 gave rise to a complex multiplicity of signals [the ABC system was identified in the spectrum of **(23)**] in the range 7-8 δ. In derivatives of **(1)** and of **(21)** the free phenolic groups appeared in the range from 12.85 to 13.90, but in 4-O-demethoxyl-7-O-methyldaunomycinone **(36)** the third phenolic proton was found at 12.22 δ. The C-9 hydroxyl group appeared at 4.41 δ and at 4.58 in **(384)**a and in **(21)** respectively, at 4.95 δ in **(23)**, but at 3.75 δ in **(22)** and at 4.1 δ in 7-O-trifluoroacetyldaunomycinone.

The $^1H$ n.m.r. spectra of methyl α-daunosaminide **(40)**, the N,O-diacetate **(41)**, and triacetyldaunosamine **(42)** allowed the identification of all the hydrogen atoms in daunosamine and its derivatives as well as of their relative configurations on the basis of the values of the coupling constants. The equatorial anomeric proton gave a signal at 4.81 δ in **(40)**, and at 4.75 in **(41)**, in both derivatives being $[J_{1e,2a}+J_{1e,2e}]$ = 5.0 Hz, while in the anomeric mixture **(42)** H-1e was at 6.17 δ and H-1a at 5.71 δ. The axial H-3 appeared at 4.22 δ in **(40)** at 4.46 δ in **(41)** ($J_{2a,3a}$ = 12.0 hz; $J_{2e,3a}$ = 5.5 Hz), and at 4.3 δ in **(42)**. This proton was also coupled with H-$4_e$ ($J_{3,4}$ was in the range 2.5-3.0 Hz), the latter resonating at 4.48, 5.02 and 5.0 δ in **(40)**, **(41)** and **(42)** respectively. The proton at C-5 was found in the range 3.2-4.0 δ and showed a diequatorial relationship with H-4 ($J_{4,5}$ in the range 1 to 1.5 Hz). In **(384)**a H-1′ (5.47 δ), H-3′ (4.20 δ), H-4′ (3.62 δ) and H-5′ (4.23 δ) showed the same relationships as in the above described simple daunosamine derivatives: $[J_{1'e,2'e} + J_{1'e,2'a}]$ = 5-5.5 Hz; width of H-3′, 28 Hz; $J_{3',4'}$ 12.5 Hz, $J_{4',5'}$ 1-1.5 Hz. This indicated that in **(384)**a, as in the above mentioned derivatives and in all known daunosamine glycosides, the sugar was in the C1 conformation. The data also allowed the establishment of the α-glycoside structure to N-acetyldaunomycin and, therefore, to the parent antibiotic. The equatorial orientation of H-1′ was also established by a $^1H$ n.m.r. study at 220 MHz of daunomycin in pyridine-$d_5$ solution [154].

The $^1H$ n.m.r. spectra of adriamycinone pentaacetate [15] clearly showed the presence of the $COCH_2OAc$ group, $CH_2$-14 giving rise to a pair of doublets at

4.66 and 5.00 δ ($J_{gem}$ = 16.5 Hz). Other signals were in agreement with the results already reviewed for daunomycinone derivatives.

In 13-dihydrodaunomycinone the methyl group of the modified side chain gave rise to a doublet at 1.29 δ coupled (J = 6.2 Hz) with H-13, the latter appearing as a quadruplet at 3.71 δ [155]. Carminomycinone pentaacetate lacked the methoxyl group signal but showed an additional phenolic acetate absorption at 2.33 δ [33].

$^{1}$H n.m.r. spectroscopy has been used for the establishment of stereochemistry of the glycosidic linkage in semisynthetic analogues of the antitumour anthracyclines [110]. The axial anomeric proton in β-glycosides appeared as a pair of doublets, the one being characterized by a low and the other by a high (about 10 Hz) coupling constant, whereas the equatorial anomeric proton in the α series appeared as a broad singlet with a half-band width of about 6 Hz. In addition, the H-1′ signal in the β-glycosides was also shifted to higher field values (about 0.5 δ) with respect to the α-anomers, which displayed the H-1′ signal at about 5.5 δ. The reverse phenomenon was observed for the benzylic proton at C-7, the H-7 signal appearing in the range 5.0 δ to 5.2 δ in the α series, and at about 5.5 δ in the β series. This behaviour was similar to that displayed by the methoxy groups of anomeric methyl N-trifluoroacetyldaunosaminides in which the axial methoxyl appeared at higher field (3.38 δ) than the equatorial one (β-anomer, 3.53 δ) [156]. The anomeric axial methoxyl group also resonates at higher field in the glucose series [157, 158].

The $^{13}$C n.m.r. spectra of daunomycin and adriamycin were analyzed [159] and all carbon frequencies were assigned. The chemical shifts of the hydrogen bearing carbons were established by single frequency selective heteronuclear decoupling except for C-2′ and C-8, because the shift differences between the corresponding bonded protons were too small. The assignment was possible however, by comparison with daunosamine methylglycoside. Assignment of phenolic protons in daunomycinone and adriamycinone and irradiation of each of them allowed the identification of C-5a and C-11a, which appeared in the undecoupled spectra of the two aglycones as sharp doublets of 5 Hz. Assignment of C-5 and C-12 was defined making use of their appreciable coupling, even through four bonds, to the hydroxyl protons. Of the other quaternary carbon atoms, C-12a was readily located, on the basis of its meta coupling, upon irradiation of H-2. The broad resonances due to C-6a and C-10a were assigned because only one of these was affected by removal of the perturbation due to the sugar moiety as in aglycones. The identification of C-4a was possible also on the basis of the presence of two meta couplings with H-1 and H-3. The $^{13}$C-n.m.r. spectrum of adriamycin is shown in Figure 2.

$^{13}$C-N.m.r. has recently been applied for the establishment of the biosynthetic pattern of daunomycin. $^{13}$C-Labelled sodium acetate was fed to the cultures of *S. peucetius* and produced daunomycin was converted into daunomycinone tetraacetate whose $^{13}$C-n.m.r. spectrum was recorded. The outlined.

route for anthracylinone biosynthesis (Scheme 2.1) was confirmed in this study [160].

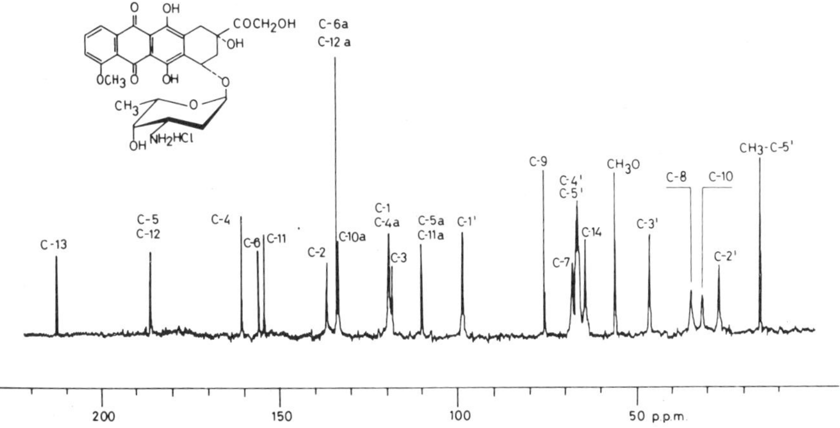


Figure 2 $^{13}C$ n.m.r. spectrum of adriamycin hydrochloride in $D_2O$ solution.

8.1.4 *Mass spectroscopy*

As previously found for other anthracyclinones [161, 162, 163, 164] mass spectrometry appeared to be a useful tool for the structure determination and for the identification of the aglycones derived from daunomycin and related glycosides [15, 128]. The fragmentation reactions of daunomycinone **(21)** (Figure 3) and of adriamycinone **(45)** after electron impact ionization are pre-

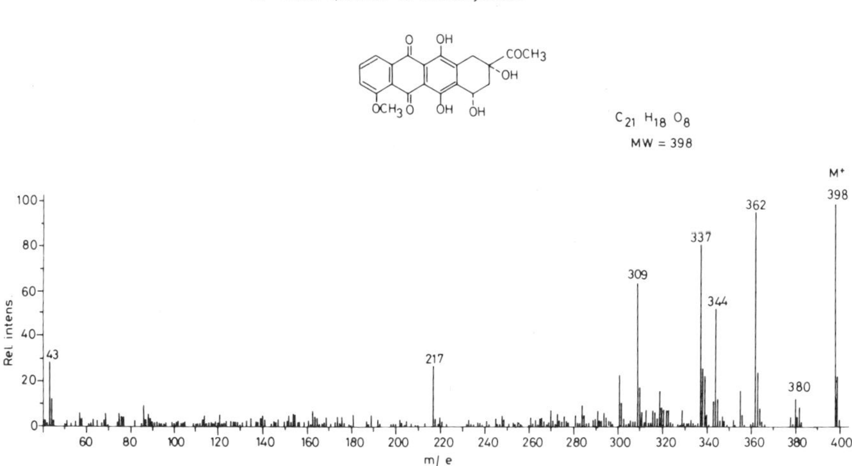


Figure 3 Electron impact mass spectrum of daunomycinone.

sented in Scheme 8.1. The molecular ion **(409)** successively eliminates two molecules of water giving rise to the peaks corresponding to the radical ions with the monohydro and bisanhydro structures **(410)** and **(412)**. Loss of the side chain takes place on the $M^{+}$-$H_2O$ ions **(410)**a and b to give the fragment with m/e 337 m.u. **(411)**, which in turn loses carbon monoxide to afford the fragment with m/e 309 m.u. Splitting of the side chain with loss of 31 m.u. takes place, in the case of adriamycinone spectrum, on fragment **(412)**b, and the resulting ion **(413)** loses carbon monoxide to give a fragment with m/e 319 m.u.

SCHEME 8.1

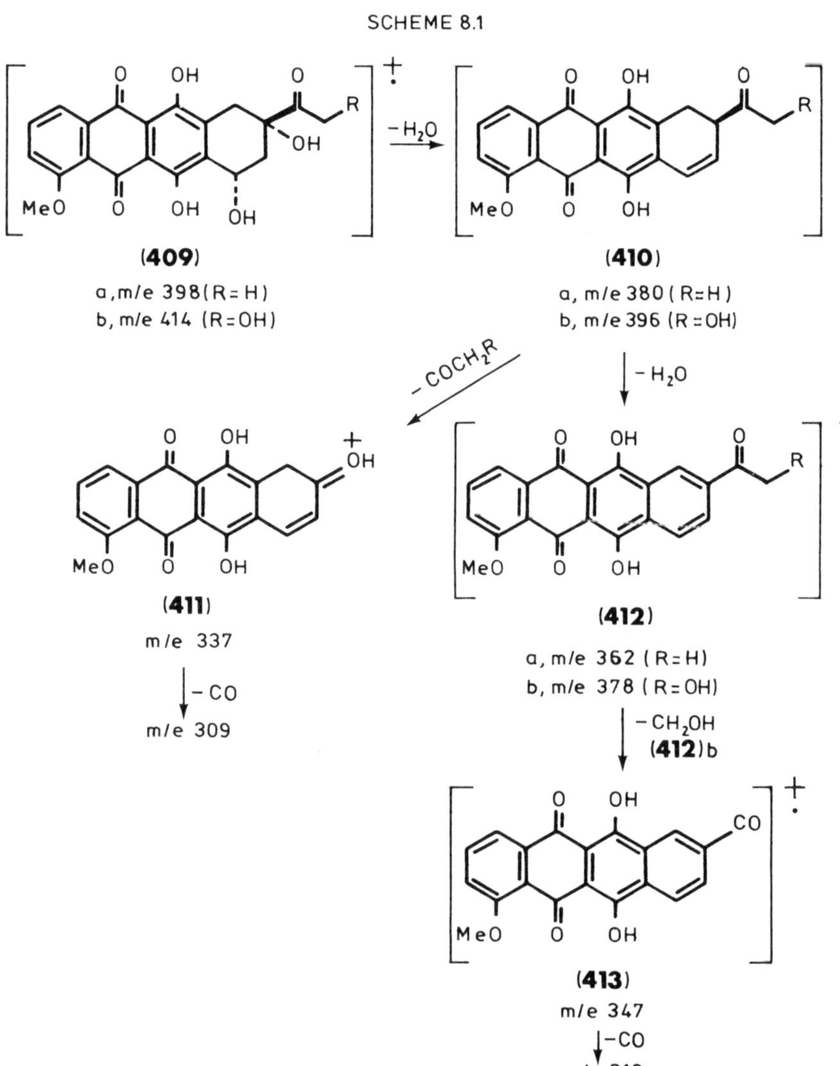

The mass spectrum of 7-deoxyadriamycinone has also been reported. As shown in Scheme 8.2, the main fragmentation reactions which start from the molecular ion **(414)** are the loss of a molecule of water to give **(415)** and the subsequent splitting of the hydroxymethylketone side chain with loss of 31 m.u. and formation of the ion **(416)**. The retro-Diels-Alder cleavage typical of 7-deoxy-anthracyclinones also occurs with formation of **(417)** [128].

SCHEME 8.2

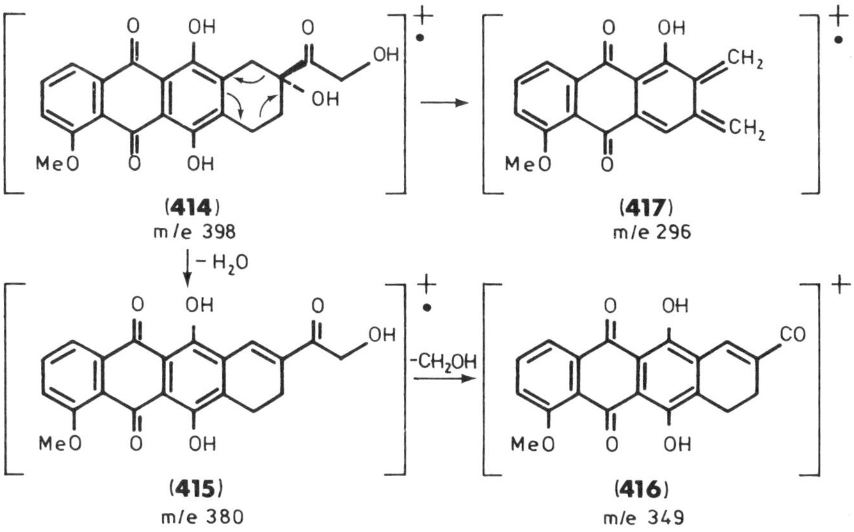

**(414)** m/e 398 → **(417)** m/e 296

**(414)** —$-H_2O$→ **(415)** m/e 380 —$-CH_2OH$→ **(416)** m/e 349

Carminomycinone is decomposed in the mass spectrometer similarly to the above mentioned aglycones, giving rise to peaks at m/e 384 ($M^+$), 366 ($M-H_2O$)$^{\cdot}$, 348 ($M-2H_2O$), 341 ($M-CH_3CO$), 333 ($348-CH_3$), 323 ($366-CH_3CO$), 305 (333-CO and $323-H_2O$), 295 (323-CO), 277 (305-CO), 249 (277-CO), and 221 (249-CO) m.u. [22, 33]. The mass spectrum of 13-dihydrodaunomycinone has been reported to show, in addition to the molecular ion at m/e 400 m.u., important fragments with m/e 382 and 364 m.u., originating from the loss of one and two molecules of water respectively. Elimination of the $CHOHCH_3$ side chain from the m/e 382 m.u. fragment has also been noticed [155].

Fragmentation subsequent to electron impact of N-acetyl, N-trifluoroacetyl and N-benzoyl derivatives of daunosamine **(39)** has been studied using specifically deuterated derivatives and high resolution measurements [156]. The fragmentation giving rise to the most abundant fragments initiates with the cleavage of the $O-C_1$ bond in the molecular radical ion **(417)** and is a generally observed process in the amino sugar derivatives. As shown in Scheme 8.3, the subsequent step is the elimination of acetaldehyde from fragment **(418)** with formation of the radical ion **(419)**, which then loses the $C_1-C_2$ moiety as a

SCHEME 8.3

(417) → (418) —$-MeCHO$→ (419) —$-CH_2{=}CHOR^1$→ (420)

$R^3O-\dot{C}H-\overset{+}{C}H-NH-CO-R^2$

(420)

neutral molecule giving the ion (**420**), one of the most abundant in the spectra of N-acyldaunosamines. The subsequent fragmentation of the ion (**420**) depends on the nature of the substituents. An interesting observation is that concerning the loss of the elements of a molecule of methanol, from 1-OMe and 4-OD in deuterated methyl β-daunosaminides, an elimination scarcely recorded in the carbohydrate field. It probably involves the boat conformation (**422**) of the molecular ion (**421**) and the formation of fragment (**423**) (Scheme 8.4).

SCHEME 8.4

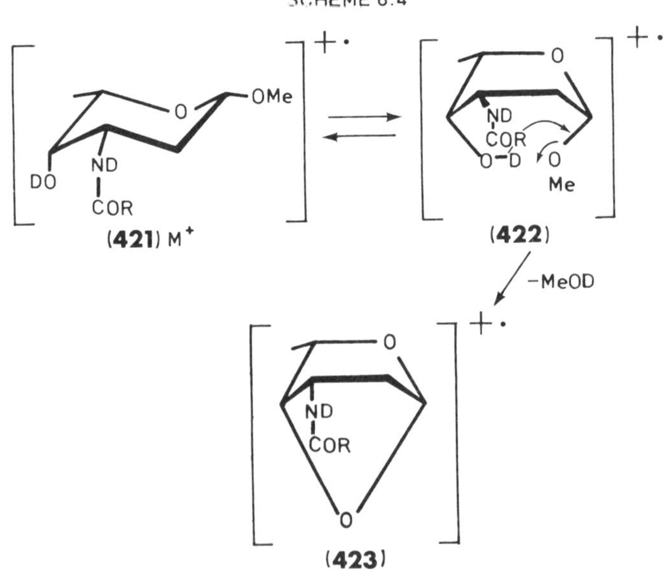

The mass spectra of peracetylated daunomycin derivatives have been recorded and analyzed for the deduction of major fragmentation pathways [166]. Field desorption mass spectrometry [167] allows characterization of intact glycosides (Figures 4 and 5).

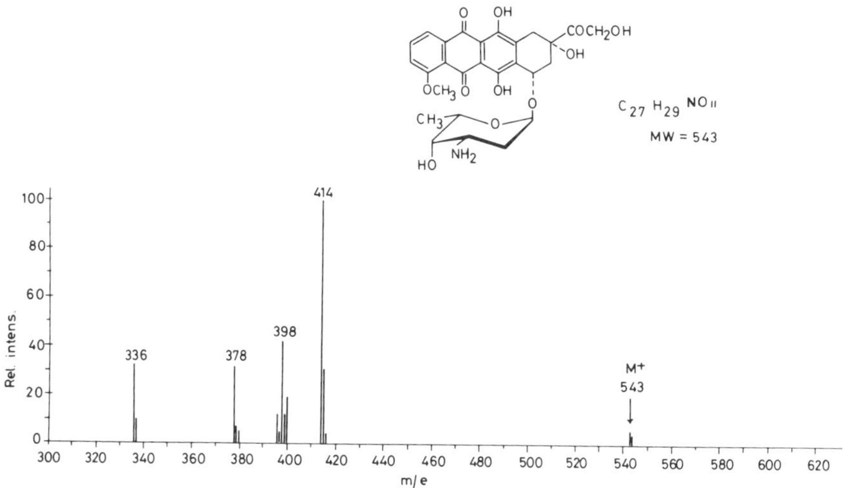


Figure 4 Field desorption mass spectrum of daunomycinone.

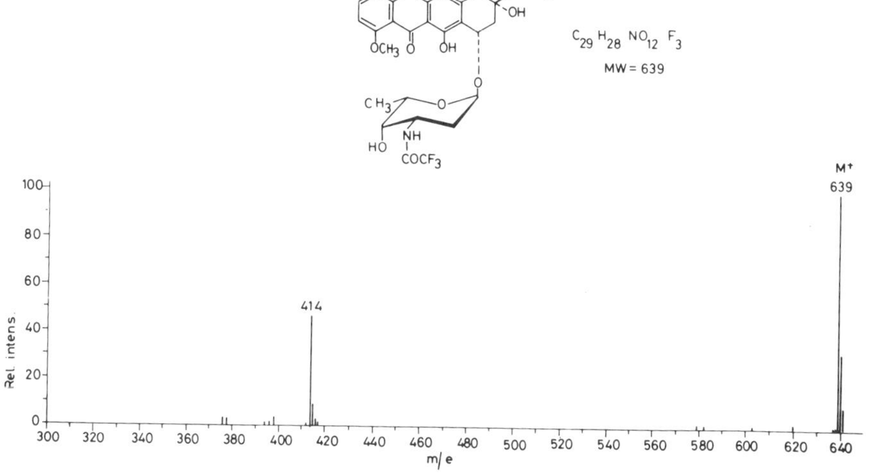


Figure 5 Field desorption mass spectrum of N-trifluoroacetyladriamycin.

8.1.5 *Other techniques*

Circular dichroism of anthracyclinones was the basis for the determination of stereochemical relationships among these compounds [167]. The Cotton effects shown in the range 270 to 390 nm were in fact found dependent only on the substitution of ring A and not on that of the anthraquinone moiety. Once the absolute configuration of daunomycinone had been established [29a], this technique was used for the extension of the discovery to the other known anthracyclinones [168], or to relate synthetic analogues to the natural algycone [37]. Similarly, the identity of absolute configuration at C-7 and C-9 of daunomycin and adriamycin and the retention of absolute configuration at C-7 during acid hydrolysis of the glycosidic linkage were established on the basis of the CD curves of the two glycosides and the corresponding aglycones [15].

N-Bromoacetyldaunomycin was suitable for X-ray analysis. The cyclohexene ring is in the 'half-chair' conformation, the displacement of C-9 from the plane of the remaining five atoms by about 0.7 Å appearing particularly evident. The sugar ring and the planar chromophore are oriented nearly perpendicularly, a property common to other molecules containing two planar systems. The distances between the quinone and the phenolic oxygen are reasonable for the presence of hydrogen bonds between the phenol hydroxy and the quinone groups. However the value for the distance 0-5 and 0-6 is 2.45 Å, and is considerably lower than that between 0-11 and 0-12, which is 2.67 Å. This would indicate a particular distribution of the electronic charges in the substituted anthraquinone chromophore [169].

Carminomycin I was also investigated by crystal structure analysis for confirmation of absolute configuration of the aglycone moiety [22, 34].

Owing to their quinone systems, both daunomycin and adriamycin give a characteristic polarographic reduction wave [128, 152]. The half-wave potential of adriamycin in pH 7.0 McIlwain buffer was found to be approximately 0.6 V [128].

## 8.2 Behaviour in aqueous solution

8.2.1 *Dimerization*

Small but reproducible changes in the spectrum of daunomycin in a buffered solution were observed upon increasing the concentration of the drug and it was concluded that deviations from the Lambert and Beer law were present at concentrations greater than $2 \times 10^{-3}$ M. The modifications of the circular dichroism spectrum of different concentrations in the wavelength range 300-600 nm reflecting intermolecular association between antibiotic molecules have been analyzed in terms of an assumed equilibrium between monomeric and dimeric species [170]. This was also based on literature examples for other dyes, such as acridine orange and proflavine, and on the fact that N-bromoacetyldaunomycin, when crystallized, was found as a dimer [169]. The plot corresponding to the equation

$$\frac{1}{\Delta\epsilon - [\Delta\epsilon_R]} = f\left(\frac{1}{R_O}\right)$$

which was derived from the assumption that at the concentrations used, the amount of dimeric species were low as compared with that of monomer, and in which $\Delta\epsilon$ is the circular dichroic absorption of the sample per molecule of daunomycin, $[\Delta\epsilon_R]$ is the molecular circular dichroic absorption of the monomer and $R_O$ is the total concentration of daunomycin, is a straight line, indicating the validity of the dimerization model. The value of 570 $M^{-1}$ was found for the association constant [170]. The dimerization process has also been studied by $^1H$ nmr spectroscopy, owing to the considerable upfield shifts of all the protons of the antibiotic, particularly those of the aromatic ring (33-36 Hz), upon increasing the concentration from $4.10^{-3}$ M to $1.5\text{-}10^{-1}$ M. Quantitative analysis of the $^1H$ nmr spectra was based however on the signal of the methoxyl group and the dimerization constant was found to be 700 $M^{-1}$, in good agreement with the CD data. It was also found that the dimerization model was not valid for the higher concentrations of the above mentioned range probably because of further association of the dimers themselves, with an association constant which was evaluated to be approximately 2 $M^{-1}$.

8.2.2 *Protolytic equilibria*

The study of the protolytic equilibria of adriamycin in aqueous media has been carried out by electron absorption and fluorescence spectrophotometry [171]. In aqueous buffered solution and in the pH range below pH 7 the only species significantly present was found to be the singly charged species (**424**) (Scheme 8.5). At pH values above pH 7, (**424**) can lose a proton either to form the neutral species (**425**) or the zwitterion (**426**). With higher pH salts such as (**427**) form. The direct evaluation of the corresponding microscopic dissociation constants was achieved by developing a method of general validity for any molecule with overlapping equilibria in which dissociation of one functional group (in this case the phenolic group) affects the electronic spectral properties of the molecule, while the other (in this case the protonated amino group) does not.

The reported values for $pk_1$, $pk_2$, $pk_3$ and $pk_4$ were respectively 8.22, 9.01, 9.36 and 10.10. The values for the macroscopic constants were found to be $pK' = 8.15$ and $pK'' = 10.16$.

SCHEME 8.5

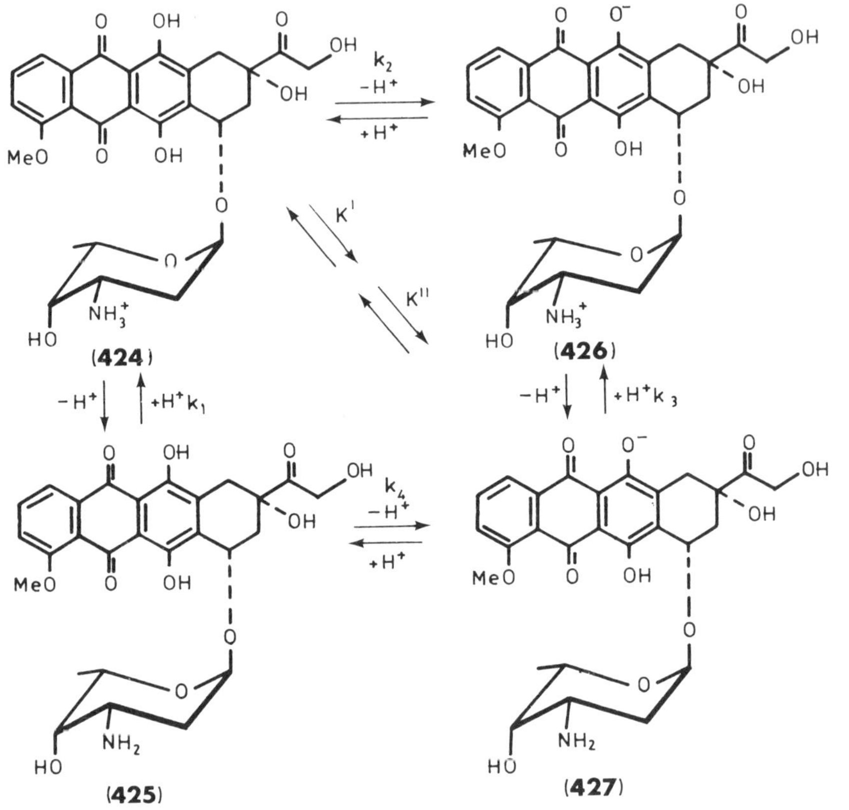

## 8.3 Complexes with small ions and molecules

The effects of different salts on the visible spectrum of daunomycin were described in the paper of Di Marco and his coworkers concerning a variety of physico-chemical interactions of the antibiotic [152]. Salts such as NaCl, KCl, $CdSO_4$, CsCl, $SnCl_2$, and $ZnCl_2$ displayed no appreciable effect. Increasing concentrations of sodium citrate and ammonium sulphate caused a decrease in daunomycin absorbancy without showing any modification of the absorption maxima. On the other hand, the visible spectrum of the antibiotic was profoundly altered by appropriate concentrations of aluminium, iron II, iron III, copper and magnesium salts, as well as by sodium acetate. Similar results were obtained with N-acetyldaunomycin. The same authors tested different purine and pyrimidine derivatives for their influence on the visible spectrum of daunomycin. Whereas pyrimidine derivatives appeared to exert no effect, a shift of the absorption maximum from 475 to 505 nm was caused by purine derivatives such as, for instance, adenine and guanine, albeit at high concentrations (above $10^{-2}$ M).

The formation of a 1:2 copper to daunomycin complex was shown by spectrophotometric titration of daunomycin with $CuSO_4$. The complex was, however, found to be a thermodynamically weak metal-ligand system, and unstable in the presence of human plasma [172].

## 8.4 Complexes with biological macromolecules

Complex formation of the antitumour anthracyclines and DNA has been the object of extensive studies, this macromolecule being currently considered as the main receptor of the antibiotic at the cell level [1, 173]. The interactions of daunomycin and related antibiotics with DNA and other biological receptors are dealt with in the subsequent part (Part D, this volume) with particular reference to the DNA interaction model as deduced by X-ray diffraction techniques and to the mechanism of action at the cellular level. Therefore only a summarized description of the other techniques used, with special reference to those applied to the study of new semisynthetic analogues, will be reported here. The studies of the interactions of the antitumour anthracyclines with other tissue constituents will also be mentioned, the knowledge of these interactions being a prerequisite for a better understanding of the pharmacological properties of the drugs.

### 8.4.1 *Complexes with nucleic acids*

(a) *Spectrophotometric studies.* The first spectrophotometric study of the molecular association of daunomycin with nucleic acids was reported by Calendi *et al.* [152]. The addition of increasing amounts of DNA to a daunomycin solution led to a decrease in the absorbance together with a shift of the absorption maxima. In the visible part of the spectrum the maximum of absorption of the complex was found at 505 nm, and maximal variation was observed when a molar ratio DNA-P: daunomycin of about 7:1 was reached. High ratios of DNA-P to daunomycin were also found to prevent the colour change observed when the daunomycin solution was made alkaline. Similar results were obtained, albeit at higher DNA concentrations, with N-acetyldaunomycin, and also when denatured DNA was used. DNA digested overnight with the enzyme deoxyribonuclease did not promote any modification of the visible spectrum of daunomycin. The absorption spectrum characteristic of free daunomycin was restored when the DNA complex was submitted to the action of the enzyme. Interestingly, a DNA nucleoprotein preparation from rat hepatoma also affected daunomycin absorption at 475 nm. An interaction of daunomycin with RNA could also be detected.

Adriamycin behaved similarly to daunomycin, the highest effect of DNA on the visible spectrum of this antibiotic being reached at a molar ratio DNA-nucleotide to adriamycin between 8 and 9. The effect was not appreciably reversed by NaCl up to a concentration 2M [1].

The spectrophotometric method was used for the study of the interaction of a number of semisynthetic derivatives with DNA. The perturbation of the chromophore was qualitatively similar but quantitatively different for the different compounds [174]. The derivatives at the side chain carbonyl function such as daunomycin oxime, semicarbazone and thiosemicarbazone exhibited an effect which was very similar to that of the parent drug. In contrast, DNA exerted a weak effect on derivatives modified in the sugar moiety. Use of the Scatchard method [175] for the evaluation of the stability constant and of the apparent number of binding sites showed, for instance, that β-D-glucosaminyl-daunomycinone (**298**) and N-acetyldaunomycin (**384**)a exhibited a stability constant respectively 46 and 183 times smaller than the one shown by daunomycin ($K = 3.3 \times 10^6 M^{-1}$) [176].

Spectral tritations were also performed by others, with the aim of deriving the binding isotherms for daunomycin and some peptide derivatives thereof [177], or of the evaluation of the thermodynamic parameters of the complex in different experimental conditions [178].

Complexation with DNA caused disappearance of the typical fluorescence spectrum of daunomycin [152] and of adriamycin [1]. This property was used for the evaluation of the DNA binding ability of daunomycin derivatives [179, 180]. The affinity of 4-demethoxydaunomycin (**323**) for DNA was found to be of the same order of magnitude as that of daunomycin, but a substantially lower interaction was found in the case of 4-demethoxy-1′-epidaunomycin and for the 7(R), 9(R) analogues. Configurational analogues were found to give rise to anomalous binding isotherms.

The circular dichroism spectrum of daunomycin appeared to be profoundly altered in the presence of DNA. The maxima of the two positive absorption bands at 350 and 450 nm were shifted to longer wave lengths and the intensity of the same bands showed an enhancement. The negative absorption, centred at 290 nm was shifted at 320 nm and its intensity was also increased. This modified spectrum was ascribed to intercalated daunomycin and was considered to be a consequence of geometrical change of the antibiotic molecule or of the interaction with the electrostatic field of DNA or with nucleotide transitions [181].

Circular dichroism of complexes of daunomycin and other antitumour antibiotics with DNA in the 220-300 nm range indicated that the different compounds showed different binding modes and that the CD spectra are not, *per se,* diagnostic for intercalation, owing to the complexity of the results [182]. Changes in the CD spectrum of N-acylated daunomycin derivatives upon addition of DNA were compared with those exhibited by the daunomycin-DNA complex [177].

The absorbancy of daunomycin at 475 nm was lowered by a RNA preparation from rat liver (essentially ribosomal RNA) indicating the ability of the antibiotic to bind to this biopolymer [152]. The hypochromic effect of different RNA's, and in particular with a double-stranded RNA, on daunomycin has also been shown [183]. However circular dichroic spectra indicated that the electronic structure of the daunomycin molecule was altered more profoundly by double stranded than by single stranded RNA.

(b) *Polarographic studies.* The presence of DNA inhibited the reduction of daunomycin at the dropping mercury electrode [152]. In a more detailed study [184] it was shown that the effect of DNA on the polarographic wave of daunomycin was similar to that occurring when DNA was added to more or less related antibiotics such as the galirubins and nogalamycin. On the other hand the polarographic wave of aglycones $\eta$-pyrromycinone, aklavinone, daunomycinone, and other anthraquinones was not affected by DNA. This clearly indicated, in agreement with other studies, that the aglycones, although possessing the necessary planarity and the same anthraquinone chromophore as the glycosides, do not form the intercalation complex with DNA typical of the latter, because of the absence of the aminosugar moiety.

(c) *Equilibrium dialysis.* Equilibrium dialysis was compared with the spectroscopic method for the determination of the stability constant of the DNA complex of daunomycin and adriamycin, and the two procedures gave essentially similar results [176]. This technique was also used by Barthelemy-Clavey *et al.* [181] in their study of the DNA-daunomycin complex. These authors found, for the intercalation complex, $K_{ass} = 7.3 \times 10^5 M^{-1}$. They also found a high value of the stability constant ($K = 6.3 \times 10^5 M^{-1}$) for the complex with denatured DNA, indicating that the double helical conformation is not a strict requirement for the formation of an intercalation complex.

In a more recent study the results obtained with the equilibrium dialysis method on daunomycin, adriamycin and twelve of their derivatives or analogues have been reported [185]. As shown in Table 8.2, the stability of the complex of $\alpha$-glycosides was higher with the native than with the denatured form of DNA. As regards the $\beta$-glycosides, both data were available only for one compound, whose association constant with native DNA was of the same order as the one with denatured DNA. The ionic strength of the buffer and the physical characteristics of the DNA used were found to affect the value of the stability constant, and this explains the differences in the said parameters recorded in the literature. The binding data were, however, in agreement with the biological potency of the compounds, as will be shown in the last Chapter of this article. The presence of a hydroxyl group at C-6′, as in 6′-hydroxydaunomycin, decreased the stability of the complex, and the same occurred upon substitution at C-14. The latter finding is noteworthy, because following the generally accepted models of the intercalation complex, the C-9 side chain should not be directly involved in the process of intercalation [1, 186] (see also Part D). The modifications at C-4′ do not affect appreciably the stability of the complex which is however greatly lowered in the 1′-epianalogues (β-anomers). For the 7(R), 9(R) analogue of 4-demethoxydaunomycin the low binding properties are clearly related with the change in stereochemistry of the aglycone moiety, because the 4-demethoxy analogues are known to form stable complexes with DNA [179].

**Table 8.2**

Binding parameters of anthracycline derivatives with calf thymus DNA. Dialysis for 72 hrs. at 25° in pH 7.0 Tris plus NaCl 0.15 M

| Compound | Native DNA | | Heat-denaturated DNA | |
|---|---|---|---|---|
| | $K_{ass} \cdot 10^{-5}$ | n | $K_{ass} \cdot 10^{-5}$ | n |
| Daunomycin | 4.5 | 0.16 | 1.6 | 0.17 |
| | 4.9* | 0.17* | | |
| 4′-Epi-daunomycin | 3.8 | 0.15 | 1.4 | 0.17 |
| 4′-Epi-daunomycin,β-anomer | 0.5 | 0.13 | 0.4 | 0.17 |
| 4′-Deoxydaunomycin | 3.1 | 0.14 | – | – |
| 6′-Hydroxydaunomycin | 2.0 | 0.15 | – | – |
| 14-Morpholinodaunomycin | 2.1 | 0.15 | – | – |
| 4-Demethoxy-7,9-epi-daunomycin | – | – | 0.1 | 0.25 |
| Adriamycin | 3.7 | 0.18 | 1.5 | 0.21 |
| | 6.2* | 0.20* | | |
| Adriamycin, β-anomer | – | – | 0.2 | 0.26 |
| 13-Dihydroadriamycin (adriamycinol) | 3.4 | 0.13 | 1.4 | 0.15 |
| 4′-Epi-adriamycin | 3.6 | 0.18 | 1.3 | 0.23 |
| 4′-Deoxyadriamycin | 4.4 | 0.17 | – | – |
| Adriamycin-14-octanoate | 1.3* | 0.18* | – | – |
| Adriamycin-14-glycolate | 2.2 | 0.13 | – | – |

*Dialysis for 48 hrs and 0.03 M NaCl.

Equilibrium dialysis has also been used in a study of the stereochemical requirements of new analogues of the antitumour anthracyclines [147]. In this study the stability of the DNA complex with 9-deacetyldaunomycin and with 9-epi-9-dacetyl-daunomycin was measured. The association constant shown by the former ($2.2 \times 10^5 M^{-1}$) was distinctly higher than the one shown by the latter ($0.8 \times 10^5 M^{-1}$), indicating that the beta-orientation of the C-9 OH group is less favourable to the stabilization of the complex itself. If this is due to the absence of the suggested interaction of the C-9 alpha-hydroxyl group with the first DNA phosphate away from the intercalation site [186] or to a modification induced on the conformation of ring A which lowers the affinity of the compound for DNA remains to be established.

(d) *Calorimetric measurements.* It has been shown that the binding of daunomycin to DNA is an exothermic process [187]. Microcalorimetric measurements allowed the evaluation of an enthalpy of intercalation of approximately −6.5 Kcal/mole and of an entropy of intercalation of approximately +7.7 e.u., providing useful information for the interpretation of the binding process. For adriamycin the value of the enthalpy for the intercalation was found to be approximately −5.1, but the corresponding $\beta$-anomer showed a much smaller value (approximately −0.9), in agreement with the lower affinity displayed by the 1′-epiderivatives for DNA when compared with the compounds with the natural $\alpha$-configuration [180].

(e) *Other methods.* A number of general methods, currently used in the study of the interaction of small molecules with double helical DNA, were applied in the investigations of the complex of DNA with the antitumour anthracyclines. These methods include thermal denaturation (melting curves), viscosimetry, sedimentation rate, flow-dichroism and hydroxyapatite column chromatography.

The effect of different concentrations of daunomycin on thermal denaturation of double-stranded DNA was monitored by means of optical rotation measurements by Calendi *et al.* [152]. Two main facts were observed, one being the higher melting temperature of the complex in comparison with DNA alone, the other the nearly complete renaturation upon cooling of the complex. Thermal denaturation was followed spectrophotometrically at 260 nm by Barthelemy-Clavey *et al.* [181] who compared different DNA's without, however, finding any specificity of the antibiotic for the base composition of DNA. In the already mentioned paper by Di Marco and his group [176], the thermal denaturation curve of native calf thymus DNA in the presence of daunomycin or of some related compound was determined. Adriamycin showed the highest increase of the melting temperature while 13-dihydrodaunomycin (daunorubicinol), N-guanidinoacetyl daunomycin, and 7-O-(D-glucosaminyl)-daunomycinone gave a somewhat lower effect. N-Acetyldaunomycin appeared to afford only a slight stabilization of the double helix towards thermal denaturation. A high $\Delta$Tm value was instead found for 4-demethoxydaunomycin while its $\beta$-anomer allowed an increase of Tm (midpoint of the thermal denaturation curve) very similar to that shown by daunomycin itself, indicating the favourable effect of the substitution of the 4-methoxyl group with a hydrogen atom as regards the stabilization of the DNA complex [179]. In a more recent study the 4′-epianalogues of adriamycin and daunomycin were found to behave identically as the parent compounds. The $\beta$-anomers were instead much less effective in increasing the Tm value than the corresponding $\alpha$-glycosides [180].

Other parameters of molecular DNA were studied for the investigation of complexes with the antitumour anthracyclines. These were the buoyant density in CsCl gradients, the sedimentation constant, both being decreased upon complexation and intrinsic viscosity of the DNA solution, this parameter being increased upon complexation. The said effects are a consequence of the fact that the complex between the DNA double helix and the drug behaves as a more elongated, stiffer rod in solution, and are considered important diagnostic features of an intercalation complex [152, 189, 190, 191].

Viscosimetric measurements have been used in the study of the DNA complexing properties of new semisynthetic daunomycin analogues. The effects of daunomycin derivatives on the viscosity of native calf thymus DNA were in agreement with the relative affinities measured by other methods [174], but were not easily accounted for by single models, also because of the difficulty in the rationalization of the hydrodynamic behaviour of complex macromolecules in solution. Different factors, related to structural features of the drug molecules, appeared to be involved as suggested by the different curves obtained for the different compounds when the ratio of intrinsic viscosity of DNA complexes with daunomycin related compounds to that of DNA alone was plotted against the ratio of bound molecules to total DNA nucleotides [176]. Viscosimetry measurements were also more recently shown to give results in agreement with those obtained by equilibrium dialysis experiments in the investigations concerning adriamycin related compounds [185, 180] and the 9(S) and 9(R) 9-deacetyldaunomycins [147]. This technique was also applied in the study of N-aminoacyl derivatives of daunomycin [177].

Removal and reversal of supercoils in circular double-stranded DNA is a characteristic property of intercalating agents [192], and the phenomenon can be monitored by either sedimentation rate [192] and viscosimetric [193] titration. Adriamycin was found to behave like daunomycin [194], while 1′-epiadriamycin showed a less typical behaviour indicating either a lower stability of the intercalation complex or a different mode of binding with DNA [180]. Flow dichroism, hydroxyapatite column chromatography, the nitrocellulose filter retention method, and displacement of methyl green from its complex with DNA have been used for the study of DNA complexes of daunomycin and its derivatives [195, 177, 196, 174].

### 8.4.2 *Complexes with other biological macromolecules*

Data begin now to be available on the interaction of the antitumour anthracyclines with biological macromolecules different from the nucleic acids. Proteins, phospholipids and mucopolysaccharides have been found to bind the drugs. The methods used for the investigations concerning these complexes included equilibrium dialysis, spectrophotometry, solvent partition and other techniques.

(a) *Proteins.* Japanese workers [197] have studied the binding of daunomycin to nuclear non-histone proteins from rat liver. The existence of this binding was deduced from previous studies on the interaction of the drug with chromatin from rat liver. Protein was isolated starting from the chromatin and different amounts (10-180 $\mu$g/ml) of the non-histone fraction were dialyzed against daunomycin (100 $\mu$M). Fluorimetric measurements indicated that the amount of daunomycin bound increased with increasing concentrations of protein until a maximum (4.45 nmoles/mg protein) was reached. This behaviour was related with aggregation of nuclear non-histone proteins occurring at the highest concentrations. The specificity of this binding was demonstrated by the lower (ten times more) binding capacity shown by other protein species such as histones, phosphoproteins, catalase, and fibrinogen. The significance of this type of interaction when occurring *in vivo*, as regards, for instance, the regulation of gene expression related with the synthesis of macromolecules essential to cell proliferation, remains to be established.

Different observations have favoured the hypothesis that the antimitotic activity of daunomycin may also involve phenomena not based on a direct action on DNA synthesis, such as for instance a perturbation of spindle fibre function [198]. The interaction of daunomycin with calf brain tubulin was therefore studied by spectroscopic and other techniques [199]. The quenching of both tubulin and daunomycin fluorescence as a consequence of the interaction was used to establish the stoichiometry and the thermodynamic parameters of the association reaction. In particular the stability constant of 37° was found to be $2.2 \times 10^3$l/mol, ten times smaller than the stability constant of the vinblastine-tubulin association ($2 \times 10^4$). Difference spectroscopy measurements confirmed the direct interaction occurring between the protein and the drug and indicated an interaction between the hydroxyl groups of the daunomycin chromophore and tubulin, apparently through formation of hydrogen bonds or salification of the phenolic groups.

In a study concerning the interaction of adriamycin with human red blood cells the binding of the drug by permeable erythrocyte ghosts and by spectrin, a membrane protein component, was investigated. Also, on the basis of morphological observations, the above mentioned protein was suggested as a binding site for adriamycin. Equilibrium dialysis experiments carried out with the isolated protein indicated a positively cooperative interaction and the presence of 100 adriamycin binding sites per moles of spectrin (M.W. 250,000), with stability constant $8.7 \times 10^3 M^{-1}$. Spectrin appeared, therefore, to be probably involved in the cell surface transformation of erythrocytes induced by the drug, a phenomenon implicating biomembranes in the pharmacodynamic behaviour of the antitumour [200].

(b) *Phospholipids.* Although phospholipids are not, strictly speaking, macromolecular species, their complex structure and their tendency to form molecular aggregates and associations with other cell constituents allows inclusion in this subsection. When adriamycin was distributed between a hydrophilic and a lipophilic phase in the presence of different lipids and at pH 7.2, negatively charged lipids such as cardiolipin (diphosphatidyglycerol), phosphatidylserine, phosphatidylinositol an phosphatidic acid induced the nearly complete transfer of the drug into lipophilic phase. This behaviour was not shown by neutral lipids and was explained by the formation of a complex of electrostatic nature between the antibiotic and the acidic phospholipids. Because cardiolipin is an important component of mitochondrial membrane these bindings could be of some interest in connection with the alteration of heart mitochondria as a component of adriamycin cardiotoxicity [201].

(c) *Mucopolysaccharides.* Adriamycin has been found to bind to heparin and chondroitin sulphate on the basis of spectrophotometric measurements. The interaction between the drug and the sulphated mucopolysaccharides induced a bathochromic shift and hypochromicity in the visible spectrum of the antibiotic. Binding curves derived from spectrophotometric titrations allowed the conclusion that the binding sites of the biopolymers could be identified with the anionic groups of the sulphonic and uronic acid residues. However, the contribution of a parallel alignment of the chromophoric moieties along the polymeric structure to the stabilization of the complex was proposed [202]. This property of adriamycin can be of relevance in tissue fixation and the mechanism of action of the drug, especially if account is taken of recent findings concerning the presence and function of sulphated mucopolysaccharides in normal and tumour tissues [203].

## 8.5 Assay in tissues and body fluids

Radioisotopic and fluorimetric methods have been used for the quantitative determination of daunomycin and related compounds in studies aimed to establish the pharmacokinetic behaviour of the antitumour anthracyclines. Fluorimetric techniques have also been coupled with thin layer chromatography (TLC) in order to afford separate assays of drugs and metabolites. High performance liquid chromatography (HPLC) has been introduced more recently for the separation of the drugs and their metabolites in biological fluids. These refined analytical studies, which also include a radioimmunoassay and a polarographic technique, document a wide interest related with the clinical applications of the antitumour anthracyclines and with the assessment of their mechanism of action.

### 8.5.1 *Radioisotopic studies*

Tritium labelled daunomycin was first used for tissue distribution and excretion studies in normal rats by Rusconi *et al.* [204]. The radioactive antibiotic used had been prepared by the Wilzbach technique and was therefore generally (but not uniformly) labelled with tritium (it should be noted here that specifically tritiated daunomycin or adriamycins are not yet available). After intravenous administration of 4 mg/kg the compound appeared to be rapidly taken up by tissues with the exception of brain. The amount of radioactivity in spleen, lymph nodes, and bone marrow, increased in the interval from 2 to 8 hours after the administration. Total excreted tritium at 96 hrs was 35–

50% of dose, most of which (30–40% of dose) was recovered in the faeces. Distribution and excretion of [$^3$H]daunomycin in normal and tumour bearing mice was then investigated [205]. After the intravenous administration, its behaviour in different organs was comparable to that found in rats. Low levels, as compared with other tissues, were found in tumours. In human patients the use of [$^3$H]daunomycin allowed deductions useful for the determination of treatment schedules [206].

The pattern of distribution of [$^3$H]adriamycin in mice was similar to that observed in rats and mice treated with [$^3$H] daunomycin, but the latter appeared to be more rapidly excreted. No difference was found between normal and S-180 tumour bearing mice [207]. In mice bearing spontaneous mammary carcinoma higher blood tissue levels of radioactivity were recorded after administration of labelled adriamycin than after labelled daunomycin, both dosed i.v. at 5 mg/kg. Significant levels of tritium, equivalent to 1 μg of antibiotic/g of fresh tissue, were still present in the tumour a week after the treatment with three doses of 2.5 mg/kg at 12 hour intervals of [$^3$H]adriamycin [208]. In humans [$^3$H]adriamycin was rapidly fixed in body tissues, with the exception of brain. After a single i.v. dose of 0.5 mg/kg, plasma levels, after an initial rapid fall, remained constant at approximately 1 μg/ml for at least 7 days. Urinary excretion of tritium for the first 7 days was 22.7% of the dose administered, faecal excretion being as high as 45% of dose for the same period. Treatment schedules were proposed on the basis of these findings [209].

Tritium labelled daunomycin was also used for the evaluation of the uptake of the antibiotic by HeLa cells in culture. The uptake was completed after 20 min exposure to the drug and was proportional to the external concentration (range 0.25 ro 2.0 μg/ml) of labelled antibiotic. It was also found that 50% inhibition of labelled uridine incorporation into RNA was reached when the amount of antibiotic present in the cells corresponded to one molecule of daunomycin per 62.5 to 111 DNA-nucleotide phsophate residues [210].

Evaluation of plasma radioactivity in rats treated with [$^3$H] adriamycin indicated two exponential components for the decay curve which was fitted in a two compartment model. Tissue levels were in agreement with the proposed model [211].

The first report concerning the use of [$^{14}$C]adriamycin and [$^{14}$C]daunomycin in pharmacokinetic investigations described the excretion and the distribution, as determined by whole body radioautograms, or radioactivity in rats after single i.v. doses of 4 mg/kg of the labelled antibiotics. At 96 hours after treatment 80% of dose of both drugs was recovered in the excreta, [$^{14}$C] adriamycin derived radioactivity being present principally in liver, skeletal muscle, lymphatic and glandular tissues, gastrointestinal contents and renal tubules, [$^{14}$C] daunomycin derived radioactivity in liver, gastrointestinal contents, kidney cortex, glandular and lymphatic tissues, and hepatic channels [212].

8.5.2 *Fluorimetric Studies*

A fluorimetric assay of daunomycin involving extraction of the drug from serum and urine with n-butanol was reported to allow the detection of concentrations as low as 0.06 μg/ml. Fluorescence was measured in the n-butyl extract at 589 nm after excitation at 483 nm. A combination of paper or thin-layer chromatography, and fluorimetry failed to detect metabolites in serum and urines of mice and rats up to 6 hours after the intraperitoneal administration of the drug. Urinary recovery of unchanged daunomycin was 20% of dose in rats at 72 hours and 3.8% in mice at 6 hours after administration. In mice, the serum concentration of daunomycin fell to 0.2 μg/ml at 30 min after a 5 mg/kg dose and remained almost constant up to the sixth hour [213].

The application of the fluorimetric technique and its comparison with a radioisotopic method for the estimation of tissue distribution and disposition of intravenously administered daunomycin in mice (15 mg/kg) was reported by Bachur *et al.* [214]. The fluorometric procedure involved homogenization of tissues with 0.3 N HC1 in 50% ethanol followed by centrifugation. The emission of fluorescence of the extracts using an activation wavelength of 470 nm was compared with that of a series of daunomycin standards made in 0.3 N NCl in 50% ethanol and that of control tissue extracts made in the same way from untreated mice. The recovery of daunomycin was found to approach 100% with a lowest limit of detection in the range from 5 to 50 ng/g of tissue. For the radioactivity measurements both tissue extracts and residues of mice treated with tritium labelled daunomycin were used, The highest levels of fluorescence were found in the heart, lung, liver, spleen and kidney during the first 12 hours after administration and remained elevated thereafter in the spleen, liver and kidney. Two general rates of removal of the drug from tissues were recorded: a 'short' half life of 1.5-4 hours in some tissues, heart, lung, kidney, and a 'long' one in some of these (e.g. lung) or in others, as in the brain, liver, spleen, and skeletal muscle. Comparison of the level of radioactivity and fluorescence at 24, 48 and 77 hours indicated differences which became greater with increasing time, the levels of tritium being higher than fluorescence. The authors considered it most likely that the fluorescent moiety of the drug was destroyed but that the radioactivity was retained and measured. Substantial radioactivity was also found incorporated into the insoluble material in all tissues assayed. For example, in the heart acid-alcohol insoluble fraction 0.52 μg of $^{3}$H-daunomycin equivalents per g of fresh tissue were found at 24 hours after the administration, this amount not being lowered at 72 hours.

Another comparative study of the fluorescence assay method and the use of tritiated daunomycin was concerned with the pharmacokinetics of this drug in man [215]. Both methods allowed the detection of amounts as low as 10 ng of drug/ml of plasma or urine, Different results were obtained with the two methods, apparently as a consequence of tritium exchange or of metabolism. More reliably, fluorescence measurements indicated a short plasma half-life of

0.75 hours and a long plasma half-life of 55 hours.

The fluorescence assay method was also applied for the quantitative estimation of daunomycin metabolites, either as single compounds (e.g. daunorubicinol) or as groups of compounds with similar polarity (e.g the 'aglycones' and the 'polar metabolites' fractions). Separation of drug and metabolites was carried out by TLC followed by elution with 50% ethanol in 0.3 N HCl. This procedure permitted, for instance, the determination of biliary excretion and tissue distribution of daunomycin and of its metabolites in rats [216]. Daunorubicinol was the predominant compound present in the bile, followed by daunomycin and by the glycuronides. In most of the tissues examined 8 hours after the i.v. injection of the drug, the fluorescent species present were, in decreasing level of concentration, daunomycin, daunorubicinol, aglycones, and polar metabolites. Aglycones were the major fluorescent fraction in the brain.

Bachur *et al.* [217] also applied the above mentioned methods to the evaluation of the behaviour of daunomycin and adriamycin in the rabbit, which is the best animal model for the study of drug-induced cardiomyopathy. For drug analysis tissues and plasma were homogenized with ice-cold chloroform-methanol and the extracts were submitted to TLC for separation of drug and metabolites. Fluorescence assays were performed as already mentioned. After i.v. injection of 5 mg/kg both drugs were cleared from the plasma at apparent first order rate for two hours, after which the disappearance rate decreased. Daunorubicinol was the main fluorescent compound excreted in the bile and in the urine within 8 hours after administration of daunomycin, while both adriamycin and adriamycinol were present in the bile and urine in rats treated with adriamycin. Tissue contained daunomycinol as the major fluorescent drug derivative in the former case but adriamycin was predominant in the latter. Only liver and kidney contained significant aglycone concentrations.

The pharmokinetic evaluation of adriamycin in cancer patients was carried out according to the methods outlined above [218]. In order to afford a more reliable separate assay of drug and metabolites in plasma, their relative amounts were determined by hydrolysis to the corresponding aglycones and chromatographic separation of the same. Urinary fluorescent components were separated in fractions by TLC and quantified separately. Adriamycin showed a biphasic disappearance from plasma, the long half-life being 16.7 hours (26.7 hours for total drug fluorescence) and the short half-life 1.1 hours (1.9 hours for total drug fluorescence). Cumulative urinary excretion in 5 days accounted for only 5.5% of the administered dose. The prolonged drug levels found in plasma after a single injection were in agreement with the reported high efficacy of the intermittent high-dosage schedule used in clinical practice.

Plasma levels of adriamycin derived fluorescence, as determined by the method reported above [215], were used for compartmental analysis in patients treated with the drug. Disappearance from plasma followed a double exponential function whose characteristics were used for the calculation of the dimension of a two compartment open model [211].

Fluorimetric assays, differing however from the above mentioned methods in the extraction procedures, were applied in investigations concerning the pharmacokinetics of daunomycin [219] and of adriamycin [220] in laboratory animals, the evaluation of the transformations of the two antibiotics in perfused isolated dog hearts preparations [221], and the distribution of daunomycin, N-acetyldaunomycin and adriamycin in the hamster [222]. In the latter study substantial amounts of aglycone-like products were found to be present in different organs, including the heart, after the administration of daunomycin and adriamycin, but not after administration of the N-acetylated derivatives, and this finding was correlated with the cardiac toxicity exhibited by the non-acetylated antibiotics. However Bachur *et al.* were not able to confirm these results, the most likely cause for the differences observed being attributed to the different recovery procedures used [223].

An adriamycin assay based on acid ethanol extraction of blood or tissues, followed by heating in order to convert the antibiotic to the aglycone, adriamycinone, recovery of the latter by solvent extraction and TLC on impregnated glass fibre, and fluorimetric measurement, was found to afford approximately 92% recovery of the drug. The method was applied to the estimation of plasma levels in cancer patients. The presence of metabolites in plasma was also recorded [224].

An interesting modification of the fluorimetric assay for daunomycin and adriamycin in animal tissue has been developed by Schwartz [225]. This method was based on previous observations from Rusconi [226] that $Ag^+$ salts cause the release of daunomycin from the binding to DNA. According to this method cells or tissue homogenates were treated with a concentrated solution of silver nitrate and the resulting mixture extracted with iso-amyl alcohol. The iso-amyl alcohol extracts were used for the fluorimetric measurement with excitation wavelength at 490 nm and emission wavelength at 560 nm. Blank values appeared substantially lowered by the protein precipitating property of the silver salt when the results were compared with those obtained by extraction of the biological material with formamide [227] or hydrogen chloride-containing ethanol [214]. It was also shown by chromatographic methods that no formation of aglycones was found during the analytical procedure and that final recovery in optimized conditions was almost quantitative from the dialyzed DNA complex of the drugs and was in the range 74 to 100% from different rat tissues and L 1210 ascites cells. In some cases, in which a colour quench was proved, internal quenching corrections were performed by adding known amounts of drug to the organic phase. In these studies the amount of drugs was in the range of 4 to 40 μg per gram of fresh tissue. In the case of the L-1210 cells the concentration of 0.2 μg/50 mg cells was regarded as the lower limit of sensitivity. As an example the uptake of daunomycin and adriamycin by L-1210 cells in mice treated with 1 mg/kg of either drug was measured. Retention of daunomycin was higher than that of adriamycin, consistent with the greater effectiveness of the former on nucleic acid synthesis in L-1210 ascites in animals but not in agreement with the greater therapeutic effectiveness of the latter against the tumour.

8.5.3 *Other methods*

(a) *Radioimmunoassay* (RIA). An RIA procedure has been developed for the estimation of the antitumour anthracyclines, capable of detecting as little as two picomoles of the antibiotics per ml. Different animal species were used (rabbit, monkey, goat) for immunization by injecting adriamycin conjugates with human serum albumin or with hemocyanin. N-(p-Hydroxyphenylacetyl) adriamycin was labelled with $^{125}I$ and used as the labelled hapten in the assays which were performed by the double antibody technique. The antisera could not distinguish among daunomycin, N-acetyldaunomycin, daunomycin benzoylhydrazone and adriamycin. Application of the method of pharmacokinetic investigations in laboratory animals was also shown to give results in agreement with those reported in the isotopic and fluorimetric studies [228].

(b) *High-Pressure Liquid Chromatography* (HPLC). An HPLC method for the separation of adriamycin, adriamycinol and adriamycinone in urines of adriamycin treated cancer patients coupled with the use of RIA to determine the amounts of isolated compounds has been developed [229]. Urine extracts [217] were submitted to reverse-phase HPLC using a linear gradient elution technique, and the collected fractions were analyzed by RIA as described above. Four out of five patients showed a higher concentration of adriamycin than adriamycinol in the urine. This behaviour appeared to be different from that observed in the rabbit. In this animal species adriamycinol was the predominant urinary drug derived component after adriamycin administration.

A different HPLC method has been proposed by other authors [230]. The method involved extraction of plasma, to which an internal standard was added, with a mixture of methylene chloride-isopropanol, separation of the drug and metabolites on a silica microsphere column and detection of the components in the eluted peaks by visible absorption. The method was applied to the estimation of daunorubicinol and daunomycin in the plasma of rabbits treated i.v. with 5 mg/kg of daunomycin. Adriamycin was used as internal standard and the lower limit of sensitivity was 10 ng/ml. A HPLC separation of anthracycline glycosides is shown in Figure 6.

(c) *Polarography.* Adriamycin was detected in plasma because of its reduction at the dropping mercury electrode. The sample required no prior treatment and the sample could be utilized for other clinical tests. The polarographic method showed, however, a limit of detection of 400 ng/ml and all the known metabolites of the antibiotic gave similar reduction waves. A number of other antineoplastic agents were found not to interfere with the measurement [231].

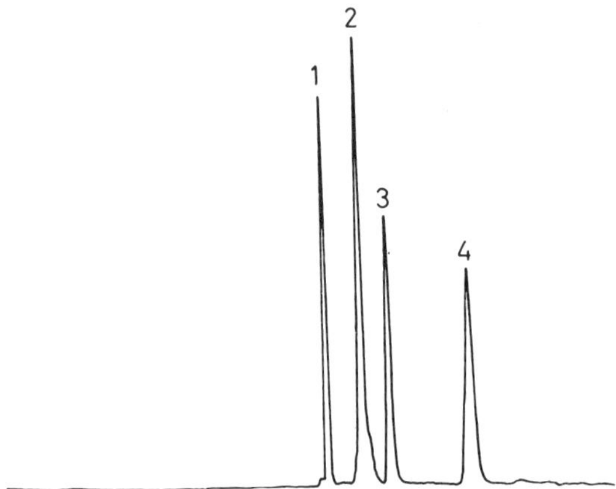


Figure 6 High-pressure liquid chromatography of a mixture of 13-dihydro adriamycin 1, adriamycin 2, 13-dihydrodaunomycin 3, and daunomycin 4. (reverse phase system).
Column: Waters Microbondapak C-18 (1 ft × 3.9 mm i.d.).
Mobile phase: 31/69 acetonitrile/aqueous phosphoric acid pH 2.
Flow rate: 1 ml/min.
Pressure: 1300 psi.

## 9 BIOCHEMICAL TRANSFORMATIONS

The antitumour anthracyclines can be metabolized in animal bodies, in tissue preparations, and in microbial cultures. Metabolism of daunomycin and adriamycin in laboratory animals and in man has been investigated in order to contribute to the understanding of pharmacological properties and of pharmacokinetic behaviour of the drugs.

Knowledge of chemical reactions involved in metabolic disposition may be helpful in the design of new analogues and comparative studies may help explain or predict pharmacological or toxicological differences among established drugs and new related compounds. Microbial transformations are of interest as a general method for the conversion of the antitumour anthracyclines or their derivatives to new bioactive, but hopefully less toxic, compounds.

Another interesting aspect inherent in the study of microbial transformations is the awareness that enzyme reactions which take place in higher animals are often also carried out by microbes, which therefore appear useful both as models for the study of metabolic transformations as well as sources of relevant enzymes or metabolites.

### 9.1 Drug metabolism studies

The two major metabolic transformations of daunomycin and adriamycin in laboratory animals and in man are represented by the reduction of the side chain carbonyl group to a secondary alcohol and the reductive hydrolysis of the sugar moiety with formation of 7-deoxyglycones (Scheme 9.1). The enzyme catalyzing the first reaction has been named daunomycin reductase, and is an aldoketo reductase of a very ubiquitous nature. The reductive splitting of the benzylic glycosidic bond is, in contrast, rather unique and no other examples of enzyme catalysis of this otherwise chemically very facile reaction are described. The aglycone-like compounds thus formed are in turn substrates of more common metabolic reactions, such as O-demethylation and conjugation.

#### 9.1.1 *The 'Aldehyde Reductase' reaction*

Daunorubicinol (daunomycinol, 13-dihydrodaunomycin) and adriamycinol (13-dihydroadriamycin) have already been mentioned in the previous section as major metabolites of, respectively, daunomycin and adriamycin in different animal species and in cancer patients. Daunorubicinol, a more polar compound than daunomycin in different TLC systems, was first detected by Bachur and Cradock [232] after incubation of rat tissue slices with daunomycin. Both labelled and unlabelled samples of the antibiotic were used. All the tissues tested (brain, lung, liver, heart, intestine, kidney and skeletal muscle) had the capacity to convert daunomycin to the metabolite, the kidney appearing the most active. Aglycone-like less polar metabolites were also formed. In a subsequent study [233] rat tissue homogenates were investigated and it was shown

SCHEME 9.1

(1) R=H; (2) R=OH

(4) R=H; (364) R=OH

(25) R=H; (428) R=OH

(22) R=H; (46) R=OH

(429) R=H; (430) R=OH

(431) R=H; (432) R=OH

(R=H)

(433)

(434) R=H; (435) R=OH

(436) R=H; (437) R=OH

that the conversion of daunomycin to daunorubicinol was catalyzed by a soluble enzyme present in the supernatant after high speed centrifugation of the homogenates. With both liver and kidney extracts, reduced triphosphopyridine nucleotide (NADPH), but not other cofactors, stimulated the production of the metabolite. It was also concluded, on the basis of the intracellular location and of the presence in different tissues, that the enzyme responsible for this conversion, daunomycin reductase, was a constitutive enzyme performing some other normal function in the animal tissues, In the same study it was also shown that aglycone-like metabolites were formed under the action of microsomal fractions mainly in the liver cell preparations.

Daunorubicinol was eventually isolated from the urine of patients treated with daunomycin in amounts sufficient to allow the determination of structure [30]. This was essentially based on the lack of the ketone absorption in the infrared, on the chromatographic behaviour of the compound and of its aglycone, and on the mass spectrum of the latter, showing a molecular weight increased by two mass units in respect to daunomycinone.

Bachur and his co-workers have carried out a detailed study of the enzyme involved in the conversion of daunomycin to daunorubicinol. A method for the quantitative estimation of daunomycin reductase in the tissue was established [234, 235]. The method was based on incubation of the tissue preparations with daunomycin, followed by extraction, hydrolysis of substrate and product to the corresponding aglycones, separation of the latter compounds by column chromatography and final fluorometric quantitation. Rat kidney exhibited a high level of enzyme activity which was, however, also present in human erythrocytes. Isolation and purification of the enzyme from rat liver afforded a homogeneous protein with a molecular weight approaching 40,000. The isolation and purification procedure involved an extraction-centrifugation step, ammonium sulphate fractionation, chromatography on DEAE cellulose and then on hydroxyapatite columns and gel filtration. The purification of enzyme activity was 2330 fold. Aminoacid composition, optimum pH and kinetic constants toward various substrates were given [236]. Characterization of the enzyme was completed in a more recent publication [237]. A range of carbonyl compounds, mainly aldehydes, were found to be substrates for the enzyme. These included both natural compounds such as lactaldehyde, glyceraldehyde, glyceraldehyde-3-phosphate, glucuronate and glucuronolactone, and xenobiotic aldehydes amongst which 4-carboxybenzaldehyde appeared to be the best substrate. Optimum pH for these substrates was however pH 6.0, while daunomycin was more rapidly reduced at pH 8.5 N-Acetyldaunomycin behaved as the former substrates, indicating that the free amino group was involved in a unique pH optimum. Adriamycin was reduced 20 times less efficiently than daunomycin. Barbiturates were inhibitors of daunomycin reductase which was confirmed as a non inducible enzyme. Daunomycin reductase appeared to be a member of the class of NADPH linked aldehyde reductases, a group of ubiquitous enzymes whose involvement, not only in detoxification reactions, but also in physiological metabolism is still incompletely understood. It was also noticed that the not too distantly related classical alcohol dehydrogenase was unable to use the antibiotics as substrates. A barbiturate-sensitive daunomycin reductase was also purified from rat liver by other authors [238].

### 9.1.2 *The Reductive Glycosidase reaction*

The anthracycline glycosides are cleaved in most tissues to the aminosugar moiety and the 7-deoxyaglycones by a reaction which formally involves the addition of two hydrogen atoms in place of the C7-O bond.

Formation of a daunomycinone-like compound upon incubation of daunomycin with rat liver or rat kidney preparations was first observed by Di Marco *et al.* [239]. Metabolic conversions of daunomycin to aglycone-like products were easily detected because of their low polarity by chromatographic analysis, by several groups [204, 205, 207, 232, 233]. A detailed study of the products of daunomycin and adriamycin metabolism in rat liver and kidney and in hamster liver homogenates was carried out by Asbell *et al.* [240]. Using a combined TLC-fluorimetry assay these workers showed that daunomycin was transformed anaerobically by liver homogenates to give two major metabolites, 7-deoxydaunomycinone (22) and 7-deoxy-13-dihydrodaunomycinone (**429**). The latter was formed in higher amounts than the former and NADPH was found to be required for the reaction to occur. With kidney homogenate (**429**) was still the main product, together with daunorubicinol (**4**) in anaerobic conditions, but the latter was the only detected product under aerobiosis. Daunomycinone (**21**), 13-dihydrodaunomycinone (**25**) and (**22**) were also substates and gave, in anaerobic conditions, compound (**429**). Adriamycin behaved similarly, giving rise to 7-deoxyadriamycinone (**45**) and 7-deoxy-13-dihydroadriamycinone (**430**) under the action of liver homogenates. Identification of structure of the new metabolites is possible through the preparative conversion of daunomycin and adriamycin to the metabolites under the action of crude rat liver homogenates. On the basis of infrared spectra, mass spectrometric measurements and 100 MHz $^{1}H$ n.m.r. spectroscopy, the structures of the metabolites were unequivocably established [241].

Yesair *et al.* [242] have proposed a mechanism for the reductive glycosidase reaction. As indicated in Scheme 9.2 the intermediate (**438**) could be converted to the 7-deoxyaglycone, the proton being furnished directly by NADH.

SCHEME 9.2

(**1**) R = H
(**2**) R = OH

(**438**)
R = H,OH

(**22**) R = H
(**46**) R = OH

### 9.1.3 *The overall metabolic sequence*

Daunorubicinol aglycone-like compounds, and more polar metabolites (aglycone conjugates) were always present near daunomycin in the excreta and tissues of rats treated with this drug [216]. In the rabbit, daunorubicinol was the main metabolite of daunomycin but significant amounts of polar metabolites were found [217]. In this species adriamycin was converted to adriamycinol to a large extent. The concentrations of the metabolites were, however, lower than those of the parent drug in all tissues and in urine, the metabolite being predominant in the bile. The metabolite, adriamycinol, was isolated from enzyme reaction mixtures, prepared upon incubation of adriamycin with rabbit liver or kidney extracts, or from rabbit bile and urine, and identified *inter alia* by the absence of the carbonyl absorption at 1720 $cm^{-1}$ in the infrared and mass spectrum of the aglycone, 13-dihydroadriamycinone [217].

Scheme 9.1 shows the metabolic degradation of daunomycin (**1**) and of adriamycin (**2**) in laboratory animals and in man [243, 244]. The following aglycone derived metabolites were identified in human urine after daunomycin treatment; 13-dihydrodaunomycinone (**25**), 7-deoxy-daunomycinone (**22**), 7-deoxy-13-dihydrodaunomycinone (**430**), 4-demethyl-7-deoxy-13-dihydro-daunomycinone (**431**), 4-demethyl-7-deoxy-13-dihydro-daunomycinone-4-O-sulphate (**434**), 4-demethyl-7-deoxy-13-dihydrodaunomycinone-4-O-$\beta$-D-glucuronide (**436**), and 7-deoxy-13-dihydrodaunomycinone-13-O-$\beta$-D-glucuronide (**433**). As pointed out by the authors [243], (**4**) was the major component of the urine (45% of total drug-related fluorescence). The parent drug accounted for 23% of the total and the conjugates (**432**), (**433**), (**435**) accounted for an equal percentage of drug related fluorescence. Compound (**434**) was the major conjugated metabolite. Combined (**22**), (**25**), (**429**) and (**431**) represented about 8% of the drug fluorescence in urine, (**431**) being the predominant species. It appeared clearly that the products derived from the reaction catalyzed by daunomycin reductase were the most abundant, the cleavage of the glycosidic bond by reductive or hydrolytic glucosidases being the reaction responsible for the formation of the aglycone-like compounds. Conjugate forms of the latter appeared to be major metabolites. Conjugates of the glycosides (**1**) and (**4**) had been found, however, in rat bile [216].

Adriamycin and its metabolites extracted from the urine of patients treated with the drug were separated by chromatography on silicic acid columns. The following compounds were isolated (in order of increasing polarity): 13-dihydroadriamycinone (**428**), which was identified by comparison with a sample obtained by sodium borohydride reduction of adriamycinone; 7-deoxy-13-dihydroadriamycinone (**430**), also identified by direct comparison with the product obtained from (**2**) by catalytic hydrogenation followed by reduction as above; 4-demethyl-7-deoxy-13-dihydroadriamycinone (**432**), identified on the basis of the absence of the carbonyl absorption at 1720 $cm^{-1}$ and of the aromatic methyl ether absorption at 1210 $cm^{-1}$ in the infrared, by mass spectroscopy and by diazomethane O-methylation to **(46)**; adriamycin **(2)** and adriamycinol **(364)**, the latter being identified also by direct comparison with the product obtained by sodium borohydride reduction of adriamycin; 4-demethyl-7-deoxy-13-dihydroadriamycinone-4-O-sulphate **(435)**, characterized, after enzymic hydrolysis with arylsulphatase or with acid, by direct comparison with **(432)**; 4-demethyl-7-deoxy-13-dihydroadriamycinone 4-O-β-D-glucuronide **(437)**, also characterised after hydrolysis with β-glucuronidase or acid to **(432)**. In total, 60% of urinary recovered fluorescence was represented by metabolites and the remainder was unchanged drug. These results indicate a fairly extensive metabolism of the drug, notwithstanding the lower rate of formation of **(364)** from **(2)** under the action of tissue aldehyde reductase. The authors also pointed out the further complexity related to the possibility of the presence of chemical breakdown products of adriamycin and non-fluorescent metabolites. In fact recovery of adriamycin fluorescence in bile and urine from a patient was about 60% of the administered dose [244]. In a recent study the above mentioned adriamycin metabolites were also detected in the plasma of patients under adriamycin treatment. The aglycone fraction, mainly **(430)** (tentative identification) accounted for nearly half of plasma fluorescence, indicating a remarkable activity of the reductive glycosidase. Individual variations were found in patients as regards the quantitative aspects of metabolism [244a]. These observations, as well as others previously made with daunomycin [218], [245], [264] were not useful for relating metabolic aspects with pharmacology of the antitumour anthracycline. Indeed, the results of the metabolic studies have not fulfilled the expectations concerning the explanation of the different efficacy of daunomycin and adriamycin and the establishment of prognostic parameters regarding the clinical response to therapy. However, knowledge of the metabolic fate and disposition of the clinically useful antitumour anthracyclines has allowed a basis for rationalization of treatment schedules and has furnished useful information for the design of new analogues.

### 9.2 Microbial transformations

In the last three years different reports, either as patents or as publications, have appeared concerning the modification of anthracycline derivatives under the action of microbial cultures. The following reaction types were described: (i) the reduction of the side chain carbonyl group to a secondary alcohol, (ii) the reductive deglycosidation of dehydroxylation at the C-7 benzylic position, (iii) reduction of the C-10 ketone grouping in steffimycinone, and (iv) N-acetylation.

#### 9.2.1 *Reduction of the side-chain carbonyl group*

Microbial reduction of daunomycin to daunorubicinol was first reported by Florent *et al.* [247] who found that the transformation could be carried our strains by *Streptomyces lavendulae, S. roseochromogenes, Corynebacterium Simplex, Bacterium cycloxydans.* It was subsequently reported that the above mentioned strains were also capable of converting carminomycin (**3**) to 13-dihydrocarminomycin, a previously undescribed anthracycline glycoside [248]. The new compound and the corresponding aglycone (4-demethyl-13-dihydro-daunomycinone or 13-dihydrocarminomycinone) were characterized by their electronic and infrared spectra. The conversion was also carried out with strains belonging to other *Streptomyces* species (*S. caeruleorubidus* and *S. bifurcus*) when adjuvant compounds such as antifolic agents, sulphadrugs, and barbiturates were added to the culture, or using a strain belonging to the new species *Streptomyces atroviolaceus.* As already mentioned in Section 2 of this Chapter, 13-dihydrodaunomycin has also been isolated as a metabolite of Streptomyces strains, the corresponding aglycone also being coproduced in the cultures [23, 24]. In the case of the *S. peucetius* related strains, it was not established whether these compounds were derived by reduction of the carbonylic precursors, or if the 13-dihydro derivatives were the precursors of the more oxidized species in the biosynthetic pathway [1]. However, daunomycin was converted into 7-deoxy-13-dihydrodaunomycinone (**429**), when the daunomycin fermentation broths were allowed to stand in anaerobic conditions [249]. Compound (**429**) was also formed with (**22**), as a minor product, when daunomycinone was submitted to the action of a crude enzyme preparation of *S. steffisburgensis* [250]. The reaction appeared to be catalyzed by a NADPH linked ketoreductase.

Two reports concerning the selective reduction of the side chain carbonyl group in daunomycin and its derivatives have been published recently. In the first, the conversion of daunomycinone (**21**) to (**25**) by means of the washed mycelium of a strain of *S. aureofaciens* in a buffered solution containing sucrose was described [155]. In the second one Aszalos and his associates at the N.C.I. Frederick Cancer Research Center reported the results of a screening carried out with different microorganisms for their ability to modify anthracycline structures. This work was aimed at the production of new compounds for antitumour testing. Selective reduction of the side chain ketone grouping in (**1**) and in N-acetyldaunomycin, affording respectively (**4**) and N-acetyl-13-dihydrodaunomycin (N-acetyl-daunorubicinol), was carried out by a number of microbial isolates, but a strain of *Corynebacterium equi* was used for the preparative experiments. Full characterization of the products was performed, yields were however, not given [251].

### 9.2.2 *Reductive deglycosidation and dehydroxylation*

When daunomycin and five other anthracycline derivatives were incubated in anaerobic or microaerophilic conditions with certain organisms such as *Aeromonas hydrophila, E. coli,* and *Citrobacter freundii,* the substrates were extensively transformed by the microbial cultures to give, predominantly, the corresponding 7-deoxy aglycones [252]. Daunomycin was converted into **(22)** in approximately 40% yield. Steffimycin, steffimycin B and the aglycone, steffimycinone, all gave 7-deoxysteffimycinone as the major degradation product and similar results were obtained with nogalamycin and cinerubin A. This indicated that the reaction could take place over a wide range of variations both in the sugar and in the aglycone moieties. Some degree of anaerobicity was a strict requirement for this transformation to occur and this was interpreted by the hypothesis of an induction-repression phenomenon involving oxygen tension. The absence of the anthracyclinones from the transformation appears to exclude their intermediate formation during the generation of the 7-deoxy compounds. Further catabolism of the 7-deoxyaglycones was also found to occur.

Other interesting results were obtained with a dialyzed cell-free extract of *A. hydrophila*, used as the crude enzyme source. These indicated that conversion of steffimycin to 7-deoxysteffimycinone occurred only in the presence of a reduced pyridine nucleotide and that NADH was superior over NADPH as a component of the incubation mixture [252]. The enzyme was subsequently purified 97 fold and characterized as an acidic protein with molecular weight approximately 35000. The assay method was based on the reductive conversion of steffimycin to 7-deoxysteffimycinone which was measured by high pressure liquid chromatography and detection by absorbance at 254 nm. The purified enzyme was strongly inhibited by molecular oxygen but not by cyanide or EDTA [253].

Daunomycin **(1)** was also converted in 66% yield to 7-deoxydaunomycinone by a cell-free extract of *Streptomyces steffisburgenis* grown aerobically on a tryptone-yeast extract-glucose medium. This conversion showed the same cofactor as the reaction catalyzed by *A. hydrophila* enzyme, NADH being required for the reaction to occur with dialyzed extract [250]. The same crude-cell-free extract was able to reduce the side-chain ketone of **(22)** to give **(429)**, as already mentioned above. Compound **(22)** was one of the aglycone type metabolites isolated from *S. peucetius* and related strains [1], and both **(22)** and **(429)** were formed when daunomycin fermentation broths were allowed to stand overnight at pH 7.5 without agitation [249]. These findings indicated the presence of the reductive glycosidase also in the anthracycline producing strains.

As for the mechanism of this interesting new biochemical reaction, mention has already been made of a proposed sequence (Scheme 9.2) in subsection 9.1.2 dealing with the corresponding mammalian enzymic reaction. Wiley *et al.* [254], in their study concerning *inter alia*, the conversion of steffimycinol **(440)** to 7-deoxy-steffimycinol **(441)** by *A. hydrophila*, propose a similar mechanism involving the peri-aromatic hydroxyl in the process ultimately leading to reduction.

### 9.2.3 *Reduction of a C-10 ketone*

In a programme based on the use of anthracycline-antibiotic producing microorganisms as agents for the modification of anthracycline derivatives, other than those produced by the organism, Wiley *et al.* [253] have found that steffimycinone **(439)** is reduced at the C-10 carbonyl group to give steffimycinol **(440)** by cultures of *S. nogalater* and *S. peucetius* var. *caesius* and by cell-free extracts of *S. nogalater* (Scheme 9.3). The yields were in the order of 32–34% and NADPH was a cofactor for the conversion. The reduction appeared to be stereospecific because only one isomer was isolated, but the configuration at C-10 in **(440)** was not determined.

SCHEME 9.3

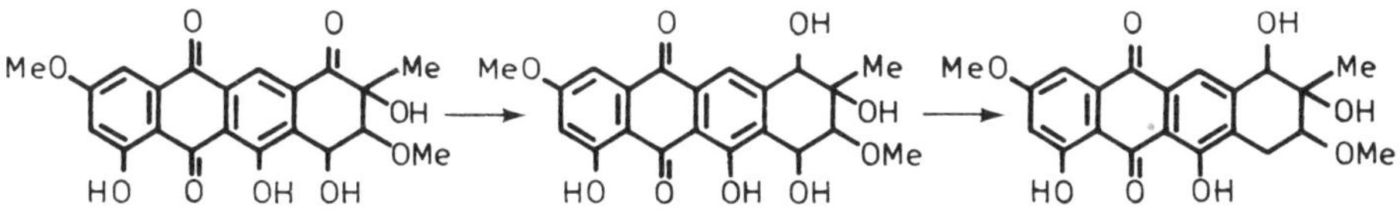

**(439)** → **(440)** → **(441)**

### 9.2.4 *N-Acetylation*

The only microbial transformation of daunomycin which has not its counterpart in mammalian systems is the N-acetylation of **(1)** and **(4)**. This transformation has recently been reported as carried out by a strain of *Bacillus cereus var. mycoides* aerobically incubated with the said compounds [254].

## 10 STRUCTURE ACTIVITY RELATIONSHIPS

The relationships between chemical structure and biological activity are of considerable importance for the establishment of molecular requirements for action and, therefore, for the development of new analogues. Presently available knowledge allows a reasonable awareness of the consequences of chemical modification on biological activity, although the consequences are better studied taking account of pharmacokinetic and metabolic transformations, which are presently incompletely known for the parent compounds and practically unknown for most of the new analogues.

The chemical modifications discussed in this section are concerned with both structural and stereochemical details of the anthracycline molecule and include the new analogues obtained semisynthetically from the natural compounds, such as those modified in the side chain or at the amine function, as well as those obtained by glycosidation of the natural aglycone with daunosamine related sugars or by coupling of daunosamine, or a stereoisomer thereof, with new aglycones prepared by total synthesis or by chemical modification of daunomycinone.

### 10.1 Side-chain modifications

Whatever their biosynthetic relationships, daunomycin, dihydrodaunomycin and adriamycin represent a group of metabolites differing only in the stage of oxidation in the C-9 side chain. The activity of the compounds is shown in Table 10.1. The higher efficacy of adriamycin in the test when compared with daunomycin indicates the importance of the C-9 side chain for the pharmacological behaviour of these compounds. At the present stage of our knowledge, these differences are not explained on the basis of the activity at the molecular level nor at the cellular level, where daunomycin appears more active than adriamycin because of a higher rate of uptake in the cells [255]. The observed differences should therefore be related to different pharmacokinetic properties and different metabolism, although a differential effect on other pharmacological parameters, as for instance the immunological response, has been reported [256]. As shown in Table 10.1, 13-dihydrodaunomycin displayed outstanding antitumour activity in the P 388 test in mice, although the optimal dose was higher than for other drugs. In other experimental tumours of mouse, such as sarcoma 180 (solid) and Gross leukemia, 13-dihydrodaunomycin showed a slightly lower effect than daunomycin [257]. In the same study, derivatives at the side chain ketone function, such as daunomycin semicarbazone, thiosemicarbazone and oxime were found to be endowed with a much lower activity, both in laboratory animals and in cultured cells, in agreement with the findings of American authors [137].

**Table 10.1** Antitumour activity of anthracyline glycosides on P 388 experimental leukemia in mice[a].

| Compound[b] | Optimal dose[c] (mg/kg) | T/C[d] % |
|---|---|---|
| Daunomycin | 1.0 | 173 |
| Adriamycin | 2.0 | 238 |
| β-Dihydrodaunomycin | 4.7 | 232 |

*a*) Means of two experiments performed under the auspices of N.C.I., N.I.H., Bethesda, Md., USA.
*b*) As the hydrochloride.
*c*) Treatment i.p. on days 1 to 9.
*d*) Average survival time expressed as percent of controls.

The effect of substitution at C–14 on antitumour activity is presented in Table 10.2. Adriamycin acetate and octanoate are representative compounds of a number of 14-acyl derivatives of adriamycin which were shown to retain significant levels of antitumour activity [143, 144, 259]. This observation is in contrast with the lower affinity for DNA shown by the octanoate in comparison with adriamycin [185]. It should, however, be noted that this ester is hydrolyzed *in vivo* in different tissues [143]. In the 14-amino analogues the biological potency appeared substantially reduced with respect to adriamycin, but at optimal doses significant antitumour activity was still retained [145].

**Table 10.2** Antitumour activity of adriamycin analogues modified at C-14 on sarcoma 180 ascites in mice [258].

| Compound | Optimal dose mg/kg | T/C % |
|---|---|---|
| Adriamycin | 2 | 210 |
| Adriamycin 14 -acetate | 2 | 252 |
| Adriamycin 14-octanoate | 2 | 250 |
| 14-(N-morpholino)-daunomycin | 25 | 226 |
| 14-(N′-methyl) piperazino daunomycin | 25 | 226 |

Out of the new derivatives obtained semisynthetically from biosynthetic daunomycin only daunomycin benzoylhydrazone (rubidazone) has been currently developed to a clinical stage [260].

Among the new analogues obtained upon oxidative degradation of the C-9 side chain, the acid (**397**)a and the corresponding methyl ester (**397**)b appear to be very moderately effective as antitumour agents against P 388 lymphocytic leukemia in mice [131]. On the other hand a significant level of activity is still present in the 9-deacetyl daunomycins (**393**) and (**395**) with respectively 9(S) and 9(R) configuration, the one showing the natural configuration being the most active of the two (Table 10.3). The higher selectivity of the 9(S) epimer could be related either with the possibility of interaction of the C-9 hydroxyl group with a phosphate group of the DNA double helix as proposed by Pigram *et al.* [186], or with the greater stability of a preferred conformation for intercalation induced by the hydrogen bond between OH-9 and O-7 when in a *cis*-relationship.

**Table 10.3** Effect of the modification at C-9 on antitumour activity and on affinity towards DNA [147].

| Compound | Activity on P 388 leukemia (a) | | Binding constant with calfthymus DNA |
|---|---|---|---|
| | Optimal dose (mg/kg) | T/C % | $(M^{-1}.10^{-5})$ |
| Daunomycin | 1.0 | 171 | 4.5 |
| Adriamycin | 2.0 | 180 | 3.7 |
| 9-Deacetyldaunomycin | 12.5 | 228 | 2.2 |
| 9-Deacetyl-9-epidaunomycin | 6.25 | 171 | 0.8 |

a) Treatment i.p. on days 1 to 9.

## 10.2 Derivatives at the amine function

N-Acetyldaunomycin exhibited a weaker antitumour activity than the non-acetylated compound at a 40 times higher dosage on L-1210 leukemia in mice [137]. This was in agreement with the previous results, showing that the free amino-group of the daunosamine moiety was essential for the exhibition of significant antitumour activity [1]. Other N-substituted daunomycin derivatives displayed even lower, or no activity at all, even at high dosages (64 mg/kg and higher) [137]. On the contrary, N-trifluoroacetyl derivatives appear to be endowed with significant antitumour activity although at higher dosages when compared with the free aminoglycosides [146].

A different class of N-substituted analogues is represented by the N-peptide derivatives of daunomycin. It was found that activity on P 388 leukemia of such compounds as (**384**)l and (**384**)m was lower than that of daunomycin, in agreement with the lower inhibition of RNA polymerase and the higher rate of dissociation of the DNA complex with the analogoues in comparison to the DNA complex with daunomycin [141].

### 10.3 Analogues containing other aminosugars

All three configurational isomers of daunomycin modified at C-3′ and C-4′ but possessing the 5′(S) configuration (L-sugars) as in the parent drugs, are now known. As shown in Table 10.4 only the L-*arabino* isomers retained the full antitumour efficacy of the parent glycosides on L-1210 leukemia in mice. The activity was still present in the *L-ribo* series, which, however, appeared endowed with a lower potency, but disappeared in the *L-xylo* analogues. The reasons for these variations in biological potency are not known, because no information is available on other parameters such as the stability of the DNA complex, the activity on nucleic acid synthesis and drug metabolism. It has been found that although the *arabino* isomers displayed an antimitotic effect in cultured cells which was of the same order of magnitude as the one shown by the parent compounds [77], 3′,4′-diepidaunomycin appeared distinctly less effective than daunomycin [119].

**Table 10.4** Antitumour activity of configurational isomers of daunomycin and adriamycin on L 1210 leukemia in mice [258, 261]. Single i.p. treatment on day 1.

| Compound | Configuration of the sugar moiety | Optimal dose mg/kg | T/C % |
|---|---|---|---|
| Daunomycin | L-lyxo | 4 | 150 |
| Daunomycin 4′-epi- | L-arabino | 4 | 143 |
| Daunomycin, 3′-epi- | L-xylo | 33[a] | 100 |
| Adriamycin | L-lyxo | 5 | 166 |
| Adriamycin, 4′-epi- | L-arabino | 5 | 150 |
| Adriamycin, 3′,4′-diepi- | L-ribo | 5 | 139 |

[a]Max. dose tested. (Istituto Nazionale per la Cura e lo Studio dei Tumori, Milan, Italy).

Modifications in sugar substitution have also resulted in different effects on biological activity. In general the introduction of an hydroxyl group at C-6′ depresses the antitumour activity as well as toxicity. This lower degree of potency could not be known *a priori* from the available knowledge about the biochemical mode of action of the antitumour anthracyclines. On the other hand the 4′-deoxy analogues displayed considerable antitumour activity thus indicating, in agreement with the observations concerning the 4′-epi analogues, that the position 4′ can be modified without loss of biological potency or, as was the case with the 4′-deoxy analogues, with an increase in activity (Table 10.5).

**Table 10.5** Activity of analogues of the antitumour anthracyclines with different modifications in the sugar moiety on L 1210 leukemia in mice [78, 261]. Single i.p. treatment on day 1.

| Compound | Optimal dose (mg/kg) | T/C % |
|---|---|---|
| 4′-Epi-6′-hydroxyadriamycin | 40 | 137 |
| 3′,4′-Diepi-6′-hydroxydaunomycin | 17.2[a] | 150 |
| 4′-Deoxydaunomycin | 8 | 187 |
| 4′-Deoxyadriamycin | 4 | 177 |

[a]Max. dose tested.

## 10.4 The 4-demethoxy analogues

An interesting modification of the antitumour anthracyclines is the substitution of the 4-methoxyl group with a hydrogen atom. Position 4 is hydroxylated in all known biosynthetic anthracyclines and total synthesis appears to be the only source of the 4-unsubstituted derivatives. 4-Demethoxydaunomycin as well as the corresponding adriamycin analogues are endowed with very high biological potency, their activity being comparable with that of the parent compounds at doses eight to ten fold lower (Table 10.6). The outstanding antitumour activity of 4-demethoxy analogues has also been demonstrated in other experimental tumour systems [40, 121]. An important property of 4-demethoxydaunomycin is the activity after oral administration [262]. It has also been found that the compound is more effective in stabilizing the DNA double helix to heat denaturation than daunomycin, but no substantial difference in the values of the stability constants of the drug-DNA complex of the two drugs was observed [179]. Recent work has shown that the 4-demethoxy analogue was taken up at a higher rate and in greater amount than the parent compound in cultured cells and that the two compounds were not equally distributed in the different organs when administered to the mouse [263]. 4-Demethoxy-4′-epiadriamycin, an analogue bearing two modifications (both compatible with a high level of biological activity), one on the chromophore moiety and the other in the sugar residue, also showed outstanding antitumour properties [121].

**Table 10.6** Antitumour activity of 4-demethoxy-analogues on L-1210 leukemia in mice [40, 121, 258]. Single i.p. treatment on day 1.

| Compound | Optimal dose (mg/kg) | T/C % |
|---|---|---|
| 4-Demethoxydaunomycin | 0.5 | 150 |
| 4-Demethoxyadriamycin | 0.5 | 166 |
| 4-Demethoxy-4′-epiadriamycin | 0.5 | 166 |
| 4-Demethoxy-1′-epidaunomycin | 8 | 150 |
| 4-Demethoxy-7,9-diepidaunomycin | 8[a] | 100 |
| 4-Demethoxy-7,9,1′-triepidaunomycin | 10[a] | 100 |

[a]Max. dose tested.

### 10.5 β-Glycosides

The anthracycline analogues exhibiting the β-configuration of the glycosidic linkage (1′-epicompounds) are unnatural because all known biosynthetic anthracyclinone glycosides are α-glycosides. No antitumour activity was shown by 1′-epiadriamycin at dosages up to 10 mg/kg body weight on sarcoma 180 ascites in mice [258]. 1′,4′-Diepidaunomycin displayed a weak activity at 20 mg/kg, the corresponding adriamycin analogue appearing somewhat less active than the α-anomer in the said test system. The β-anomer of 4-demethoxydaunomycin displayed good activity at a dose which was 16 times higher than that of the corresponding α-anomer but only twice that of daunomycin itself (Table 10.6). Inspection of molecular models showed that the β-anomers could intercalate between adjacent base pairs in the DNA double-helix, However, in the lower energy conformation obtained by minimizing non-bonded interactions around the C7-O and the glycoside linkages, the distance between the amino group and the second DNA phosphate away from the interaction site was larger for the β-anomers, in agreement with the lower stability constant of the DNA complex and with the reduced bioactivity [185].

### 10.6 The 7(R), 9(R) analogues

Compounds with the unnatural configuration at C-7 and C-9 were devoid of biological activity. For instance 7(R),9(R)-demethoxydaunomycin showed no activity on L-1210 leukemia in mice up to a dosage level of 8 mg/kg. The corresponding β-anomer was inactive at 10 mg/kg in the same test (Table 10.6). These results were confirmed on Gross leukemia in mice and non-toxic effects were detected at the doses tested [40]. These observations are in agreement with the low affinity of these stereoisomers for DNA [179]. The presence of activity in the 7(S), 9(R) stereoisomer of 9-deacetyl daunomycin, reported above indicates the importance of the absolute stereochemistry at C-7 for biological activity.

## ACKNOWLEDGEMENTS

The author expresses his thanks to A. Vigevani and B. Gioia, Farmitalia, Milan, for the n.m.r. and mass spectra reported in Figures 2 to 5, and Dr. L. Malspeis, the Ohio State University, and Dr. E. M. Acton of Stanford Research Institute, Cal., for preprint copies of papers cited in ref. 130 and 133.

## REFERENCES


[1] A. Di Marco and F. Arcamone, *Arzneim. Forsch.*, **25**, 368 (1975).

[2] F. Arcamone, *Chim. Ind.* (Milan), **59**, 281 (1977).

[3] S. A. Waksman 'The Actinomycetes', The William and Wilkins Co., Baltimore, 1959, Vol. I; S. A. Waksman, *The Actinomycetes,* The Ronald Press Co., New York, 1967.

[4] H. Brockmann, *Fortschr. Chem. Org. Naturstoffe,* **21**, 127 (1963).

[5] F. Arcamone, A. Di Marco, M. Gaetani and T. Scotti, *Giorn. microbiol.,* **9**, 83 (1961).

[6] A. Di Marco, M. Gaetani, P. Orezzi, B. M. Scarpinato, R. Silvestrini, M. Soldati, T. Dasdia and L. Valentini, *Nature,* **201**, 706 (1964).

[7] G. Cassinelli and P. Orezzi, Giorn. *Microbiol.*, **11**, 167 (1963).

[8] S. Pinnert, J. Preud'homme and G. H. Werner, *C.R. Acad. Sci.*, **257**, 1813 (1963).

[9] A. Di Marco, *Path. Biol.,* **15**, 897 (1967).

[10] F. Arcamone, G. Franceschi, P. Orezzi, G. Cassinelli, W. Barbieri and R. Mondelli, *J. Amer. Chem. Soc.*, **86**, 5334 (1964).

[11] F. Arcamone, G. Cassinelli, P. Orezzi, G. Franceschi and R. Mondelli, *J. Amer. Chem. Soc.,* **86**, 5335 (1965).

[12] C. Tan and A. Di Marco, *Proc. Amer. Ass. Cancer Res.,* **6**, 64, abstr. 253 (1965).

[13] J. Bernard, R. Paul, M. Boiron, C. Jacquillat, R. Maral *Recent Results in Cancer Research* (Rubidomycin), Springer Verlag, 1969, Vol. 20.

[14] F. Arcamone, G. Cassinelli, G. Fantini, A. Grein, P. Orezzi, C. Pol and C. Spalla, *Biotech. Bioeng.,* **11**, 1101 (1969).

[15] F. Arcamone, G. Franceschi, S. Penco and A. Selva, *Tetrahedron Letters,* 1007 (1969).

[16] A. Di Marco, M. Gaetini and B. M. Scarpinato, *Cancer Chemother. Rep.,* **53**, 33 (1969).

[17] G. Bonadonna, S. Monfardini, M. De Lena, F. Fossati-Bellani and C. Beretta, *Cancer Res.,* **30**, 2572 (1970).

[18] S. K. Carter, A. Di Marco, M. Ghione, I. H. Krakoff and G. Mathe, *International Symposium on Adriamycin,* Springer Verlag, 1972.

[19] S. K. Carter, *J. Nat. Cancer Inst.,* **55**, 1265 (1975).

[20] R. H. Thomson, *Naturally Occurring Quinones,* Academic Press, p. 536 (1971).

[21] Z. Vanek, J. Tax, I. Komersova, P. Sedmura and J. Vokoun, *Folia Microbiol.,* **22**, 139 (1977).

[22] G. R, Pettit, J. J. Einck, C. L. Herald, R. H. Ode, R. B. Von Dreele, P. Brown, M. L. Brashnikova and G. F. Gause, *J. Amer. Chem. Soc.*, **97**, 7387 (1975).

[23] J. Lunel, J. Preud'homme, Ger. Offen. 1, 911, 240; *C.A.* **72**, 20603 (1970).

[24] F. Arcamone, G. Cassinelli, S. Penco and L. Tognoli, Ger. Offen. 1, 923, 885; *C.A.* **72**, 131086 (1970).

[25] G. Cassinelli, A. Grein, P. Masi, A. Suarato, L. Bernardi, F. Arcamone, A. Di Marco, A. Casazza, G. Pratesi and C. Soranzo, *J. Antibiotics* (Tokyo), **31**, 178 (1978).

[26] Y. Takahashi, H. Nagasawa, T. Takeuchi, H. Umezawa, T. Komiyama, T. Oki, T. Inuri, *J. Antibiotics* (Tokyo), **30**, 622, (1977).

[27] G. B. Fedorova, *Antibiotiki,* **15**, 403 (1970).

[28] P. F. Willey, F. A. MacKellar, E. L. Caron, and R. B. Kelly, *Tetrahedron Letters,* 663 (1968).

[29] a) F. Arcamone, G. Franceschi, P. Orezzi, S. Penco, and R. Mondelli, *Tetrahedron Letters,* 3349 (1968).
b) F. Arcamone, G. Cassinelli, G. Franceschi, P. Orezzi and R. Mondelli, *Tetrahedron Letters,* 3353 (1968).
c) F. Arcamone, G. Cassinelli, G. Franceschi, R. Mondelli, P. Orezzi and S. Penco, *Gazz. Chim. Ital.,* **100**, 949 (1970).

[30] N. R. Bachur, *J. Pharmacol. Exp. Ther.,* **177**, 573 (1971).

[31] H. Hartmann and E. Lorenz, *Z. Naturforsch,* **7A**, 360 (1952).

[32] R. U. Lemieux and E. von Rudloff, *Can. J. Chem.,* **33**, 1711 (1955).

[33] M. I. Brazhnikova, V. B. Zbarsky, V. I. Ponomarenko and N. P. Potapova, *J. Antibiotics* (Tokyo), **27**, 254 (1974).

[34] M. C. Wani, H. L. Taylor, M. E. Wall, A. T. McPhail and K. D. Onan, *J. Amer. Chem. Soc.,* **97**, 5955 (1975).

[35] G. Schroeter, *Ber.* **54**, 2242 (1921).

[36] C. Dufraisse and R. Horclos, *Bull. Soc. Chim. France,* **3**, 1880 (1936).

[37] J. P. Marsh, Jr., R. H. Iwamoto, and L. Goodmann, *Chem. Commun.,* 589 (1968).

[38] C. M. Wong, D. Popien, R. Schwenk and J. Te Raa, *Can. J. Chem.,* **49**, 2712 (1971).

[39] C. M. Wong, R Schwenk, D. Popien and T. Ho, *Can. J. Chem.,* **51**, 466 (1973).

[40] F. Arcamone, L. Bernardi, P. Giardino, B. Patelli, A. Di Marco, A. M. Casazza, G. Pratesi and P. Reggiani, *Cancer Treat. Rep.,* **60**, 829 (1976).

[41] F. Arcamone, L. Bernardi, B. Patelli, P. Giardino, A. Di Marco, A. M. Casazza, C. Goranzo and G. Pratesi, *Experientia*, in press.

[42] D. G. Miller, S. Trenbeath and C. J. Sih, *Tetrahedron Letters,* 1637 (1976).

[43] J. B. Brewster and C. J. Ciotti, *J. Amer. Chem. Soc.,* **77**, 6214 (1955).

[44] R. D. Gleim, S. Trenbeath, R. S. D. Mittal, and C. J. Sih, *Tetrahedron Letters,* 3385 (1976).

[45] P. W. Raynolds, M. J. Manning and J. S. Swenton, *Tetrahedron Letters,* 2283 (1977).

[46] J. Heimann-Trosien, *Ber.* **90**, 1448 (1957).
[47] W. W. Lee, A. P. Martinez, T. H. Smith and D. W. Henry, *J. Org. Chem.*, **41**, 2296 (1976).
[48] K. E. Pfitzner and J. G. Moffat, *J. Amer. Chem. Soc.*, **87**, 5670 (1965).
[49] T. H. Smith, A. N. Fukiwara, D. W. Henry and W. W. Lee, *J. Amer. Chem.*, **98**, 1969 (1976).
[50] A. S. Kende, Y. Tsay and J. E. Mills, *J. Amer. Chem. Soc.*, **98**, 1967 (1976).
[51] T. Ross Kelly, R. N. Goerrner, Jr., J. W. Gillard and B. K. Prazak, *Tetrahedron Letters,* 3869 (1976).
[52] T. Ross Kelly, J. W. Gillard and R. N. Goerrner, Jr., *Tetrahedron Letters,* 3873 (1976).
[53] F. Farina and J. C. Vega, *Tetrahedron Letters,* 1655 (1972).
[54] T. Ross Kelly, J. W. Gillard, R. N. Goerner, Jr., and J. M. Lyding, *J. Amer. Chem. Soc.*, **99**, 5513 (1977).
[55] H. H. Inhoffen, H. Muxfeldt, H. Schaefer and H. Kramer, *Croat. Chem. Acta,* **29**, 329 (1967).
[56] H. Muxfeldt, *Angew. Chem.*, **74**, 825 (1962).
[57] V. H. Powell, *Tetrahedron Letters,* 3462 (1970).
[58] A. J. Birch and V. H. Powell, *Tetrahedron Letters,* 3467 (1970).
[59] A. S. Kende, J. Belletire, T. J. Bentley, E. Home and J. Airey, *J. Amer. Chem. Soc.*, **97**, 4425 (1975).
[60] A. S. Kende, D. P. Curran, Y. Tsay and J. E. Mills, *Tetrahedron Letters,* 3537 (1977).
[61] N. N. Lomakina, I. A. Spiridonova, Yu. N. Shrinker and T. F. Vlassova, *Khim. Prir. Soedin.*, **9**, 101 (1973), C.A. **78**, 14817 (1973).
[62] R. Bognar, F. Sztaricskai, M. F. Munk and J. Thomas, *J. Org. Chem.*, **39**, 2971 (1974).
[63] A. C. Richardson, *Carbohyd. Res.*, **4**, 422 (1967).
[64] R. D. Guthrie and D. Murphy, *J. Chem. Soc.*, 6956 (1965).
[65] H. H. Baer, K. Capek and M. C. Cook, *Can. J. Chem.*, **47**, 89 (1969).
[66] H. H. Baer, *Ber.* **93**, 2865 (1960).
[67] H. H. Baer, *J. Amer. Chem. Soc,*, **83**, 1882 (1961).
[68] H. H. Baer and T. Neilson, *Can J. Chem.*, **43**, 840 (1965).
[69] H. H. Baer, and F. Kienzle, *Can. J. Chem.*, **43**, 3074 (1965).
[70] J. P. Marsh, Jr., C. W. Mosher, E. M. Acton and L. Goodmann, *Chem. Commun.*, 973 (1967).
[71] B. Iselin and T. Reichstein, *Helv. Chim. Acta.*, **27**, 1146 (1943).
[72] D. Hort and W. Weckerle, *Carbohyd. Res.*, **44**, 227 (1975).
[73] A. Klemer and Y. Rodemeyer, *Ber.*, **107**, 2612 (1974).
[74] S. Hanessian, *Carbohyd. Res.*, **2**, 86 (1966).
[75] C. M. Wong, T. Ho, and W. P. Niemxzura, *Can. J. Chem.*, **53**, 3144 (1975).

[76] H. J. Jakobsen, E. H. Larsen, P. Madsden and S. Lawesson, *Arkiv Kemi*, **24**, 519 (1965).
[77] F. Arcamone, S. Penco, A. Vigevani, S. Redaelli, G. Franchi, A. Di Marco A. M. Casazza, T. Dasdia, F. Formelli, A. Necco and C. Soranzo, *J. Med. Chem.*, **18**, 703 (1975).
[78] F. Arcamone, S. Penco, S. Redaelli and S. Hanessian, *J. Med. Chem.*, **19**, 1424 (1976).
[79] S. K. Gupta, *Carbohyd. Res.*, **37**, 381 (1974).
[80] W. W. Lee, H. Y. Wu, J. E. Christensen, L. Goodman, and D. W. Henry, *J. Med. Chem.*, **18**, 768 (1975).
[81] D. C. Jordan and P. E. Reyonds, in *Antiobiotics* (J. W. Corcoran and F. E. Hahn, eds.), Vol. **3**, p. 705, Springer Verlag, 1975.
[82] W. W. Lee, H. Y. Wu, J. J. Marsh, Jr., C. W. Mosher, E. M. Acton, L. Goodman and D. W. Henry, *J. Med. Chem.*, **18**, 767 (1975).
[83] H. Y. Wu, W. W. Lee, T. H. Smith and D. W. Henry, 172nd Nat. Meeting A.C.S., Aug. 29-Sept. 3, 1976, S. Francisco, Cal. Abstr. CARB 098.
[84] F. Sztaricskai, L. Pelyvas, H. Bognar and Gy. Bujtas, *Tetrahedron Letters*, 1111 (1975).
[85] K. Heyns, M. Lim, J. I. Park, *Tetrahedron Letters*, 1477 (1976).
[86] D. M. Clode, D. Horton and W. Weckerle, *Carbohyd. Res.*, **49**, 305 (1976).
[87] J. C. Sowden and H. L. O. Fischer, *J. Amer. Chem. Soc.*, **69**, 1048 (1947).
[88] G. B. Howarth and J. K. N. Jones, *Can. J. Chem.*, **45**, 2253 (1967).
[89] I. W. Hughes, W. G. Overend and M. Stacey, *J. Chem. Soc.*, 2846 (1949).
[90] A. Bargiotti, G. Cassinelli, G. Franchi, B. Gioià, E. Lazzari, S. Redaelli, A. Vigevani, F. Arcamone and S. Hanessian, *Carbohydr. Res.*, **58**, 353 (1977).
[91] J. Kovar, V. Dienstbienova, and J. Jary, *Coll. Czech. Chem. Commun.*, **32**, 2498 (1967).
[92] P. J. Beynon, P. M. Collins and W. G. Overend, *J. Chem. Soc.* (C), 272 (1969).
[93] E. H. Williams, V. A. Szarek and J. K. N. Jones, *Can. J. Chem.*, **47**, 4467 (1969).
[94] F. Arcamone, A. Bargiotti, G. Cassinelli, S. Penco and S. Hanessian, *Carbohydr. Res.*, **46**, C 3 (1976).
[95] J. K. Christensen and L. Goodman, *J. Amer. Chem. Soc.*, **83**, 3827 (1961).
[96] S. Hanessian, M. M. Pompipom and P. Lavallee, *Carbohydr. Res.*, **24**, 45 (1972).
[97] A. Bargiotti, G. Cassinelli and F. Arcamone, *Ger. Offen.* P2,752,115 (Jan. 22, 1977).
[98] B. T. Lawton, W. A. Szarek and J. K. N. Jones, *Carbohyd. Res.*, **10**, 456 (1969).

[99] G. N. Bollenback, *Methods Carbohyd. Chem.*, **2**, 326 (1963).
[100] L. W. Wiggins, *Methods Carbohyd. Chem.*, 2, 188 (1963).
[101] D. Horton and W. Weckerle, *Carbohyd. Res.*, **46**, 227 (1976).
[102] I. Pelyvàs, F. Sztaricskai, R. Bognàr and G. Biutàs, *Carbohyd. Res.*, **53**, C 17 (1977).
[103] H. H. Baer and F. F. Z. Georges, *Carbohyd. Res.*, **55**, 253 (1977).
[104] G. Wulff and G. Röhle, *Angew. Chem.*, **13**, 157 (1974).
[105] R. U. Lemieux, *Adv. Carbohyd. Chem.*, **9**, 1 (1954).
[106] S. Penco, *Chim. Ind.*, (Milan) **50**, 908 (1968).
[107] W. L. Evans, D. D. Reynolds and E. A. Tolley, *Adv. Carbohyd. Chem.*, **6**, 27 (1951).
[108] W. W. Zorbach and K. V. Bhat, *Adv. Carbohyd. Chem.*, **21**, 273 (1966).
[109] E. M. Acton, A. N. Fujiwara and D. W. Henry, *J. Med. Chem.*, **17**, 659 (1974).
[110] F. Arcamone, S. Penco and A. Vigevani, *Cancer Chemotherapy Rep.*, Part 3, **6**, 123 (1975).
[111] W. G. Overend, in 'The Carbohydrates' (W. Pigman and D. Horton, eds.), Academic Press, New York and London, Vol. **1A**, p. 279, 1972.
[112] G. Cassinelli, French Patent 2, 183, 710 (Dec. 21, 1972).
[113] R. J. Ferrier, *Adv. Carbohyd. Chem.*, **20**, 67 (1965).
[114] F. Arcamone and G. Cassinelli, U.S. Patent 4,020,270 (Apr. 26, 1977).
[115] F. Arcamone, A. Bargiotti, G. Cassinelli, S. Redaelli, S. Hanessian, A. Di Marco, A. M. Casazza, T. Dasdia, A. Necco, P. Reggiani and L. Supino, *J. Med. Chem.*, **19**, 733 (1976).
[116] P. J. L. Daniels, A. K. Mallams, and J. J. Wright, *Chem. Commun.*, 675 (1973).
[117] F. J. Krouzer and C. Schaerch, *Carbohyd. Res.*, **27**, 372 (1973).
[118] S. Hanessian and J. Bonoub, *Carbohyd. Res.*, **44**, C14 (1975).
[119] F. Arcamone, A. Bargiotti, A. Di Marco and S. Penco, *Ger. Offen.* 2618822 (Nov. 11, 1976); *C.A.* **86**, 140416 (1977).
[120] A. Di Marco, A. M. Casazza, F. Giuliani, G. Pratesi, F. Arcamone, L. Bernardi, G. Franchi, P. Giardino, B. Patelli and S. Penco, *Cancer Treat. Rep.*, **62**, 375 (1978).
[121] F. Arcamone, L. Bernardi, B. Patelli and S. Penco, Belg. Pat. 842,930 (Oct. 1, 1976); *C.A.* **87**, 8501 (1977).
[122] H. Brockmann and B. Franck, *Chem. Ber.*, **88**, 1972 (1955).
[123] D. L. Kern, R. H. Bunge, J. C. French and H. W. Dion, *J. Antibiotics* (Tokyo), **30**, 432 (1977).
[124] T. H. Smith, A. N. Fujiwara and D. W. Henry, *172nd Nat. Meeting of ACS*, Aug. 29–Sept. 3, 1976, S. Francisco, Cal., Abstr. MEDI-88.
[125] H. S. El Khadem, D. L. Swartz and R. C. Cermak, *J. Med. Chem.*, **20**, 957 (1977).

[126] F. Arcamone, W. Barbieri, G. Franceschi and S. Penco, *Chim. Ind.* (Milan), **51**, 834 (1969).
[127] F. Arcamone, G. Franceschi and S. Penco, Ger. Offen. 1,917,874 (Nov. 6, 1969); *C.A.* **73**, 45799 (1970).
[128] F. Arcamone, G. Cassinelli, G. Franceschi, S. Penco, C. Pol, S. Redaelli and A. Selva, in 'International Symposium on Adriamycin' (S. K. Carter, A. Di Marco, M. Ghione, I. N. Krakoff and G. Mathé, eds.), p. 9, Springer Verlag, Berlin, 1972.
[129] S. Penco, G. P. Vacario, A. Angelucci and F. Arcamone, *J. Antibiotics* (Tokyo), **30**, 773 (1977).
[130] B. R. Vishnuvajjala, T. Kataoka, F. D. Lazer, D. T. Witiak and L. Malspeis, *J. Lab. Comp.*, **14**, 77 (1978).
[131] C. Tong, W. W. Lee, D. R. Black and D. W. Henry, *J. Med. Chem.*, **19**, 395 (1976).
[132] T. R. Smith, A. N. Fujiwara, D. W. Henry and W. W. Lee, *J. Amer. Chem. Soc.*, **98**, 1970 (1976).
[133] C. R. Chen, M. Tan Fong, A. N. Fujiwara, D. W. Henry, M. A. Leaffer, W. W. Lee and T. H. Smith, *J. Lab. Comp.*, **14**, 111 (1978).
[134] G. Jolles and G. Ponsinet, Ger. Offen. 2,202,690 (July 27, 1972); *C.A.* **77**, 164320 (1972).
[135] A. Suarato, P. Masi, L. Bernardi and F. Arcamone, *Gen. Offen.*, P2,804, 099 (Jan. 31, 1978).
[136] R. Pettit, Arizona State University, Temple, Arizona, USA: personal communication.
[137] K. Yamamoto, E. M. Acton and D. W. Henry, *J. Med. Chem.*, **15**, 872 (1972).
[138] G. Jolles, Ger. Offen. 1,803,892 (May 29, 1969; *C.A.* **71**, 70907 (1969).
[139] G. Jolles, Ger. Offen. 2,327,211 (May 28, 1963; *C.A.* **82**, 171381 (1975).
[140] Rhône-Poulenc, Belg. Pat. 839,540 (Sept. 23, 1976).
[141] D. W. Wilson, D. Grier, R. Reimer, J. D. Bauman, J. F. Preston and E. J. Gabbay, *J. Med. Chem.*, **49**, 381 (1976).
[142] J. Bouchandon and J. Jolles, Ger. Offen, 1,813,518 (July 10, 1969); *C.A.* **71**, 91866 (1969).
[143] F. Arcamone, G. Franceschi, A. Minghetti, S. Penco, S. Redaelli, A. Di Marco, A. M. Casazza, T. Dasdia, G. Di Fronzo, F. Giuliani, L. Lenaz, A. Necco, and C. Soranzo, *J. Med Chem.*, **17**, 335 (1974).
[144] B. Patelli, L. Bernardi, F. Armacone and A. Di Marco, Ger. Offen. 2,627,146 (Dec. 30, 1976); *C.A.* **86**, 190419 (1977).
[145] F. Arcamone, L. Bernardi, B. Pateli and A. Di Marco, Ger. Offen. 2,557,537 (July 8, 1976); *C.A.* **85**, 177886 (1976).
[146] M. Israel, E. J. Modest and E. Frei III, *Cancer Res.*, **35**, 1365 (1975).
[147] S. Penco, F. Angelucci, A. Vigevani, E. Arlandini and F. Arcamone, *J. Antibiotics* (Tokyo) **30**, 1722 (1977).

[148] P. Masi, A. Suarato, P. Giardino, L. Bernardi and F. Arcamone, *Gen. Offen.*, P2,735,455 (Aug. 5, 1977).

[149] L. Bernardi, P. Masi, A. Suarato and F. Arcamone, *Belg. Pat.*, 860,782 (Nov. 20, 1977).

[150] J. H. Birkinshaw, *Biochem. J.*, **59**, 485 (1955).

[151] H. G. Brazhnikova, V. B. Zbarskiy, M. M. Kudinova, L. I. Muravyeva, V. I. Potomarenko and N. P. Potapoya, *Antibiotiki,* **18**, 678 (1973).

[152] E. Calendi, A. Di Marco, M. Reggiani, B. Scarpinato, and L. Valentini. *Biochim. Biophys. Acta.*, **103**, 25 (1965).

[153] F. Arcamone, G. Cassinelli, A. Di Marco and M. Gaetani, U.S. Patent 3,590,028 (June 29, 1971).

[154] R. H. Iwamoto, P. Lim and N. S. Bhacca, *Tetrahedron Letters,* 3891 (1969).

[155] K. Karnetova, J. Mateju, P. Sedmera, J. Vokoun, and Z. Vanek, *J. Antibiotics* (Tokyo), **29**, 1199 (1976).

[156] A. Vigevani, B. Gioia and G. Cassallini, *Carbohyd Res.*, **32**, 321 (1974).

[157] V. Casu, M. Reggiani and G. G. Gallo and A. Vigevani, *Tetrahedron Letters*, 803 (1968).

[158] S. A. Barker, J. Homer, M. C. Keith and L. F. Thomas, *J. Chem. Soc.*, 1538 (1963).

[159] A. Arnone, G. Fronza, R. Mondelli and A. Vigevani, *Tetrahedron Letters,* 3349 (1976).

[160] R. C. Paulick, M. L. Casey and H. W. Whitlock, *J. Amer. Chem Soc.*, **98**, 3370 (1976).

[161] H. Budzikiewicz, C. Djerassi, and D. H. Williams, in 'Structure elucidation of natural products by mass spectrometry', Holden-Day Inc., San Francisco, London, Amsterdam, Vol. 2 (1964), p. 241.

[162] R. I. Reed and W. K. Reid, *Tetrahedron,* **19**, 1817 (1963).

[163] H. Brockmann, J. Niemeyer, H. Brockmann, Jr., H. Budzikiewicz, *Chem. Ber.*, **98**, 3785 (1965).

[164] H. Brockmann, J. Niemeyer and W. Rode, *Chem. Ber.*, **98**, 3145 (1965).

[165] P. P. Roller, M. Sutphin and A. A. Aszalos, *Biomed. Mass Spectrim.*, **3**, 166 (1976).

[166] H. D. Beckey and H. R. Schulten, *Agnew. Chem.*, **14**, 403 (1975).

[167] H. Brockmann, Jr., and M. Legrand, *Tetrahedron Letters,* 395 (1963).

[168] H. Brockmann, H. Brockmann, Jr. and J. Niemeyer, *Tetrahedron Letters,* 4719 (1968).

[169] R. Angiuli, E. Foresti, L. Riva di Sanseverino, N. W. Isaacs, O. Kennard, W. D. S. Motherwell, D. L. Wamplu and F. Arcamone, *Nature New Biol.*, **234**, 78 (1971).

[170] V. Barthelemy-Clavey, J. C. Maurizot, J. L. Dimicoli and P. Sicard, *FEBS Letters,* **46**, 5 (1974).

[171] R. J. Sturgeon and S. G. Schulman, *J. Pharmac. Sci.,* **66**, 958 (1977).

[172] K. Mailer, and D. H. Petering, *Biochem. Pharmacol.,* **25**, 2085 (1976).

[173] A. Di Marco, F. Arcamone and F. Zunino, in 'Antibiotics' (J. W. Corcoran and F. E. Hahn, eds.), vol. III, p. 101. Springer-Verlag, Berlin, Heidelberg, New York, 1974.
[174] A. Di Marco, F. Zunino, R. Silvestrini, C. Gambarucci and R. A. Gambetta, *Biochem. Pharmacol.*, **20**, 1323 (1971).
[175] G. Scatchard, *Ann. N.Y. Acad. Sci.*, **51**, 660 (1949).
[176] F. Zunino, R. Gambetta, A. Di Marco and A. Zaccara, *Biochim. Biophys. Acta*, **277**, 489 (1972).
[177] E. J. Gabbay, D. Grier, R. E. Fingerle, R. Reimer, R. Levy, S. W. Pearce, and W. D. Wilson, *Biochemistry*, **15**, 2062 (1976).
[178] Y. M. Huang and D. R. Phillips, *Biophys. Chem.*, **6**, 363 (1977).
[179] F. Zunino, R. Gambetta, A. Di Marco, G. Luoni and A. Zaccara, *Biochim. Biophys. Res. Comm.*, **69**, 744 (1976).
[180] F. Zunino, R. Gambetta, A. Di Marco, A. Valcich, A. Zacarra, F. Quadrifoglio and V. Crescenzi, *Biochim. Biophys. Acya.*, **476**, 38 (1977).
[181] V. Barthelemy-Clavey, J. Maurizot and P. J. Sicard, *Biochimie*, **55**, 859 (1973).
[182] D. G. Dalgleish, G. Fey, and W. Kersten, *Biopolymers*, **13**, 1757 (1974).
[183] J. Doskocil and I. Fric, *FEBS Letters*, **37**, 55 (1973).
[184] H. Berg and K. Eckardt, *Z. Naturforsch.*, **26b**, 362 (1970).
[185] E. Arlandini, A. Vigevani and F. Arcamone, *Farmaco (Pavia) Ed. Sci.*, **32**, 315 (1977).
[186] W. J. Pigram, W. Fuller and L. D. Hamilton, *Nature New Biol.*, **235**, 17 (1972).
[187] F. Quadrifoglio and V. Crescenzi, *Biophys. Chem.*, **2**, 64 (1974).
[188] A. Di Marco, A. M. Casazza, R. Gambetta, R. Supino and F. Zunino, *Cancer Res.*, **36**, 1962 (1976).
[189] W. Kernsten and H. Kernsten, *Biochem. Zeitschr.*, **341**, 174 (1975).
[190] W. Kernsten, H. Kernsten and W. Szybalsky, *Biochemistry*, **5**, 236 (1966).
[191] F. Zunino, *FEBS Letters*, **18**, 249 (1971).
[192] M. J. Waring, *J. Mol. Biol.*, **54**, 247 (1970).
[193] B. M. J. Revet, M. Schmir and J. Vinograd, *Nature New Biol.*, **235**, 10 (1971).
[194] J. M. Saucier, B. Festy and J. B. Le-Pecq, *Biochemie*, **53**, 973 (1971).
[195] F. Dall'Acqua, M. Terboievich, S. Marciani, D. Vedaldi and G. Rodighiero, *Farmaco (Pavia) Ed. Sci.*, **29**, 682 (1974).
[196] R. K. Neogy, K. Chowdhury and I. Kerr, *Biochim. Biophys. Acta*, **374**, 96 (1974).
[197] H. Hikuchi and S. Sato, *Biochim, Biophys. Acta*, **434**, 509 (1976).
[198] A. Di Marco, *Cancer Chemother. Rep. Part 3*, **6**, 91 (1975).
[199] C. Na and S. N. Timasheff, *Arch. Biochem. Biophys. Acta.*, **182**, 147 (1977).

[200] R. B.Nikkelsen, P. Lin and D. F. H. Wallach, *J. Mol. Med.*, **2**, 33 (1977).

[201] M. Duarte-Karim, J. M. Ruysschaert and J. Hildebrand, *Biochem. Biophys. Res. Comm.*, **71**, 658 (1976).

[202] M. Menozzi and F. Arcamone, *Biochem. Biophys. Res. Commun.*, **80**, 313 (1978).

[203] C. P. Dietrich, L. O. Sarupaio, O. M. S. Toledo and C. M. F. Cassaro, *Biochem. Biophys. Res. Comm.*, **75**, 329 (1977).

[204] A. Rusconi, G. Di Fronzo and A. Di Marco, *Cancer Chemother. Rep.* **52**, 331 (1968).

[205] G. Di Fronzo and R. Gambetta, *Europ. J. Clin. Biol. Res.*, **16**, 50 (1971).

[206] G. Di Fronzo and G. Bonadonna, *Europ. J. Clin. Biol. Res.*, **15**, 314 (1970).

[207] G. Di Fronzo, R. A. Gambetta and L. Lenaz, *Europ. J. Clin. Biol. Res.*, **16**, 572 (1971).

[208] L. Lenaz and G. Di Fronzo, *Tumori,* **58**, 213 (1972).

[209] G. Di Fronzo, L. Lenaz and G. Bonadonna, *Biomedicine,* **19**, 169 (1973).

[210] A. Rusconi and A. Di Marco, *Cancer Res.*, **29**, 1507 (1969).

[211] P. M. Wilkinson and G. E. Mawer, *Brit. J. Clin. Pharmacol.*, **1**, 241 (1974).

[212] R. H. Liss, D. W. Yesair, J. D. Schepis and I. C. Harenchic, AACR Abstracts, 884 (1977).

[213] J. M. Finkel, K. T. Knapp, and L. T. Mulligan, *Cancer Chemother. Rep. Part 1,* **53**, 159 (1969).

[214] N. R. Bachur, A. L. Moore, J. G. Bernstein and A. Liu, *Cancer Chemother. Rep. Part 1,* **54**, 89 (1970).

[215] D. S. Alberts, N. R. Bachur and J. L. Holtzman, *Clin. Pharmacol. Ther.*, **12**, 96 (1971).

[216] J. C. Cradock, M. J. Egorin and N. R. Bachur, *Arch. int. Pharmacodyn. Ther.*, **202**, 48 (1973).

[217] N. R. Bachur, R. C. Hildebrand and R. S. Jaenke, *J. Pharmacol. Exp. Ther.*, **191**, 331 (1974).

[218] R. S. Benjamin, C. E. Riggs and N. R. Bachur, *Clin. Pharmacol. Ther.*, **14**, 592 (1973).

[219] M. A. Picone and A. Traina, *Arzneim. Forsch.*, **20**, 88 (1970).

[220] L. Dusonchet, M. Gebbia and F. Gerbasi, *Pharmacol. Res. Comm.*, **3**, 55 (1971)

[221] R. Mhatre, E. Herman, A. Huldobro and V. Waravdekar, *J. Pharmacol. Exp. Ther.*, **178**, 216 (1971).

[222] R. M. Mhatre, E. H. Herman, V. S. Waravdekar and I. P. Lee, *Biochem. Med.*, **6**, 445 (1972).

[223] N. R. Bachur, M. J. Egorin and R. C. Hildebrand, *Biochem. Med.*, **8**, 353 (1973).

[224] K. K. Chan and P. A. Harris, *Res. Commun. Chem. Path. Pharmacol.*, **6**, 447 (1973).

[225] H. S. Schwartz, *Biochem. Med.,* **7**, 396 (1973).
[226] A. Rusconi, *Biochim. Biophys. Acta.,* **123**, 627 (1966).
[227] D. Kessel, V. Botterill and C. Wodinsky, *Cancer Res.,* **28**, 938 (1968).
[228] H. Van Vunakis, J. J. Langone, L. F. Riceberg and L. Levine, *Cancer Res.,* **34**, 2540 (1974).
[229] J. J. Langone, H. Van Vunakis and N. R. Bachur, *Biochem. Med.,* **12**, 283 (1975).
[230] R. Hulhoven and J. P. Desager, *J. Chromatograph.,* **125**, 369 (1976).
[231] L. A. Sternson and Y. Thomas, *Anal. Lett.,* **10**, 99 (1977).
[232] N. R. Bachur and J. C. Cradock, *J. Pharmacol. Exp. Ther.,* **175**, 331 (1971).
[233] N. R. Bachur and M. Gee, *J. Pharmacol. Exp. Ther.,* **17**, 567 (1971).
[234] N. R. Bachur, *Biochem. Pharmacol.,* **23**, Suppl. 2, 207 (1974).
[235] N. R. Bachur and D. H. Huffman, *Brit. J. Pharmac.,* **43**, 828 (1971).
[236] R. L. Felsted, M. Gee and N. R. Bachur, *J. Biol. Chem.,* **249**, 3672 (1974).
[237] R. L. Felsted, D. R. Richter and N. R. Bachur, *Biochem. Pharmacol.,* **26**, 1117 (1977).
[238] A. J. Turner and P. E. Hick, *Biochem. J.,* **159**, 819 (1976).
[239] A. Di Marco, G. Boretti and A. Rusconi, *Farmaco (Pavia) Ed. Sci.,* **22**, 535 (1967).
[240] M. A. Asbell, R. Schwartzbach, F. J. Bullock and D. W. Yesair, *J. Pharmacol. Exp. Ther.,* **182**, 63 (1972).
[241] F. J. Bullock, R. J. Bruni and M. A. Asbell, *J. Pharmacol. Exp. Ther.,* **182**, 70 (1972).
[242] D. W. Yesair and S. McNitt, *Z. Physiol. Chem.,* **357**, 1066 (1976).
[243] S. Takanashi and N. R. Bachur, *Proc. Amer. Assoc. Cancer Res.,* **15**, 76 (1974).
[244] S. Takanashi and N. R. Bachur, *Drug Metabolism and Disposition,* **4**, 79 (1976).
[244]a R. S. Benjamin, C. E. Riggs, Jr. and N. R. Bachur, *Cancer Res.,* **37**, 1416 (1977).
[245] D. H. Huffman, R. S. Benjaimin and N. R. Bachur, *Clin. Pharmacol. Ther.,* **13**, 895 (1972).
[246] D. H. Huffman and N. R. Bachur, *Blood,* **39**, 637 (1972).
[247] J. Florent, J. Lunel and J. Renaut, Ger. Offen. 2,546, 139 (May 28, 1975). *C.A.* **83**, 112355 (1975).
[248] J. Florent and J. Lunel, Ger. Offen. 2,610557 (Sept. 23, 1976).
[249] D. L. Kern, R. H. Bunge, J. C. French and H. W. Dion, *J. Antibiotics* (Tokyo), **30**, 432 (1977).
[250] V. P. Marshall, E. A. Reisender and P. F. Wiley, *J. Antibiotics* (Tokyo), **29**, 966 (1976).
[251] A. A. Aszalos, N. R. Bachur, B. K. Hamilton, A. F. Langlykke, P. P.

Roller, M. Y. Sheikh, M. S. Sutphin, M. C. Thomas, D. A. Wareheim and L. H. Wright, *J. Antibiotics* (Tokyo), **30**, 50 (1977).

[252] V. P. Marshall, E. A. Reisender, J. H. Johnson and P. F. Wiley, *Biochemistry,* **15**, 5139 (1976).

[253] M. McCarville and V. Marshall, *Biochem. Biophys. Res. Commun.*, **74**, 331 (1977).

[254] B. K. Hamilton, M. S. Sutphin, M. C. Thomas, D. A. Wareheim and A. A. Aszalos, *J. Antibiotics* (Tokyo), **30**, 425 (1977).

[255] R. Supino, A. M. Casazza and A. Di Marco, *Tumori,* **63**, 31 (1977).

[256] A. M. Casazza, A. M. Isetta, F. Guiliani and A. Di Marco, in *Adriamycin Review,* an EORTC Int. Symp., European Press Medikon, Ghent, Belgium, p. 123, 1975.

[257] A. Di Marco, A. M. Casazza, T. Dasdia, F. Giuliani, L. Lenaz, A. Necco and C. Soranzo, *Cancer Chemother. Rep.,* Part 1, **57**, 269 (1973).

[258] F. Arcamone, *Lloydia,* **40**, 45 (1977).

[259] L. Lenaz, A. Necco, T. Dasdia and A. Di Marco, *Cancer Chemother. Rep.,* Part 1, **56**, 769 (1974).

[260] R. Maral, G. Ponsinet and G. Jolles, *C. R. Acad. Sci.* (Paris), **275**, 301 (1972).

[261] F. Arcamone, A. Di Marco and A. M. Casazza, paper presented at the *Eighth Int. Symp. of Princess Takamatsu Cancer Res. Fund,* Tokyo, Nov. 15-18, 1977.

[262] A. Di Marco, A. M. Casazza and G. Pratesi, *Cancer Treat. Rep.,* **61**, 893 (1977).

[263] F. Formelli, A. Di Marco, A. M. Casazza, G. Pratesi, R. Supino and A. Mariani, paper presented at the 10th Int. Congr. of Chemotherapy, Zurich, Switzerland, Sept. 18-23, 1977.

# PART D

# INTERACTIONS OF DAUNOMYCIN AND RELATED ANTIBIOTICS WITH BIOLOGICAL RECEPTORS

by

**STEPHEN NEIDLE**
DEPARTMENT OF BIOPHYSICS
UNIVERSITY OF LONDON KINGS'S COLLEGE

## PART D

## CONTENTS

## 1 INTRODUCTION

The antibiotic daunomycin (**1**), isolated from strains of *Streptomyces peucetius*, is highly cytotoxic against both normal and cancerous cells. It is clinically useful in the treatment of acute lymphocytic leukemia. The 14-hydroxy derivative (**2**), known as adriamycin, is also active against leukemia; however its spectrum of activity is much greater. Thus, a variety of solid tumours have shown significant responses to adriamycin, including some that have been previously relatively unresponsive to chemotherapy [1].

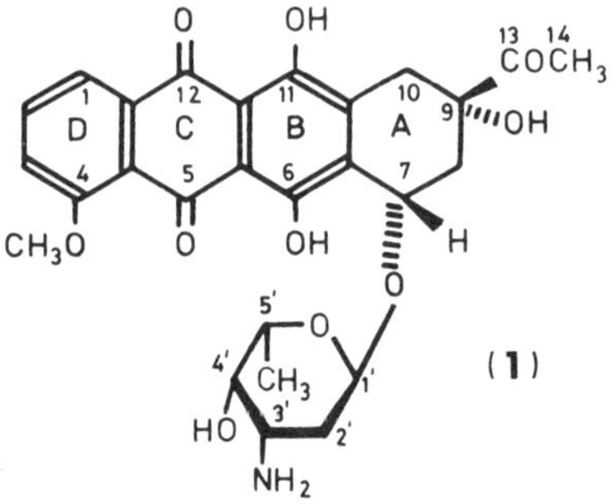

It is generally recognised [2] that the most sensitive targets for the inhibition of rapidly proliferating neoplastic cells, are those molecules involved in aspects of DNA function, especially DNA itself. It is therefore unsurprising that most clinically-useful anti-cancer compounds act against such targets. Daunomycin, adriamycin and their derivatives are believed to exert their primary effect in this way [3, 4], although it must be emphasised that a variety of others have been noted (see section 6). Indeed, in view of the multifunctional chemistry of these antibiotics, it would be surprising if the *in vivo* mechanisms of action were other than complex. Nonetheless, the most plausible hypothesis for the action of the anthracycline anti-cancer agents, remains that they act by directly blocking DNA function, by means of drug-nucleic acid (DNA) binding interactions [5, 6]. Not the least of the attractions of such a hypothesis is that there exists a large body of detailed structural information at the molecular level concerning nucleic acids, and in particular DNA [7]. This may be called upon to define receptor interactions to a level unsurpassed by almost all other classes of drugs and antibiotics.

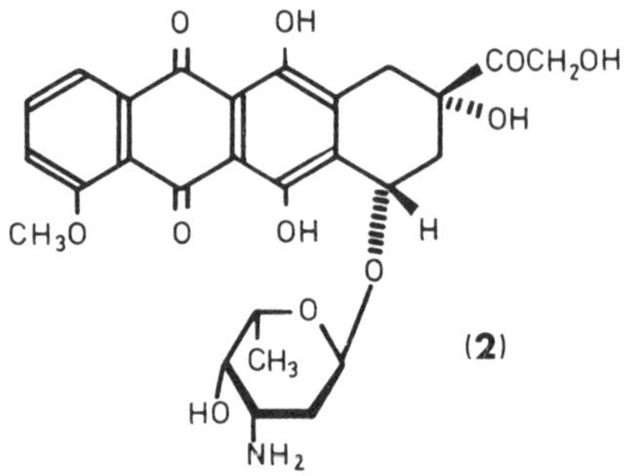

## 2 BIOLOGICAL ACTION

The *in vitro* growth of a number of normal and neoplastic cell lines is markedly inhibited by daunomycin and adriamycin [3, 8]. This inhibition is characterised by cell damage, chiefly to the nucleus. Phase contrast and electron microscopy, and audioradiography, have shown that chromosomal binding and damage is the primary effect.

Important consequences of this cellular uptake are inhibition of both RNA [9-13] and DNA [14, 15] synthesis, in both cell cultures and intact animals, as well as in cell-free systems. It is apparent from studies of isolated polymerase systems that the inhibitions are not due to drug-polymerase interactions. Thus, with *E. coli* DNA-dependent RNA polymerase [9], the inhibition is independent of polymerase concentration, and is consistent with drug-template (i.e. DNA) binding. This conclusion is in accord with results on intact L1210 mouse leukemia cells [10], which also showed that DNA and RNA metabolism were inhibited to the same extent.

A comparative analysis of the inhibitory effects of daunomycin and adriamycin on various DNA polymerases [14] has shown that the effect is most marked for the enzyme from murine sarcoma virus, with template inhibition being predominant. The binding of adriamycin to DNA, as implicated in a detailed study of the kinetics of DNA synthesis directed by DNA polymerase from T4 bacteriophage-infected *E. coli* [15], has revealed two distinct modes of enzyme inhibition, uncompetitive and competitive, at low and high drug: DNA ratios, respectively.

In general, it has been found that the extent of inhibition of nucleic acid synthesis in a suitable test system, can often be correlated with biological activity against experimental tumours. Table 2.1 details such data accumulated for a number of derivatives of daunomycin. Due to differences between test systems, not all the data are quantitatively comparable.

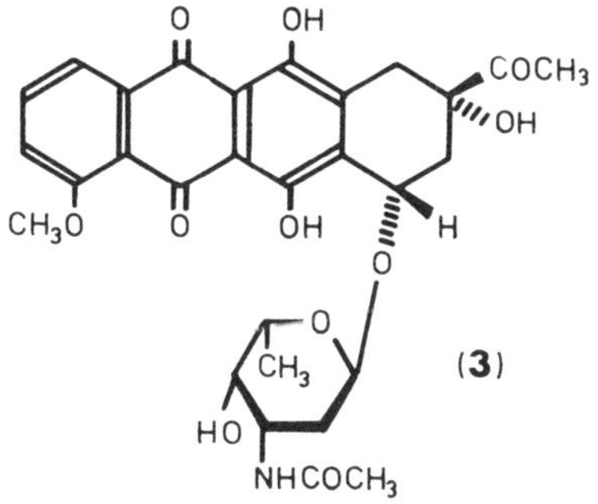

(3)

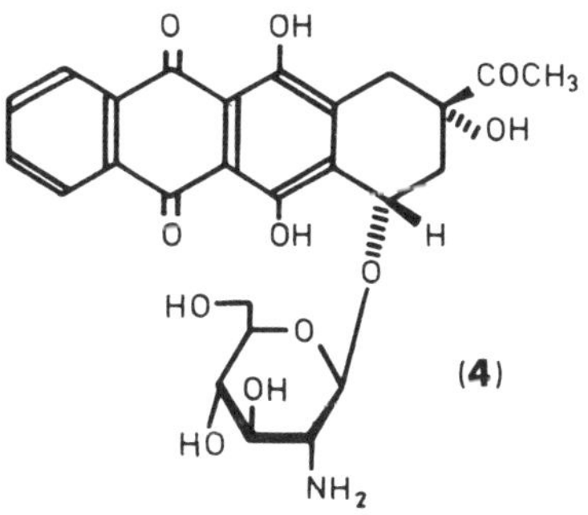

(4)

**Table 2.1** Biological Activity of some Daunomycin Derivatives

| Compound | Dose required for 50% inhibition of DNA synthesis (M × $10^6$) | Average survival time[c] for S ascites experimental tumour |
|---|---|---|
| Daunomycin (1) | 1.6[a] | 222[a] |
| Adriamycin (2) | 3.4[a] | 227[a] |
| 13-Dihydrodaunomycin | 8.8[a] | 231[a] |
| Daunomycin 13-semi-carbazone | >8.5[a] | |
| Daunomycin 13-oxime | >8.6[a] | 130[a] |
| N-Acetyl-daunomycin (3) | >8.3[a] | 100[?a, d] |
| N-Guanidine-acetyl-daunomycin | >7.6[a] | 100[a] |
| Adriamycin 14-octanoate | | 250[b] |
| Adriamycin 14-acetate | | 252[b] |
| 2-Amino-2-deoxyglucosyl-daunomycinone (4) | 8.8 | 107[a] |
| 4,-Epi-daunomycin (5) | 9[e] | 234[f] |
| β-Anomer of adriamycin | >40[e] | |
| β-Anomer of 4′-epi-daunomycin (6) | >40[e] | 126[f] |
| 4-Demethoxydaunomycin | | 264[g] |
| N-Trifluoroacetyladriamycin 14-valerate | >50[h] | >400[i] |
| Daunomycin 13-benzhydrazone (rubidazone) | 2.0[i] | |

*a* From refs, [3, 8]. *b* From ref. [4]. *c* Average survival times as percentage of controls. *d* From ref. [16]; results are for the inhibition of growth of Rous Sarcoma Virus. *e* From ref. [17]. Note that this study reports values of 6 and 8 μM for adriamycin and daunomycin 50% inhibition of RNA polymerase (contrast ref. [3]. Values given here are thus not strictly comparable with other in the table). *f* From ref. [19]: optimum dosage average survival times are given. *g* From ref. [20]. *h* From ref. [21]. *i* From ref. [22]: this represents a median percentage increase in survival time for both P388 and L1210 leukemia. *j* From ref. [18].

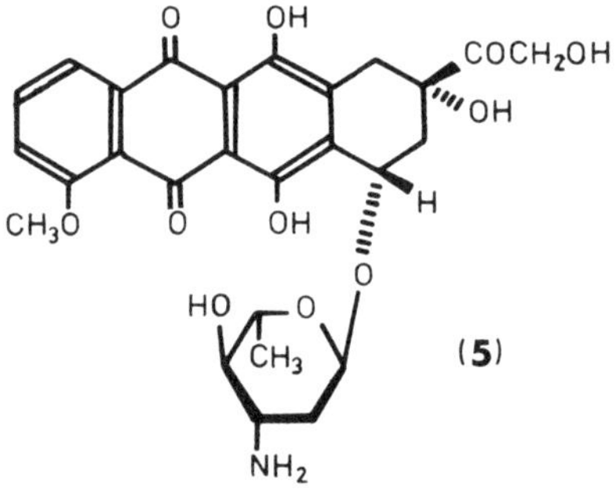

(5)

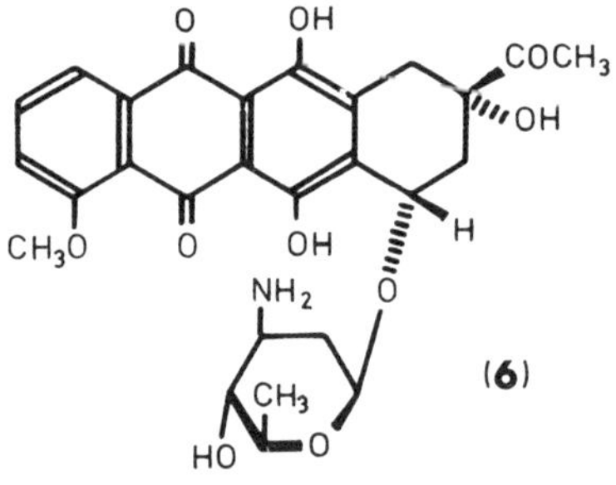

(6)

## 3 STUDIES ON NUCLEIC ACID BINDING

### 3.1 Interactions with DNA

On the basis of evidence such as that outlined above, it is generally accepted that nuclear double-stranded DNA is the prime cellular receptor for daunomycin and adriamycin. This hypothesis has prompted a large number of physico-chemical studies aimed at elucidating the nature of the binding involved. The variety of methods employed fall into two principal categories: (i) those that follow changes (chiefly spectroscopic) in antibiotic properties and (ii) those that monitor changes in the properties of the polynucleotide. At this point, a note of caution must be given: it is not apparent from the literature that all investigators have satisfactorily purified their DNA from nucleoprotein, or have sonicated the purified DNA, to obtain homogenenous DNA essential for accurate hydrodynamic and other studies. Moreover, a wide variety of buffering and ionic strength conditions have been employed. This all serves to ensure that reliable comparisons of experimental data cannot easily be made.

#### 3.1.1 *Changes in antibiotic properties*

(a) *The ultraviolet and visible absorption spectrum.* A marked decrease in the 480 nm visible absorbance of daunomycin has been observed when DNA is added, together with a shift to a higher wavelength (505nm at a DNA: daunomycin molar ratio of 7:1) [23, 24]. The maxima at 233 and 255 nm in the ultra-

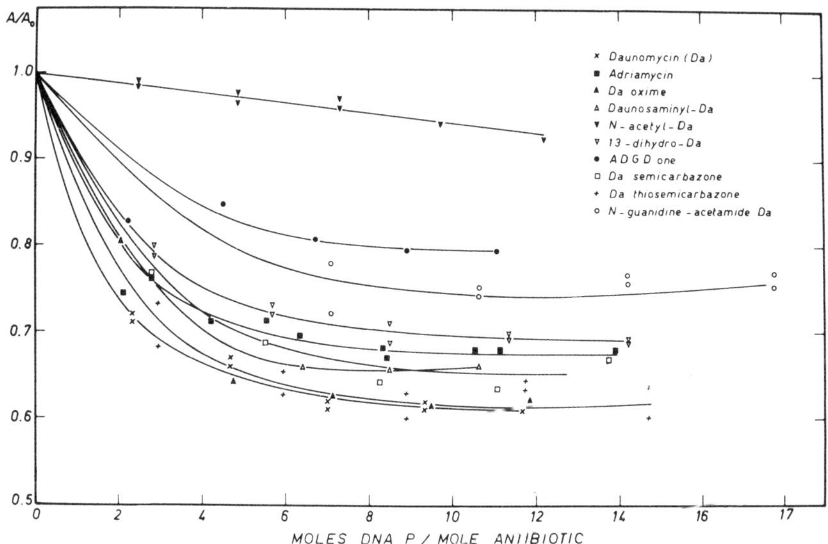


**Figure 3.1** The effect of calf thymus on the 480 nm absorption maximum of daunomycin and various derivatives. The antibiotics were at 0.5 × $10^{-4}$M concentration, buffered at pH7. AFGDone is derivative (4). (Reproduced with permission from Zunino *et al.*, *Biochem. Pharmacology*, **20**, 1323 (1971)).

violet similarly decrease in intensity, and shift in wavelength, to produce a single maximum at 257 nm. Monitoring of the 480 nm absorbance has frequently been employed when examining derivatives of daunomycin; as Figure 3.1 shows, a very wide variation of behaviour has been observed [24, 25], with daunomycin itself showing a maximal effect, and the N-acetyl derivative a minimal one.

In order to investigate these bindings quantitatively, the Scatchard plot procedure has been used [26], which essentially applies the law of mass-action to determine the binding (association) constant, and the number of binding sites per DNA nucleotide – this convenient method (albeit sometimes slightly modified) has been used to obtain these binding parameters from all the different experimental approaches discussed in this article. The Scatchard plots obtained are invariably non-linear, indicating that there is more than one distinct type of binding site on the DNA; it is, however possible, to fit a straight line to at least part of the data, and so obtain binding parameters.

(b) *Fluorescence properties.* The characteristic fluorescence of the dauno-

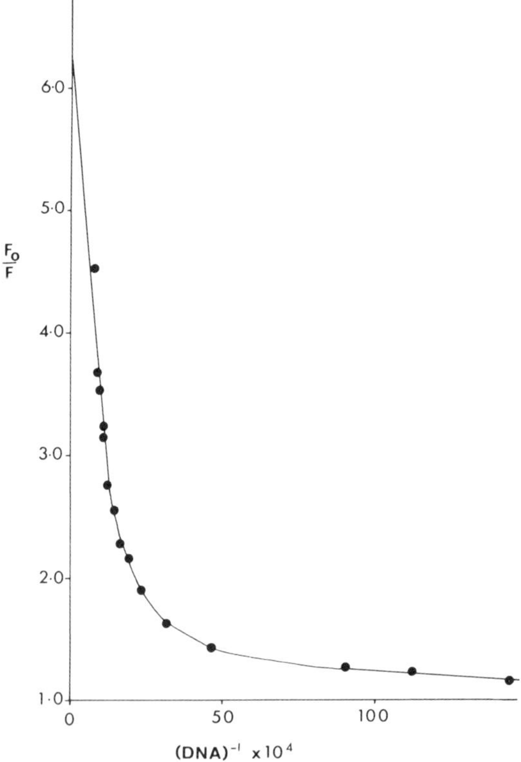


**Figure 3.2** The reduction in the fluorescence emission from daunomycin (at 555 nm) with increasing DNA concentration [43]. The drug concentration was 1.155 $\times 10^{-6}$M.;

mycin antibiotics, due to the anthracycline chromophore, is markedly quenched when binding to DNA takes place [17, 23, 27, 28] (Figure 3.2). Although the binding curves so obtained are perhaps less straightforward to analyse than the visible absorbance curves, they do have a very considerable advantage over the latter is that they can be performed with much reduced quantities of material. This is especially useful when daunomycin derivatives can be obtained only in small amounts, after lengthy syntheses.

(c) *Other changes.* Circular dichroism studies [29-31] have shown that interaction of daunomycin with DNA produces characteristic alterations in the drug's CD spectrum (such as intensification of the broad weak positive 440–480 nm band), which do vary somewhat with the drug/DNA ratio [29]. Differing behaviour with various derivatives have also been noted [30], although it is difficult to quantify these. These CD spectral alterations have been considered to be *not* comparable to those obtained with DNA and aminoacridines [29].

Other techniques have been but little-used; this is perhaps surprising since results of mechanistic significance have been obtained in these few instances where they have been employed. Polarographic studies [23] have shown that the characteristic polarographic reduction of the quinone of the chromophore, was almost completely inhibited on binding daunomycin to DNA; as we shall subsequently see, this result is of significance for a physical model of the binding. A study of the elution behaviour of daunomycin on DNA-cellulose columns has directly shown [32] that there are two distinct types of binding sites, with three-quarters of the drug being eluted by 2M sodium chloride, and the rest by 7M urea as well.

### 3.1.2 *Changes in DNA properties*

The hydrodynamic properties of nucleic acids are, in general, well understood [33]. Thus, the physical changes that occur when daunomycin and its derivatives are bound to DNA can often be correlated with a meaningful physical picture of the complex.

(a) *Intrinsic viscosity.* Complexation of DNA with increasing amounts of daunomycin causes a progressive increase in the relative viscosity of the polynucleotide [23, 24, 34]. A comparison of the effect caused by daunomycin, with that produced by the aminoacridines (such as profavine), has been made [34], and they are in general analogous. This technique has been employed in the examination of a number of derivatives of daunomycin [25] – as Figure 3.3 shows, the results qualitatively parallel those obtained from spectrophotometric analysis. An increase in viscosity such as has been observed, is correlated with 'stiffening' of the biopolymer, together with an increase in length.

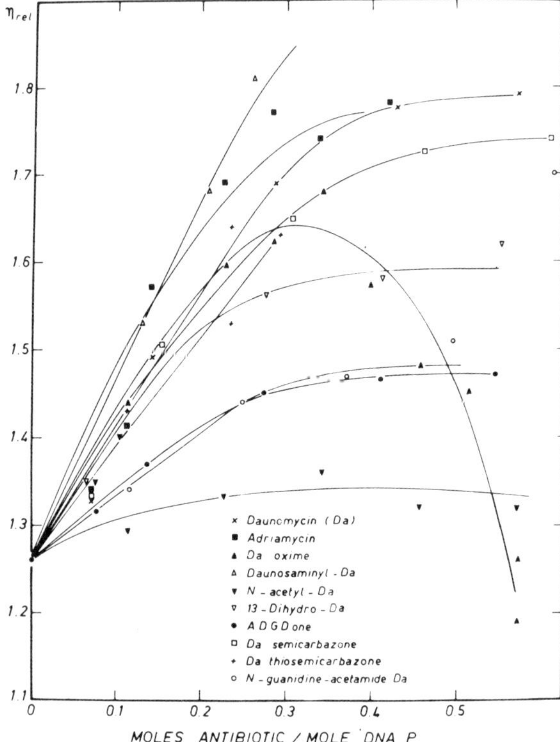


**Figure 3.3** The effect of daunomycin and various derivatives on the viscosity of DNA. (Reproduced with permission from Zunino *et al.*, *Biochem. Pharmacology*, **20**, 1323 (1971).

(b) *Buoyant density and sedimentation coefficient.* Concomitant with changes in viscosity on drug – DNA binding, these other hydrodynamic properties also show characteristic changes. The sedimentation coefficient of DNA is decreased on complex formation [23, 24], as is buoyant density in either caesium chloride or sulphate gradients [34]. This latter property indicates a change in some aspect of DNA conformation, due to the formation of a drug-DNA complex which is stable at high ionic strength.

(c) *Melting temperature.* The temperature (Tm) at which the DNA polymer molecule undergoes a thermal denaturation transition from helix to coil, has frequently been employed as a sensitive means of testing the binding of daunomycin and many of its derivatives, to DNA [4, 18, 34]. Daunomycin itself increases Tm from 70.5°C to 83.9°C [24], for a drug: nucleotide ratio of 1:10, at pH 7. The ΔTm change is dependent on this ratio, and is a manifestation of the stabilisation of the double helical structure of DNA upon drug binding.

(d) *Equilibrium dialysis.* Using tritium-labelled daunomycin, several studies have investigated the thermodynamics of DNA binding by means of equilibrium dialysis [24, 30, 35] and have obtained binding constants which are very similar to those obtained from spectrophotometric analysis. The technique has the advantage of being able to measure very low drug levels. The enthalpy change on binding daunomycin to DNA has been estimated to be an exothermic one of about −5.3 Kcal $mole^{-1}$ [35], (−6.5 Kcal $mole^{-1}$ [36] from calorimetry) at low drug: DNA ratios, comparable to values obtained for other DNA-binding drugs such as proflavine and ethidium. It appears [35] that the association constant $K_{app}$ is not markedly dependent on ionic strength.

(e) *Interaction with closed circular DNA.* A number of DNA-binding drugs have been shown to first remove and then reverse the supercoiling of closed circular supercoiled double-helical DNA [26, 37], as measured say, by changes in sedimentation behaviour [37] or viscosity [38]. Among important examples of drugs with this property are ethidium, proflavine, actinomycin, and most aminoacridines, as well as daunomycin itself.

This phenomenon is considered to be a diagnostic test for a molecule that interacts with DNA by 'intercalation', in which a planar aromatic group (the common structural fragment of all the drugs mentioned above) becomes inserted inbetween adjacent base pairs of the double helix [39], which is apparently associated with a local unwinding of the angle between these base pairs (36° in the B form of DNA [7]). It is possible with this technique to estimate the unwinding angle per drug molecule, relative to a value of 12° for ethidium [40] (assumed from model-building studies)-the value for daunomycin is 5.2°, with an apparent roughly 44% (relative to 100% for ethidium) of the drug being intercalated [37]. On the other hand [38], another study finds almost all of the drug intercalated, with a 4° unwinding angle. The obvious implications of these results for understanding the details of DNA–daunomycin interactions, will be discussed in section 4.2.

### 3.1.3 *Overview of the results from drug-DNA binding studies*

Comparative examinations of the DNA-binding ability of daunomycin and its derivatives, using the techniques outlined in the previous sections, have on the whole, vindicated the hypothesis that extent of binding can be correlated with

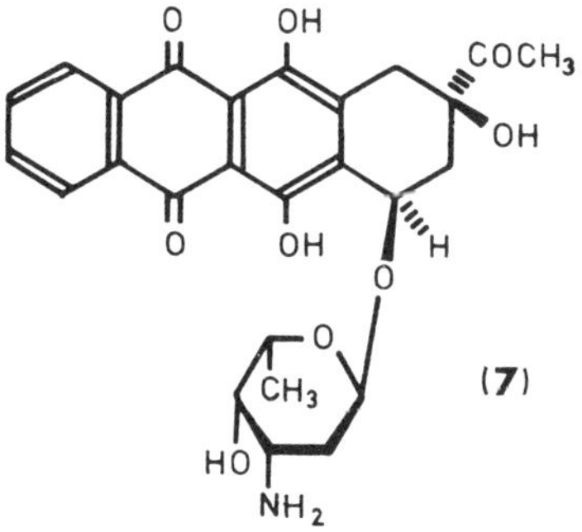

(7)

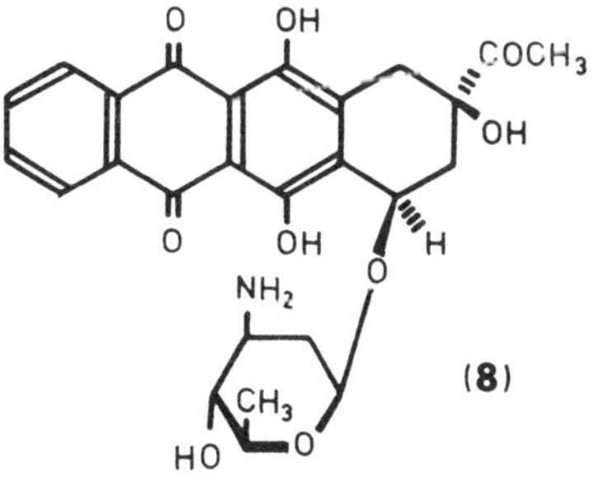

(8)

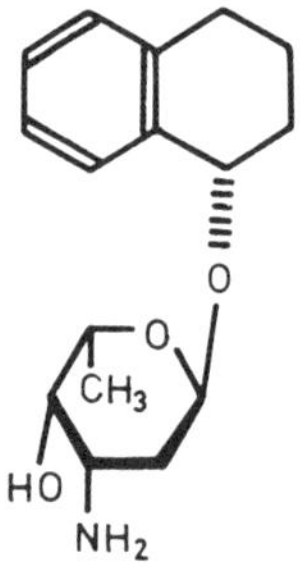

(9)

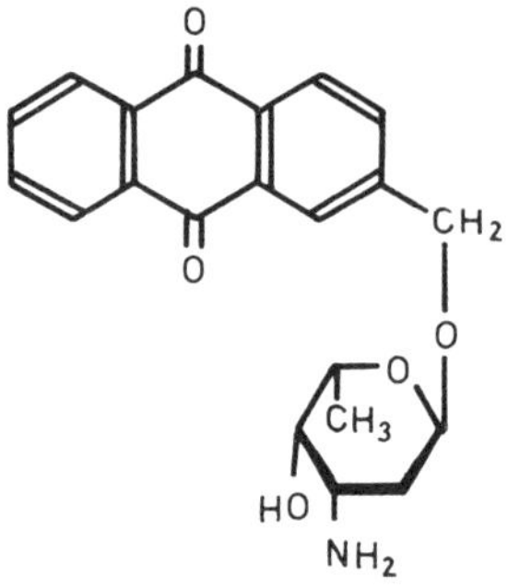

(10)

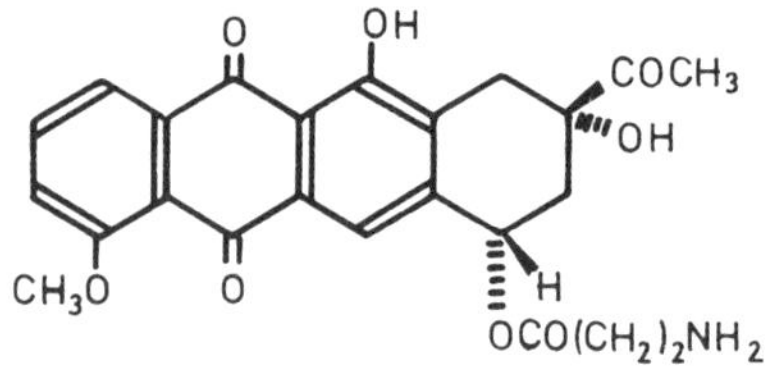

(11)

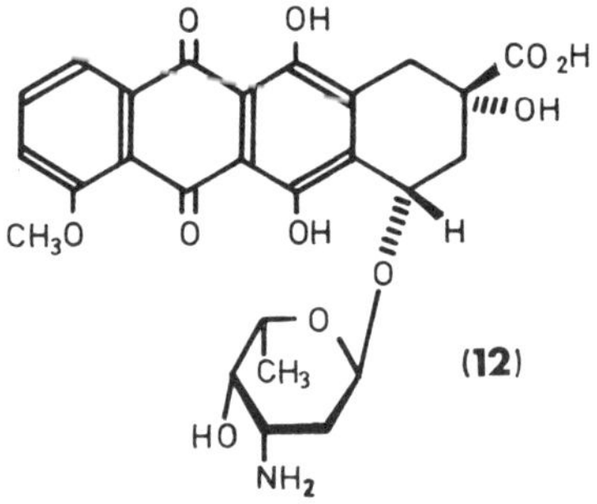

(12)

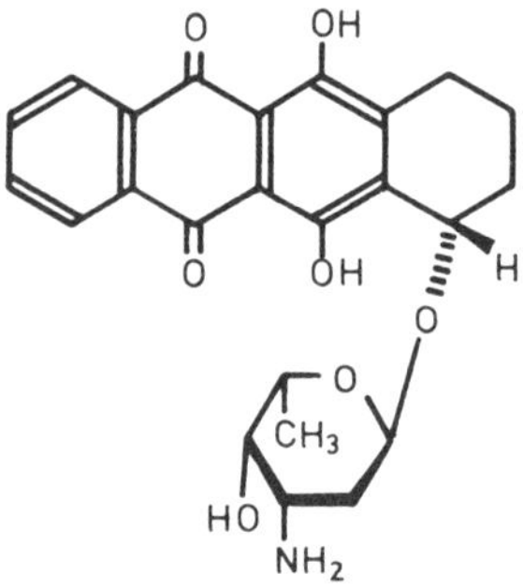

(13)

biological activity (though there are a few notable exceptions to this [22]). Perhaps a weakness of this is that the binding is measured *in vitro*, to DNA free from its intimate and regular arrangement with nucleoprotein in chromatin [41].

The reported values for the association constant of daunomycin itself and DNA (Table 3.1) show some deviation from the mean value[†] of $3.8 \times 10^6 M^{-1}$, which probably reflects differences in experimental conditions, ionic strength etc. and DNA preparations, as well as in Scatchard plot treatment of the results. Thus, when results from various derivatives, from different determinations are examined (Figures 3.4 and 3.5 and Table 3.2), they are not always quantitatively comparable; however in a qualitative sense, the differences are meaningful. There is some need for a standardised procedure to be employed for the determination of $K_{app}$. Table 3.3 gives $\Delta Tm$ data for a number of derivatives.

[†]This average excludes the high value of $9.3 \times 10^6 M^{-1}$ [30].

**Table 3.1** Apparent association constants ($K_{app}$) and number of binding sites per nucleotide ($B_{app}$).

| $K_{app}$ ($M^{-1} \times 10^6$) | $B_{app}$ | Method | Reference |
|---|---|---|---|
| a) For daunomycin | | | |
| 2.6 | 0.16 | Equilibrium dialysis | 24 |
| 3.3 | 0.18 | Spectrophotometric | 24 |
| 6.8 | 0.17 | Spectrophotometric | 30 |
| 9.3 | 0.17 | Solvent distribution | 30 |
| 2.1 | 0.16 | Equilibrium dialysis | 35 |
| 1.3 | 0.20 | Spectrophotometric | 42 |
| 3.0 | 0.18 | Spectrofluorimetric | 43 |
| 7.2 | 0.16 | Spectrophotometric | 44[†] |
| b) For adriamycin | | | |
| 2.3 | 0.19 | Spectrophotometric | 24 |
| 2.8 | 0.20 | Equilibrium dialysis | 24 |
| 2.7 | 0.09 | Spectrophotometric | 28 |
| 4.2 | 0.19 | Spectrofluorimetric | 45 |

[†]For calf thymus DNA:– this study also reported on DNA isolated from various clinical cases.
(i) normal $K_{app} = 7.4 \times 10^6 M^{-1}$; $B_{app} = 0.17$.
(ii) with acute myeloblastic leukemia. $K_{app} = 9.0 \times 10^6 M^{-1}$; $B_{app} = 0.17$.
(iii) with acute lymphoblastic leukemia. $K_{app} = 7.3 \times 10^6 M^{-1}$; $B_{app} = 0.17$.

**Table 3.2** Apparent binding constants ($K_{app}$), and number of binding sites per nucleotide ($B_{app}$), for various daunomycin derivatives.

| Compound | $K_{app}$ ($M^{-1} \times 10^6$) | $B_{app}$ | Reference |
|---|---|---|---|
| Daunomycin (**1**) | 3.8 | 0.17 | a |
| Adriamycin (**2**) | 3.0 | 0.19 | a |
| 13-Dihydrodaunomycin | 1.1 | 0.10 | 24 |
| N-Acetyldaunomycin (**3**) | $1.8 \times 10^2$ | 0.12 | 24 |
| N-Gaunidine-acetyldaunomycin | 72 | 0.09 | 24 |
| 2-Amino-2-deoxyglycosyl daunomycinone (**4**) | $7.1 \times 10^2$ | 0.09 | 24 |
| 4′-Epi-adriamycin (**5**) | 2.2 | 0.24 | 17 |
| 4′-Epi-daunomycin | 2.0 | 0.19 | 17 |
| 4-Demethoxydaunomycin | 2.4 | 0.20 | 27 |
| Daunomycin 13-benzhydrazone | 7.0[b] | 0.18 | 30 |
| Daunomycin N-$Me_2$glycine | 1.7[b] | 0.18 | 30 |

[a] Averages, from Table 3.1.
b) In this study, $K_{app}$ for daunomycin was determined to be $6.8 \times 10^6 M^{-1}$.

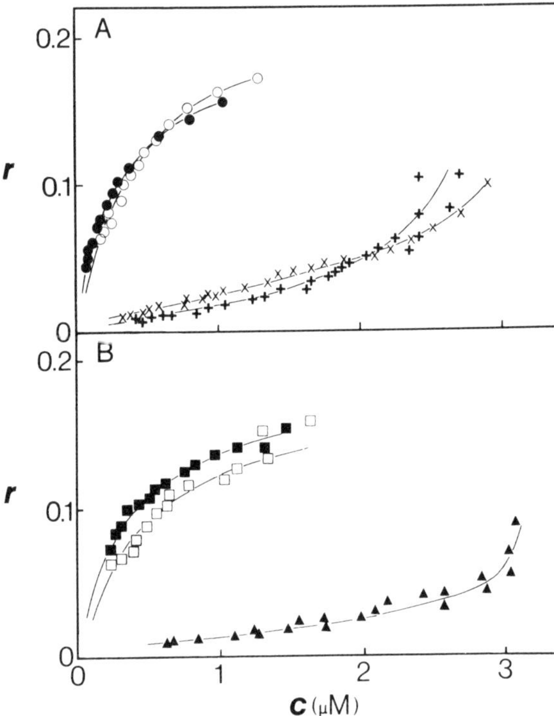


**Figure 3.4** Binding of adriamycin (A) and daunomycin (B) derivatives to calf thymus DNA from spectrofluorimetric measurements. r represents the molar ratio bound drug: total DNA nucleotides, and c the free antibiotic concentration. ● and ■ are for adriamycin and daunomycin, respectively; ○ and □ are the 4′-*epi* anomers; X and Δ are the β,4-*epi* anomers; + is β-adriamycin. (Reproduced with permission from Di Marco *et al.*, *Cancer Research*, **36**, 1962 (1976)).

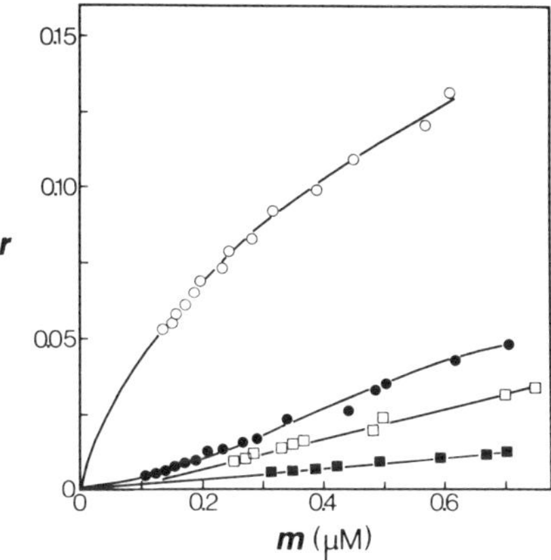


**Figure 3.5** Binding of some 4-demothoxydaunomycin derivatives to calf thymus DNA, from spectrofluorimetry. r is thenumber of drug molecules bound per nucleotide and m is the free drug concentration. o is for 4-demethoxydaunomycin: • is for the β anomer: □ is for the 7,9-bis-*epi*-derivative; ■ is for the β anomer of the 7,9-bis-*epi derivative.* (Reproduced with permission from *Biochem. Biophys. Res. Comm.*, **69,** 744 (1976)).

**Table 3.3** The change in thermal transition temperature (ΔTm) in °C, for various daunomycin derivatives[a] –

| Compound | ΔTm | Reference |
|---|---|---|
| Daunomycin | 13.4 | 24 |
| Adriamycin | 14.8 | 24 |
| 13-Dihydrodaunomycin | 9.8 | 24 |
| N-Guanidineacetyl daunomycin | 8.3 | 24 |
| N-Acetyldaunomycin | 1.0 | 24 |
| 2-Amino-deoxyglucosyl daunomycinone | 8.0 | 24 |
| 4′-Epi-daunomycin | 12.4 | 17 |
| 4′-Epi-adriamycin | 12.5 | 17 |
| β-Adriamycin | 3.0[b] | 17 |
| β-Anomer of 4′-epi--daunomycin | 4.8 | 17 |
| β-Anomer of 4′-epi-adriamycin | 7.6 | 17 |
| 4-Demethoxydaunomycin | 21 | 27 |
| 4-Demethoxy-7,9-bis-epi daunomycin (**7**) | 10 | 27 |
| β Anomer of 4-demethoxydaunomycin | 18 | 27 |
| β Anomer of 4-demethoxy-7,9-bis-epi -daunomycin (**8**) | 7 | 27 |
| Compound (**9**) | 0.5[c] | 18 |
| Compound (**10**) | 2.2[c] | 18 |
| Compound (**11**) | 6.3[c] | 18 |
| Compound (**12**) | 2.6[c] | 18 |
| N-Trifluoroacetyladriamycin 14-valerate | 0[d] | 47 |

a Relative to a Tm of 70.5° for DNA alone. b 4.5° C from ref. [45].
c Relative to ΔTm for adriamycin of 17.8° C [18].
d Relative to ΔTm for adriamycin of 11° C [47].

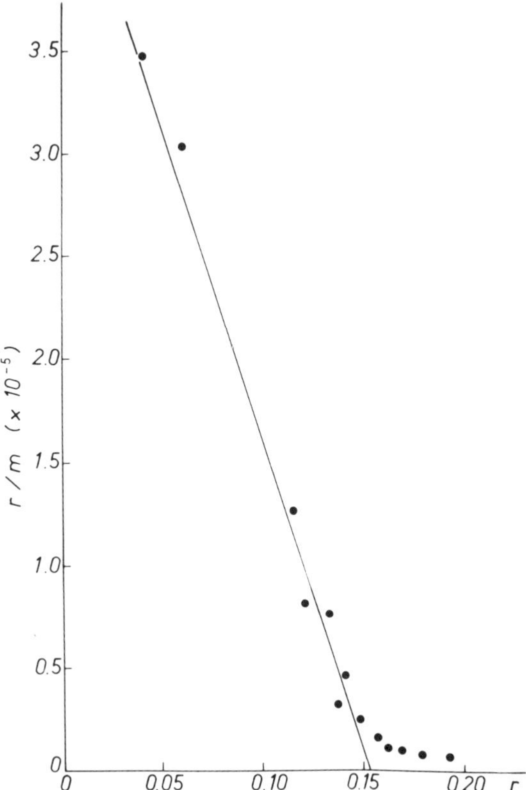


**Figure 3.6** Scatchard plot of the binding of daunomycin to calf thymus DNA, obtained from equilibrium dialysis studies. (Reproduced with permission from *Biochim. Biophys. Acta,* 277, 489 (1972)).

The Scatchard plots obtained from analysis of binding, are typically non-linear [24] (Figure 3.6), indicating more than one mode of binding (*c.f.* daunomycin elution from DNA-cellulose columns [32]), although deviations from non-linearity only occur at high (>0.15) levels of the daunomycin: nucleotide ratio [35]. These results have been interpreted as being due to initial strong binding involving intercalation, followed by weaker external binding, as has been suggested for other DNA-binding drugs [26, 39, 45]. This strong binding has an electrostatic component arising from interactions between the negatively-charged phosphate-oxygen atoms of the polynucleotide backbone, and the protonated amino group of the sugar residue (the binding is strongly dependent on ionic strength [46], $K_{app}$ decreasing with increasing NaCl concentration; however, a reverse effect has been reported [35], with $K_{app}$ increasing slightly with increases in NaCl concentration). Furthermore, N-acetylation (which serves to diminish the basicity of the nitrogen atom), markedly diminishes the ability of the drug to bind to DNA (Table 3.1), and does not significantly affect the stabilisation of the double helix to thermal denaturation (Table 3.3)†. The strong binding is also considered to involve hydrogen bonds, (as witnessed by the effect of urea on the complex [4], as well as a hydrophobic component due to stacking interactions between base pairs and the intercalated chromophore.

### 3.2 Interactions with other nucleic acids

#### 3.2.1 *Base and sequence dependence*

The influence of nucleotide base composition on the binding of daunomycin to DNA has been the subject of several investigations. Measurements of buoyant density decreases indicated a slight dependence on GC bas composition [34], which was not revealed by the degree of inhibition of DNA-dependent RNA polymerase [12], or by the analysis of melting curves of DNAs with different base compositions [45]. This contrasts with other melting curves obtained [9, 48] which show clearly that stabilisation (i.e. ΔTm) of double-helical structure increases with increasing AT content. The situation is further complicated by the considerable differences in ΔTm between poly (dA)·poly (dT) (a ΔTm of 20.4°C), and the alternating co-polymer poly (dA-dT)·poly (dA-dT), with a ΔTm of 29.5°C [48]. However, the differences in $K_{app}$ and K (the association constant of an isolated potential site), between AT and GC polymers are not great (only $K_{app}$ differs by a factor of two between the types of polymer) – this is paralleled by the DNA polymerase inhibition data given in this study [48], which also correlates with the amount of drug bound. It is considered significant though, that the two AT sequence isomers differ markedly with respect to the apparent number of binding sites ($B_{app}$) found per nucleotide residue, possibly a manifestation of differences between the secondary structures of the polynucleotides. However, an analysis of adriamycin-polynucleotide binding [28] has found, using $K_{app}$ as a criterion, that poly (dG)·poly (dC) binds seven times as strongly as poly (dA)·poly (dT). Clearly, there are major discrepancies between these various results, which can only be resolved on the basis of standardisation in experimental procedure.

The dependence of binding on sequence has been clearly shown for ethidium [49] and proflavine [50]. Both drugs, which are DNA-intercalating agents, markedly prefer to bind to pyrimidine-(3′5′)-purine sequences – thus, for dinucleoside phosphates, CpG is preferred to GpC. This finding has been rationalised on the basis of increased base pair – chromophore overlap and stacking at the intercalation site [51]. Preliminary spectrofluorimetric studies from the author's laboratory [43] indicate that daunomycin binding to defined-sequence oligomers also shows a preference, but to purine-(3′,5′)-pyrimidine sequences.

The antibiotic actinomycin binds strongly to DNA by intercalation and has

†In general, N-acetylation has a profound deleterious effect on *in vivo* anti-cancer activity, although there are exceptions to this (Section 4).

a requirement for a guanine base at the binding site [12, 26]; it does not intercalate into double-stranded poly (dA-dT)·poly (dA-dT). However, such binding does take place in the presence of daunomycin [31]; it has been suggested that the conformational changes produced in the polynucleotide by daunomycin binding somehow facilitate the co-operative intercalative binding of actinomycin, presumably at an adjacent site. Previous studies [36, 52] have shown that the two drugs occupy different, independent binding sites on DNA itself – however, as indicated above, defined-sequence polymers may well have different binding properties compared to the natural DNA. It should always be borne in mind that the results of physicochemical measurements relate to averaged DNA sequences, so that subtle effects are often masked.

### 3.2.2 *Interactions with ribonucleic acids*

Daunomycin has been reported [23] to bind to RNA, although it is not clear from this study whether the nucleic acid used was single or double-stranded – the former is probably more likely. A more recent analysis [53] has shown that daunomycin does indeed bind to authentic double-stranded RNA. In contrast to daunomycin DNA complexes, however, the binding of the drug has no effect on the thermal stability of the double helix. On the basis of this and other evidence, which suggested that polymer secondary structure was relevant for binding, it was therefore concluded that the RNA complex is not an intercalation one, but involves only external binding. This conclusion is reinforced by spectrophotometric and fluorescence polarisation studies of daunomycin binding to poly (I.C.) [42], a polynucleotide which adopts a RNA-11 like conformation [7]. It is apparent then, that a B-DNA type of conformation is essential for daunomycin binding – the seemingly abnormal 8-fold helix adopted by poly (dA-dT)·poly(dA-dT) is merely a member of a B-form sub-class [7].

Transfer RNA has been suggested [54] as a possible cellular receptor for daunomycin; in support of this, it has been reported that the drug inhibits *in vitro* protein synthesis [55]. The evidence presented [54] demonstrates that daunomycin binds strongly to the (unfractionated) tRNA used, with a $K_{app}$ of $1.2 \times 10^8 M^{-1}$, and about three binding sites per tRNA molecule. Although intercalative binding is suggested to account for these findings, it does seem relatively likely that the compact tertiary structure of tRNA would constrain the double-helical regions from unwinding. It has recently been reported that, contrary to expectation, ethidium does not form an intercalated complex, but binds in a fold of the tertiary structure, as revealed by X-ray crystallography [56]. It would not be surprising if a similar type of environment was found for daunomycin; however the relevance of tRNA as a primary, rather than a secondary daunomycin receptor, remains open to speculation.

# 4 MOLECULAR MODELS FOR DAUNOMYCIN-DNA BINDING

## 4.1 Conformation of daunomycin

The crystallographic analysis of the N-bromoacetyl derivative of daunomycin [57] verified the molecular structure and relative stereochemistry of the drug previously established on the basis of extensive chemical studies [3]. Moreover, the conformational details of daunomycin available from the crystal structure have been employed in model-building studies of the drug-DNA complex [58]. However, the N-bromoacetyl daunomycin analysis was of low accuracy, due to the exceptionally poor quality of crystals then obtained, together with a degree of disorder of some solvent atoms in the crystal.

Carminomycin I (4-hydroxydaunomycin), has been recently subjected to two independent crystal structure analyses [59-61], (as the hydrochloride monohydrate) which provide identical conformational results. Comparison of this structure with that obtained for a pyridine adduct to native daunomycin hydrochloride monohydrate, as well as with that of the N-bromoacetyl derivative, has proved instructive [62]. Examination of Figures 4.1 and 4.2 reveal an overall close correspondence between the stereochemistry of daunomycin and carminomycin I, and considerable differences in detail between these and that of the N-bromoacetyl derivative. (At a gross level, the three conformations are relatively similar.) The principal differences between daunomycin [62] and its N-bromoacetyl derivative [57] are:—

(i) the cyclohexane ring A in both cases is in a half- (or twist) chair conformation. However, as shown in Figure 4.2, in the parent compound C(8) deviates most (+0.58Å) from the mean molecular plane, whereas in the derivative, it is C(9) which deviates most significantly, by 0.70Å.

(ii) the relative disposition of the daunosamine ring with respect to the chromophore, as measured by the torsion angles around the C(7)-O(7) bond, differs in the two cases by about 20°.

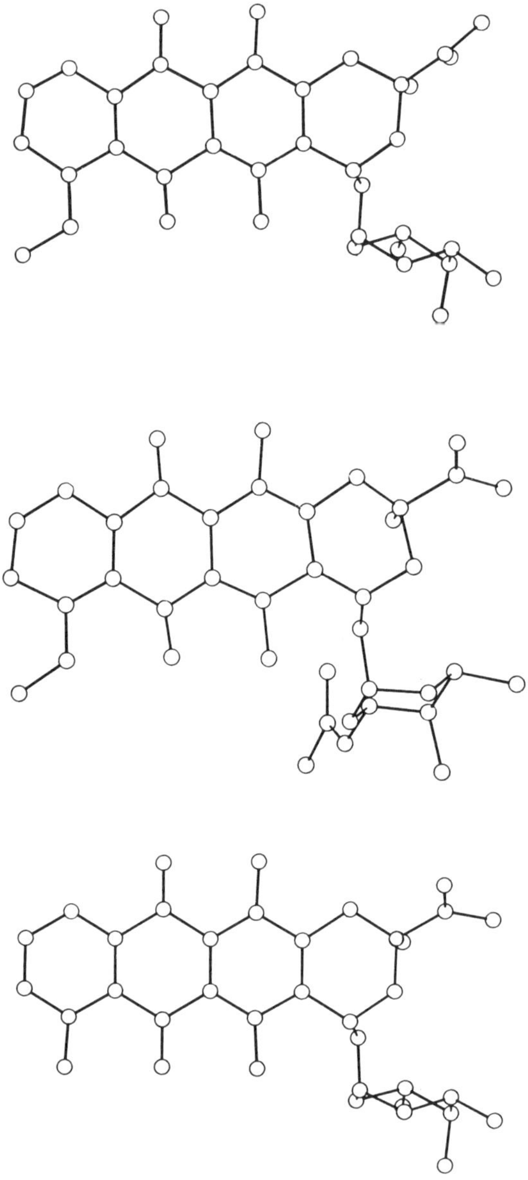

**Figure 4.1** Computer-drawn projections, looking down onto the anthraquinone plane, of (a) daunomycin, in the daunomycin-pyridine crystal structure [62], (b) N-bromo-acetyldaunomycin [57], and (c) carminomycin I, drawn from the averaged coordinates of [59-60]. (Reproduced with permission from *Biochim Biophys. Acta*, **479**, 450 (1977)).

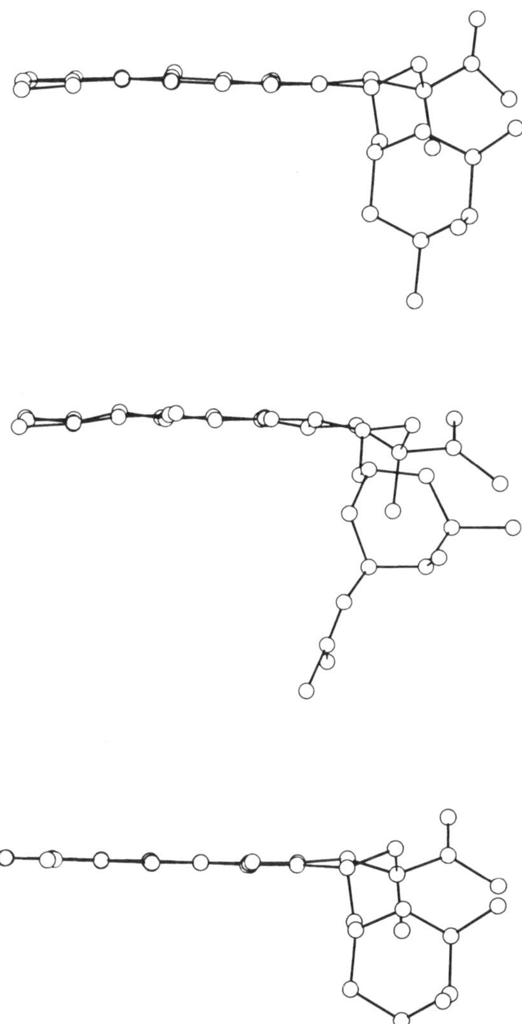

**Figure 4.2** As in Figure 3.5, but now drawn at right-angles to the anthraquinone plane. (Reproduced with permission from *Biochim. Biophys. Acta*, **479**, 450 1977)).

It is remarkable that the conformations of daunomycin and carminomycin I are so similar in the solid state at least. It has been suggested [62] that this is due to an intramolecular O(7) . . . H-O(9) hydrogen bond, which would help to minimise possible flexibility about the glycosidic bond – the analysis of carminomycin has unequivocally located the O(9) proton in the required position for such a hydrogen bond.

The ring A conformation has the daunosamine ring joined in an axial conformation and the C(13) side chain equatorial. It has been suggested [18] that an alternative ring A conformation (Figure 4.3(b)) is possible, in which the daunosamine ring becomes equatorially attached and the C(13) group axial. A molecular model for daunomycin-DNA binding has been proposed [18] on the basis of this alternative drug stereochemistry – this will be discussed further in section 4.2. It does seem unlikely that the proposed conformation isomerisation actually takes place, even during the formation of a DNA complex, the conformation shown in Figure 4.3(a) has now been found (admittedly in the solid state), in three independent crystal structures [57, 59-62], which is reasonable presumptive evidence for it being a highly favoured conformation. In addition, only conformation 4.3(a) has the intramolecular hydrogen bond. Loss of this would be energetically unfavourable.

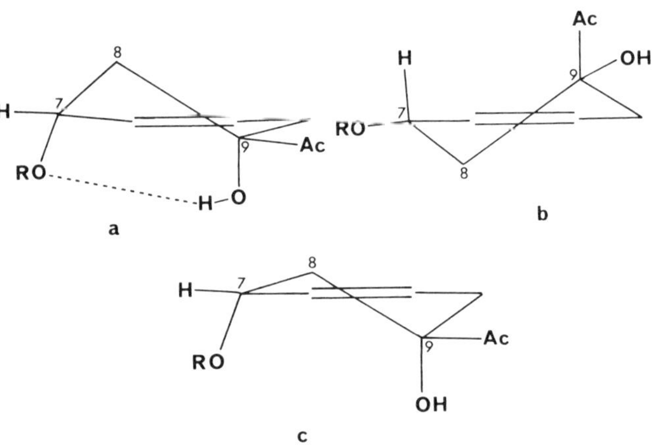


**Figure 4.3** (a) The conformation of ring A in daunomycin, as found in the crystal structure of the pyridine adduct [62]. (b) An alternative suggestion for the ring A conformation [18] (c) The ring A conformation in N-bromoacetyldaunomycin.

The existence of a preferred conformation for a flexible molecule, as indicated by X-ray studies in the solid state, must in general be treated with caution when extrapolated to the situation in solution. However, in the case of daunomycin, it is now possible to examine its conformation in three distinct crystallographic environments, which have the effect of averaging out intermolecular force contributions to the molecular conformation. So the existence of a preferred conformation is a good indication that it is the minimum energy one, and thus favoured in solution. It thus has been suggested that the conformation found for daunomycin [62] may well represent its biologically active shape (except for the flexible rotatory disposition of the C(13) side chain).

### 4.2 Daunomycin-DNA models

#### 4.2.1 *The Pigram-Fuller-Hamilton Model*

A detailed analysis has been made [58] of the X-ray diffraction patterns obtained from oriented fibres of daunomycin-DNA complexes. The patterns, which resemble those from semi-crystalline B-DNA itself, cannot be analysed to produce a three-dimensional structure *ab initio*, but like all polynucleotide fibre diffraction, can have a 'best' molecular model fitted to it. Moreover, the pattern (and indeed the resulting molecular fit), provide a visualisation averaged over the polynucleotide sequence. Subtleties of sequence-binding, and other fine detail, cannot be obtained. Nevertheless, by means of studying the changes in various parameters of the crystalline double-helix (pitch and intermolecular separation) as functions of drug: nucleotide ratios (Figure 4.4), it was possible to distinguish between different models of binding. It was observed that the only external-binding model which produced a reasonable fit to the data was one with a 40° unwinding angle, necessitating profound (and unobserved) backbone conformational changes. The unequivocal best fit was with an intercalative model with a 12° unwinding angle (Figure 4.5). The model has the aminosugar group of the drug situated in the wide groove of the double helix, assuming the drug conformation to be that found for the N-bromoacetyl derivative [57]. The anthracycline chromophore is intercalated inbetween adjacent base pairs, which open out to become 6.8Å apart. The daunomycinone is in such a position that the charged nitrogen atom forms a close contact with an anionic phosphate-oxygen atom, two phosphates away from the intercalation site – this electrostatic/hydrogen bond would undoubtedly confer much stability on the complex. An additional hydrogen bond was also suggested between the O(9) hydroxyl and the first phosphate. The data could not define the details of the nucleotide conformation at the intercalation site.

It is apparent that this model satisfactorily explains many of the observed properties of the complex, such as have been enunciated in previous sections. Thus, the binding has the required dominant electrostatic component, which is abolished on N-acetylation. The maximal binding predicted by the model of

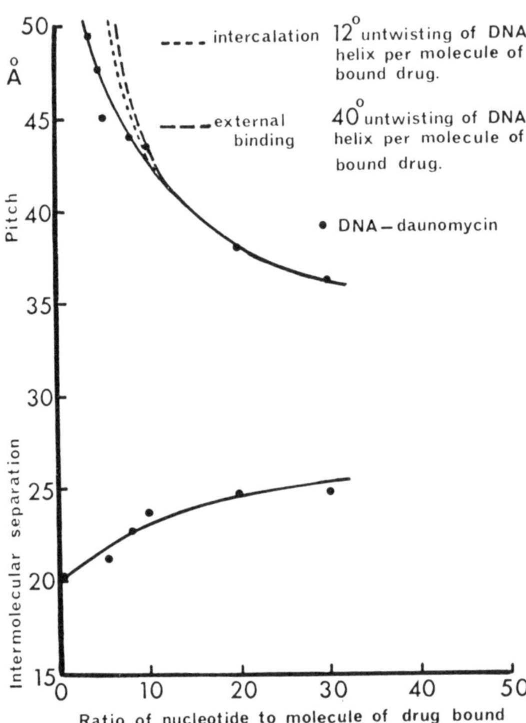


**Figure 4.4** Variation of molecular parameters as functions of the DNA: drug ratio at 92% relative humidity. The best theoretical fit to the variation of pitch is indicated for two types of model. ---, Intercalation; 12° untwisting of DNA helix per molecule of bound drug; ---, external binding, 40° untwisting of DNA helix per molecule of bound drug; •, DNA-daunomycin. (Reproduced with permission from *Nature New Biology*, 235, 17 (1972)).

one drug molecule every three base pairs (i.e. six nucleotides), is in good agreement with the $B_{app}$ values of ~0.17 drug binding sites per nucleotide residue. Hydrodynamic changes on binding (lengthening and stiffening of the double helix) are satisfactorily explained by the intercalative binding of the chromophore. Thus, it is unsurprising that this model has commanded widespread acceptance [3, 4, 5, 30], as providing significant insight into the binding process. Furthermore, as will be seen in section 5, the model and its modifications (below), are of use in understanding much of the binding data that has been obtained for many of the derivatives of daunomycin.

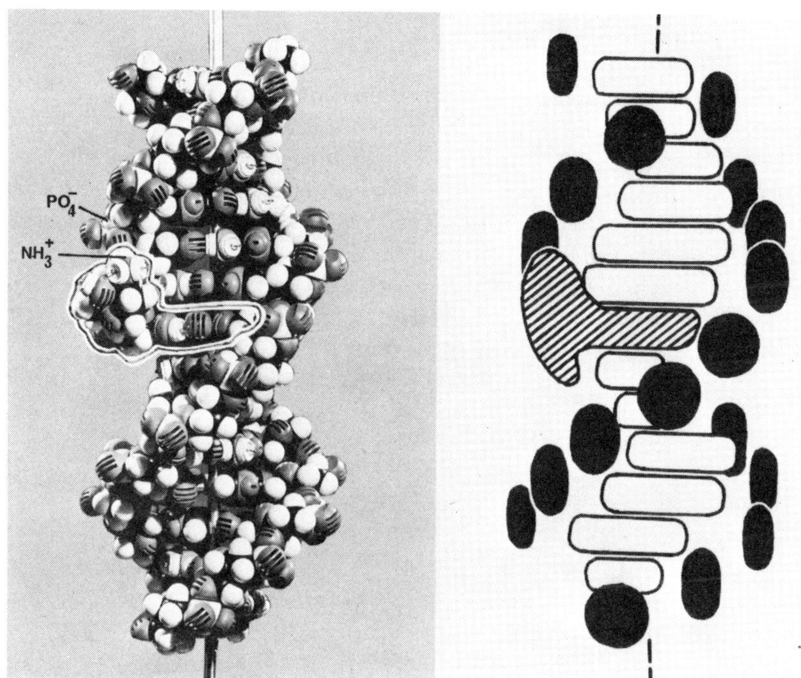


**Figure 4.5** (a) The Pigram-Fuller-Hamilton model for daunomycin-DNA binding, shown built with space-filling models. The drug molecule is outlined in white. (Reproduced with permission from *Nature New Biology*, **235**, 17 (1972)).
(b) A diagramatic representation of this model, with the drug molecule shown half-shaded, phosphate groups shaded black, and base pairs white. (Figure supplied by Professor W. Fuller).

4.2.2 *Modifications to the model*

The establishment of a preferred conformation for daunomycin [62] somewhat distinct in detail from that assumed earlier, has made relatively little difference to the fit of the drug into its DNA site (Figure 4.6). The drug still spans three phosphate groups; detailed examination now shows that the base pairs at the intercalation site necessarily become slightly skew to the helix axis. The O(9)-phosphate oxygen hydrogen bond can now be considered unlikely in view of the probable O(7)-O(9) intramolecular one. A view of the base pair – chromophore stackings (a possible arrangement being shown in Figure 4.7), shows that there is relatively little overlap of the planar groups, with ring A protruding right out of the site, mainly for steric reasons.

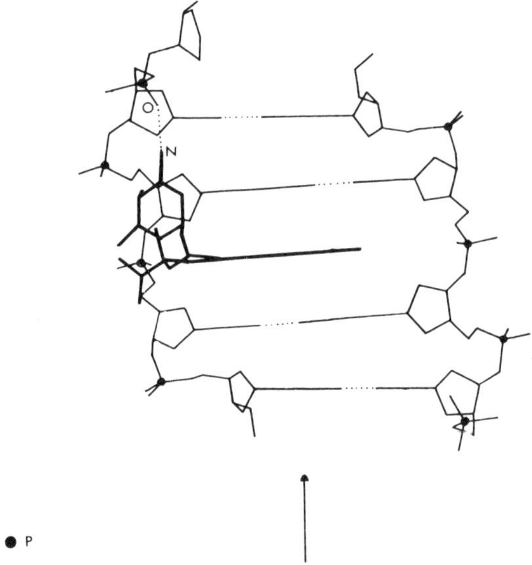


**Figure 4.6** A representation of the modified DNA-daunomycin model, with the drug molecule shown in heavy outline. Dashed lines represent hydrogen bonds. The daunomycin conformation is as described in [62]. The arrow indicates the helix axis.

The value for the unwinding angle of 12° chosen for the model is apparently in conflict with that determined from the supercoiling reversal of closed circular DNA [39], of 5.2°. However, a recent careful analysis [63] of alkaline titration studies on superhelical PM2 DNA has suggested that ethidium unwinds DNA by 26° per insertion and not the 12° assumed previously [39]. Thus, the unwinding angle for daunomycin becomes 11°, remarkably close to the value assigned in the Pigram-Fuller-Hamilton model. Support for the 26° unwinding has come

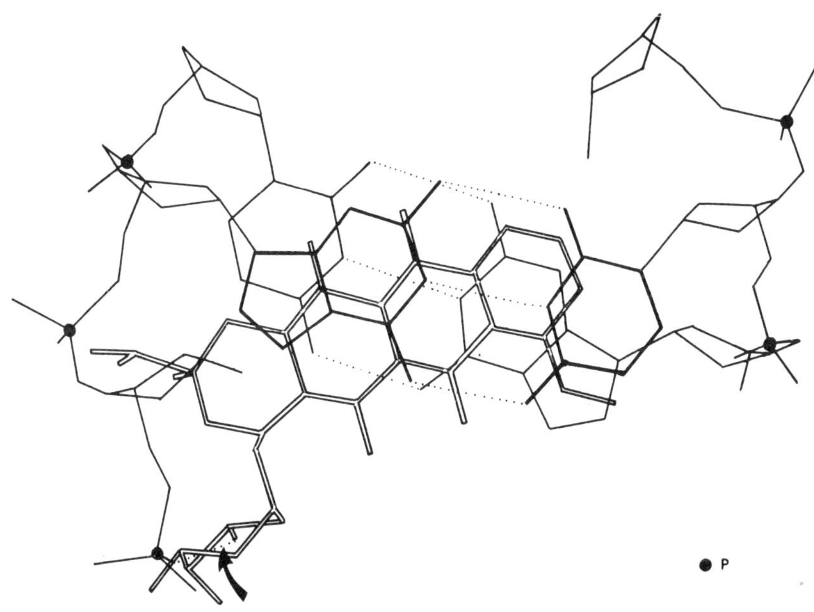


Figure 4.7 As in Figure 4.6 but now viewed looking down onto the planes of the base pairs. The upper base pair at the intercalation site is drawn in heavy outline, and the drug molecule in double outline. The arrow indicates the nitrogen-oxygen bond.

from a single-crystal X-ray structure determination of an ethidium-CpG complex [51]; this (and related structures) is considered to be a general model for the polymer situation, since a 'mini' intercalated double helix is observed [64]. The concepts of intercalation that have emerged from these structural studies suggest (i) that daunomycin belongs to a family of drugs (including proflavine) that intercalate from the wide groove of the double helix,† and (ii) the deoxyribose nucleotide sugars on each strand at the intercalation site alternate in puckering, so that they become C(3)′*endo*-(3′,5′)-C(2)′*endo* instead of the C(2)′-*endo* in B-DNA.

The recently-determined crystal structure of a proflavine-CpG complex [65] has however, cast some doubts on these conclusions, as (i) it has a 0° unwinding angle, and (ii) non-alternating sugar pucker. A further computerised model-building analysis has shown that, for dinucleoside phosphate intercalation complexes, alternate sugar puckering is not a prerequisite for intercalation; furthermore, the unwinding angle is dependent upon the steric bulk nature of

†This agrees with the model [58].

the intercalating drug [66]. Differing angles can be accommodated in the double helix, not by conformational changes in the backbone geometry, but by small alterations in the base-pair geometry. It is also apparent that insertion of the geometry of any of these drug-model double helical structures into DNA, necessitates alterations in the geometry of residues adjacent to the actual intercalation site. This conclusion is reinforced by other computerised model-building studies on proflavine intercalation in both A-and B-DNA [67, 68].

It thus appears that the present state of knowledge regarding the daunomycin-DNA model does not enable unequivocal conclusions to be drawn regarding the geometry of the backbone, other than that (i) mixed sugar puckering does not have to be invoked; (ii) the apparent 11° unwinding may well be distributed over several base pairs; (iii) there may well be a preference for binding to certain sequences, especially alternating purine-(3′,5′)-pyrimidine ones. The crystal structure of a daunomycin-oligonucleotide complex may well resolve these problems to some extent; however, it has recently been pointed out that the conformation of DNA in chromatin could differ appreciably from that of the isolated polynucleotide [41].

An alternative model for the adriamycin-DNA complex has been proposed [18], which has as its basis the alternative daunomycin conformation discussed in section 4.1, and shown in Figure 4.3(b). The positioning of the daunosamine ring equatorially to ring A of the chromophore necessitates that the amino group interacts with the phosphate group only one, instead of two base pairs away from the intercalation site. Other hydrogen bonds (Figure 4.8) have been suggested, involving the 4′- and 9-hydroxyl groups to phosphates, and the 14-hydroxyl to N7 of a purine base in an adjacent base pair. Thus a maximum number of drug functional groups are used in non-bonded contacts – as shall be seen in the next section, not all the binding data supports this hypothesis.

Further detailed examination of the modified Pigram-Fuller-Hamilton model has shown [69] that adriamycin can participate in an additional hydrogen-bonded interaction, compared to daunomycin, with the C(14) hydroxyl group positioned close to the phosphate group at the interaction site (Figure 4.9). Although the association constant data for adriamycin and daunomycin do not support stronger binding of the former, the ΔTm data suggests that adriamycin stabilises DNA slightly more than the parent compound. The fact that daunomycin is slightly more potent *in vivo* [10, 18] is considered to be due to differences in membrane transport properties [70, 71] even though, significantly, the affinity of adriamycin for isolated nuclei was appreciably higher than that of daunomycin. (The C(14) hydroxyl group on adriamycin increases the polarity and hence decreases the membrane permeability of the drug). The inhibition of DNA synthesis catalysed by T4 phage DNA polymerase shows two distinct modes of inhibition, dependent on the drug: nucleotide molar ratio [15]; these have been correlated with whether the daunosamine is N-blocked or not. Un-

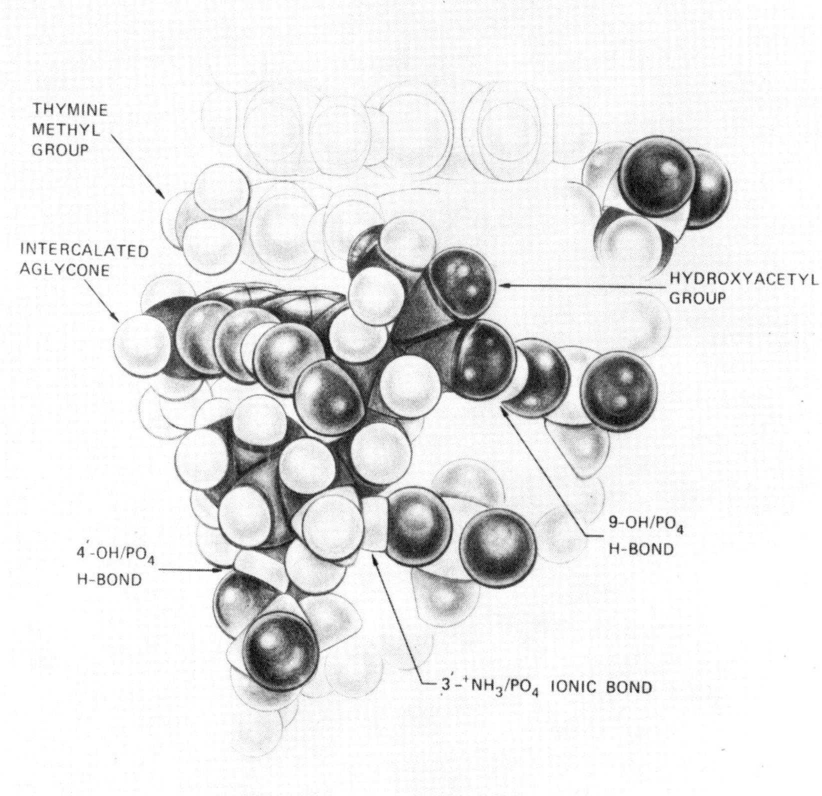


**Figure 4.8** The model for the DNA-adriamycin complex, as proposed by Henry [18]. (Reproduced with permission from *Amer. Chem. Soc. Symp. Ser.*, **30**, 15 (1976)).

blocked drug would directly interfere with polymerase binding to free 3′-OH primer ends of the polynucleotide template.

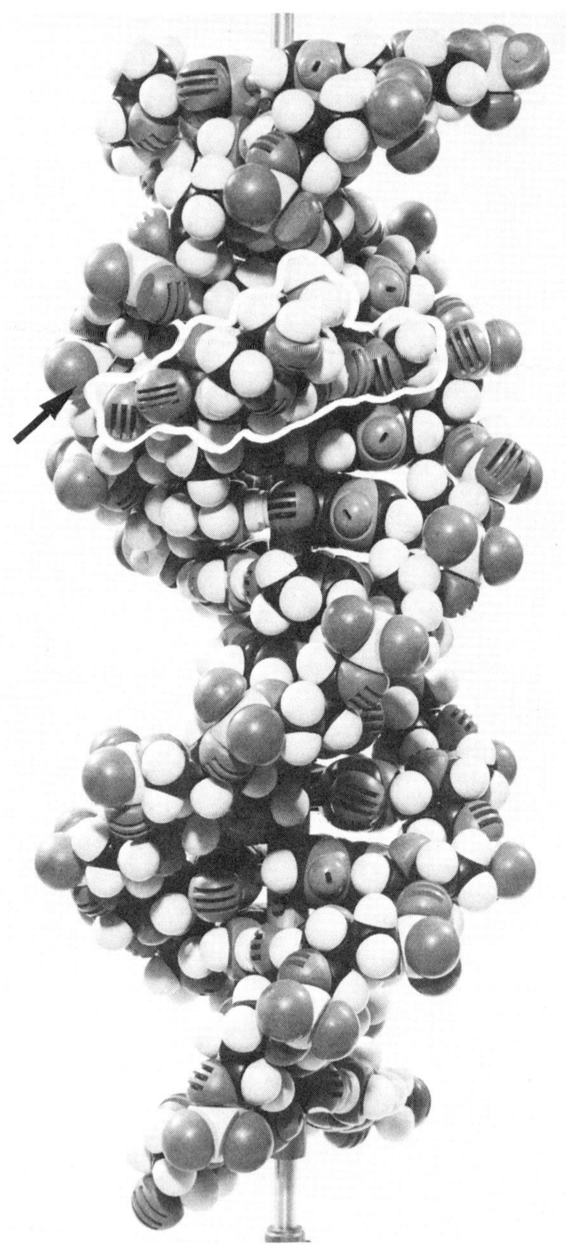

**Figure 4.9** Space-filling model of a molecule of adriamycin complexed to DNA, with the drug molecule outlined in white. The arrow indicates the location of the suggested subsidiary hydrogen bond. (Reproduced with permission from *Cancer Treatment Reports,* **61**, 928 (1977)).

## 5 PROPERTIES OF DAUNOMYCIN DERIVATIVES IN RELATION TO THE DRUG – DNA MODELS

In the absence of data to the contrary, it is necessary to assume that there are no major conformational differences between the structure of daunomycin and that of many of its derivatives, when bound to DNA.

### 5.1 Modifications of the chromophore

It is apparent [18] that a minimum size of chromophore is needed for there to be effective binding. As Table 3.3 shows, synthetic compounds with two or sometimes even three rings in the chromophore do not stabilise the DNA helix to any appreciable extent; this is correlated with the lack of appreciable nucleic acid synthesis-inhibitory properties. Thus, compound **(9)** is required in a concentration of 210 $\mu$M in order to effect a 50% reduction in RNA synthesis, compared to a concentration of 0.3 $\mu$M for daunomycin. This requirement for a minimum size for the intercalative part of the drug molecule, is entirely predictable from the binding model (see especially Figure 4.7).

Partial or complete removal of the 4-methoxy substituent on ring D would, on the basis of the binding model, be expected to result in somewhat increased penetration of the chromophore into the intercalation site, since the steric constraints due to the bulk of the methoxy group would be removed. 4-Demethoxy-daunomycin [20, 27] certainly stabilises DNA to a greater extent than the parent drug, and also has significantly higher anti-cancer activity; (Its $K_{app}$ at physiological pH is not appreciably different from that of daunomycin, since the formers pKa of 7.9 is significantly less; at lower pH, the 4-demethoxy derivative does show enhanced binding ability [72]. The 4-hydroxyl derivative carminomycin I, has also been reported [18] to have enhanced activity. It would perhaps be of interest to examine derivatives that do not have hydroxy-quinoid character, but have fully aromatised rings B and C.

### 5.2 Modifications of the A rings and its substituents

Modification of the C(9) side chain has been especially favoured in studies of daunomycin derivatives. Examination of the molecular model shows that the side-chain protrudes out from the intercalation site; thus, provided no over-bulky groups are attached, substitution here would not have profound effects on binding, although they might be somewhat deleterious. Thus, carbonyl derivatives at C(13), such as the semicarbazone or benzhydrazone do indeed have slightly inferior binding properties compared to daunomycin itself. Of course, pharmacokinetic properties of such derivatives may be superior – this is well illustrated by a series of 14-O-acyl derivatives [4, 73], such as the 14-octanoate, which shows superior anti-tumour activity in some test systems, compared to adriamycin.

It is apparent from studies [18] on compounds such as **(13)**, that the side-chain and/or the O(9) hydroxyl, are necessary for binding and activity comparable to the parent drug, the latter possibly because of its role in stabilising the molecule's conformation. Several studies [20, 27] have examined the effects of altering the stereochemistry at C(7) and C(9), which change the absolute stereochemistry at these chiral centres from 7(*S*), 9(*S*) to 7(*R*), 9(*R*) [Compounds (**7**) and (**8**)]. Such 7,9-bis-epi derivatives have low DNA-binding affinities and zero or slight biological activity. These results can be understood on the basis of the molecular model for binding since the 7,9-bis-epi derivatives, whatever their precise conformations, clearly cannot fit into the daunomycin binding site in DNA. The amino group on the sugar, in particular, cannot interact with a phosphate group as it does in daunomycin.

### 5.3 Modifications of the sugar ring

The relatively poor DNA-binding properties and lack of biological activity, of 2-amino-2-deoxy-flucosyl daunomycinone (**4**) illustrate the highly stereospecific requirement of the binding site; this derivative is distinguished by having the amino group at the 2′ instead of the 3′ position, (as in daunomycin itself). Examination of the binding model (Figures 4.5–4.) shows that the 2′ amino group cannot hydrogen-bond to a phosphate oxygen, although the 3′ hydroxy or 5′ hydroxymethyl groups might be able to do so, albeit rather less effectively than a charged 3′ amino group.

Inversion of configuration at C(1)′ to produce the β-daunomycin derivatives [17, 20, 45], results in structures that although clearly able to retain the O(7) . . . O(9) intramolecular hydrogen bond, cannot bind to DNA in the same way as daunomycin, since the N(3)′-phosphate oxygen close contact cannot be made in the same way. Thus, although accurate binding parameters could not be obtained [45], the β-anomers certainly bind considerably more weakly to DNA than the normal α ones, and have drastically reduced anti-tumour activity. It has been further suggested that the binding mechanism for the β-anomers, although undetermined, is substantially different from that of the normal isomer.

The 4′epi isomers [17, 19] are of interest in that they show comparable binding and anti-cancer activity to daunomycin and adriamycin. Moreover, they are significantly less toxic to cultured cardiac cells than daunomycin or adriamycin (the severe cumulative dose-dependent carditoxicity of these drugs [74], is a major drawback in their clinical use). The lack of effect on the binding parameters produced by 4′-epimerisation suggests that the 4′-hydroxyl group is but little, if at all, involved in the DNA-binding processes; the Pigram-Fuller-Hamilton model does indeed have this group isolated from others such that epimerisation would not alter the binding at all (contrast the Henry model).

The examination of derivatives such as compound (**11**) [18] interestingly suggests, as might be expected, that the daunosamine ring is not unique in conferring DNA-binding and biological activity on the chromophore. Rather, it appears that any side-chain at C(7) of suitable length, and with a protonated amino group at an appropriate position, would be suitable. In the light of the binding model, it is also desirable for this side-chain to be conformationally stabilised, as the sugar is in daunomycin itself.

The profound effect of N-acetylation on drug properties has already been mentioned in Section 3.1.3. It can be seen that retention of N-basicity is crucial to the DNA binding as envisaged in all the molecular models discussed. However, N-acetyldaunomycin has been reported to be not without some biological activity. More significantly, N-trifluoroacetyladriamycin 14-valerate (AD32) [18, 22, 47], which does not bind to DNA, has promising anti-tumour activity, though at dose levels ten times that of adriamycin itself. AD32 does not appear to be metabolised to adriamycin [75], nor does it become located in the nuclei of living cells [76]. It is therefore conceivable that AD32 acts by a quite different mechanism from that of other daunomycin derivatives.

## 6 OTHER POTENTIAL RECEPTORS

The possibility that daunomycin has a unique cellular receptor (i.e. DNA) is in principle, a relatively unlikely one†, especially in view of the considerable diversity of biological effects [6] that have been attributed to the drug, ranging over cardiotoxicity [74] membrane receptor binding [6, 77], DNA strand scission [78], lipid peroxidation [79], calcium transport inhibition [80] and tubulin interaction [81]. The origin of the cardiotoxic properties shown by daunomycin and its congeners, remains obscure. (It has recently been suggested that the structural similarities between the anthraquinone grouping on the drug chromophore, and the quinone residue in various coenzymes, especially co-enzyme $Q_{10}$, serve to promote the drug's inhibition of mitochondrial enzymes [82].

†Even though about 70% of the drug binds to the cell nucleus [70].

## 7 CONCLUSIONS

A question that perhaps arises after due consideration of the comparative DNA-binding properties of daunomycin and its various derivatives, is concerned with the design of a drug molecule with optimum binding properties. It is apparent that daunomycin and adriamycin themselves have been endowed by Nature (perhaps fortuitously?) with properties that have as yet been only rarely equalled, even in some respects, by human endeavour.

In spite of the almost näive lock-and-key assumptions of the DNA-daunomycin molecular model, it is remarkable how well it accords with much of the drug's DNA-binding data, as well as with its biological activity, especially since daunomycin behaviour inter- and intracellularily depends on so many factors other than its template binding. Detailed knowledge of many of these factors is to a large extent still lacking, especially concerning daunomycin – membrane interactions. It is to be hoped that together with an increased understanding of the structural organisation of DNA in cells [41] (both normal and cancerous), study of these other factors will contribute to effective rational drug design so as to achieve the goal of daunomycin derivatives more effective clinically than the parent compound, yet with fewer, undesirable side-effects.

## ACKNOWLEDGEMENTS

I am most grateful to Professors A. Di Marco and W. Fuller and Dr. D. W. Henry for permission to reproduce diagrams from their publications, and for supplying copies of them, and Dr. D. R. Phillips for information in advance of publication. My colleagues M. R. Sanderson and G. L. Taylor are thanked for much useful discussion, as are Drs. M. J. Broadhurst, D. R. Phillips, A. B. Robbins, W. A. Thomas and M. J. Waring. Studies in the author's laboratory have been supported by the Cancer Research Campaign, Pucha Products Ltd. and the Science Research Council.

## REFERENCES


[1] S. K. Carter, *Cancer Chemother. Rep. Part 3,* **6**, (2), 389 (1975).
[2] T. A. Connors, *FEBS Letters,* **57**, 223 (1975).
[3] A. Di Marco, F. Arcamone and F. Zunino, *in* 'Antibiotics, Vol. 3, Mechanism of Action of Antimicrobial and Antitumour Agents' (J. W. Corcoran and F. E. Hahn, eds.), p. 101. Springer-Verlag, Berlin (1974).
[4] A. Di Marco and F. Arcamone, *Arnzeim. Forsch,* **25**, 368 (1975).
[5] I. H. Goldberg, T. A. Beerman and R. Poon, *in* 'Cancer', (F. K. Becker, ed.), Vol. 5, p. 427. Plenum Press, New York (1977).
[6] H. S. Schwartz, *Biomedicine,* **24**, 317 (1976).
[7] S. Arnott, *in* 'Proceedings of the First Cleveland Symposium on Macromolecules', (A. G. Walton, ed.), p. 88. Elsevier, Amsterdam (1977).
[8] A. Di Marco, *Cancer Chemotherapy Rep. Part 3,* **6** (2), 91 (1975).
[9] F. Zunino, A. Di Marco, A. Zaccara and G. Luoni, *Chem. Biol. Interactions,* **9**, 25 (1974).
[10] W. D. Meriwether and N. R. Bachur, *Cancer Research,* **32**, 1137 (1972).
[11] V. Barthelemy-Clavey, C. Molinier, G. Aubel-Sadron and R. Maral, *Eur. J. Biochem,* **69**, 23 (1976).
[12] D. C. Ward, E. Reich and I. H. Goldberg, *Science,* **149**, 1259 (1965).
[13] R. Silvestrini, L. Lenaz, G. Di Fronzo and O. Sanfilippo, *Cancer Research,* **33**, 2954 (1973).
[14] F. Zunino, R. Gambetta, A. Di Marco, A. Zaccara and G. Luoni, *Cancer Research,* **35**, 754 (1975).
[15] M. F. Goodman, G. M. Lee and N. R. Bachur, *J. Biol. Chem.,* **252**, 2670 (1977).
[16] P. Chandra, F. Zunino, A. Götz, D. Gericke, R. Thorbeck and A. Di Marco, *FEBS Letters,* **21**, 264 (1972).
[17] A. Di Marco, A. M. Casazza, R. Gambetta, R. Supino and F. Zunino, *Cancer Research,* **36**, 1962 (1976).
[18] D. W. Henry, in 'Cancer Chemotherapy' (A. C. Sartorelli, ed.) *Amer. Chem Soc. Symp. Ser.,* **30**, 15 (1976).
[19] F. Arcamone, S. Penco, A. Vigevani, S. Redaelli, G. Franchi, A. Di Marco, A. M. Casazza, T. Dasdia, F. Formelli, A. Necco and C. Soranzo, *J. Med. Chem.,* **18**, 703 (1975).
[20] F. Arcamone, L. Bernardi, P. Giardino, B. Patelli, A. Di Marco, A. M. Pratesi and P. Reggiani, *Cancer Treatment Reports,* **60**, (7) 829 (1976).
[21] T. Facchinetti, A. Mantovani, R. Cantoni, L. Cantoni, C. Pantorotto and M. Salmona, *Biochem. Pharmacology,* **26**, 1953 (1977).
[22] M. Israel, E. J. Modest and E. Frei, *Cancer Research,* **35**, 1365 (1975).
[23] E. Calendi, A. Di Marco, M. Reggiani, B. Scarpinato and L. Valentini, *Biochim. Biophys. Acta,* **103**, 25 (1965).

[24] F. Zunino, R. Gambetta, A. Di Marco and A. Zaccara, *Biochim. Biophys. Acta,* **277**, 489 (1972).
[25] A. Di Marco, F. Zunino, R. Silvestrini, C. Gambaruccu and R. A. Gambetta, *Biochem. Pharmacology,* **20**, 1323 (1971).
[26] M. J. Waring, *in* 'The Molecular Basis of Antibiotic Action' (E. F. Gale, E. Cundliffe, P. E. Reynolds, M. H. Richmond and M. J. Waring), p. 191. John Wiley, London, (1972).
[27] F. Zunino, R. Gambetta, A. Di Marco, G. Luoni and A. Zaccara, *Biochem. Biophys. Res. Comm.,* **69**, 744 (1976).
[28] K. C. Tsou and K. F. Yip, *Cancer Research,* **36**, 3367 (1976).
[29] D. G. Dalgleish, G. Fey and W. Kersten, *Biopolymers,* **13**, 1757 (1974).
[30] E. J. Gabbay, D. Grier, R. E. Fingerle, R. Reimer, R. Levy, S. W. Pearce and W. D. Wilson, *Biochemistry,* **15**, 2062 (1976).
[31] T. R. Krugh and M. A. Young, *Nature,* **269**, 627 (1977).
[32] F. Zunino, *FEBS Letters,* **18**, 249 (1971).
[33] V. A. Bloomfield, D. M. Crothers and I. Tinoco, 'Physical Chemistry of Nucleic Acids', Harper and Row, New York (1974).
[34] W. Kersten, H. Kersten and W. Szybalski, *Biochemistry,* **5**, 236 (1966).
[35] Y. M. Huang and D. R. Phillips, *Biophys. Chem.,* **6**, 363 (1977).
[36] F. Quadrifoglio and V. Crescenzi, *Biophys. Chem.,* **2**, 64 (1974).
[37] M. J. Waring, *J. Mol. Biol.,* **54**, 247 (1970).
[38] J. M. Saucier, B. Festy and J.-B. Le Pecq, *Biochimie,* **53**, 973 (1971).
[39] L. S. Lerman, *J. Mol. Biol.,* **3**, 18 (1961).
[40] W. Fuller and M. J. Waring, *Ber. Bunsenges. Physik. Chem.,* **68**, 805 (1974).
[41] J. T. Finch, L. C. Lutter, D. Rhodes, R. S. Brown, B. Rushton, M. Levitt and A. Klug, *Nature,* **269**, 29 (1977).
[42] T. W. Plumbridge and J. R. Brown, *Biochim. Biophys. Acta,* **479**, 441 (1977).
[43] M. R. Sanderson and S. Neidle, unpublished results.
[44] P. J. Gray and D. R. Phillips, *Europ. J. Cancer,* **12**, 237 (1976).
[45] V. Barthelemy-Clavey, J.-C. Maurizot and P. J. Sicard, *Biochimie,* **55**, 859 (1973).
[46] F. Zunino, R. Gambetta, A. Di Marco, A. Velcich, A. Zaccara, F. Quadrifoglio and V. Crescenzi, *Biochim. Biophys. Acta,* **476**, 38 (1977).
[47] S. K. Sengupta, R. Seshadri, E. J. Modest and M. Israel, *Abstracts of American Association for Cancer Research,* **109**, 1976.
[48] D. R. Phillips, A. Di Marco and F. Zunino, *Europ. J. Biochem.,* **85**, 487 (1978).
[49] T. R. Krugh and C. G. Reinhardt, *J. Mol. Biol.,* **97**, 133 (1975).
[50] D. J. Patel and L. L. Canuel, *Proc. Natn. Acad. Sci. U.S.A.,* **74**, 2624 (1977).

[51] S. C. Jain, C.-C. Tsai and H. M. Sobell, *J. Mol. Biol.*, **114**, 317 (1977).
[52] A. Rusconi, *Biochem. Biophys. Acta,* **123**, 627 (1966).
[53] J. Doskocil and I. Fric, *FEBS Letters,* **37**, 55 (1973).
[54] R. H. Shafer, *Biochem. Pharmacology,* **26**, 1729 (1977).
[55] R. L. Momparler, M. Karon, S. E. Siegel and F. Avila, *Cancer Research,* **36**, 2891 (1976).
[56] M. Liebman, J. Rubin and M. Sundaralingham, *Proc. Natl. Sci. U.S.A.,* **74**, 4821 (1977).
[57] R. Anguila, E. Foresti, L. Rivadi Sanseverino, N. W. Isaacs, O. Kennard, W. D. S. Motherwell, D. L. Wampler and F. Arcamone, *Nature New Biology,* **234**, 78 (1971).
[58] W. J. Pigram, W. Fuller and L. D. Hamilton, *Nature, New Biology,* **253**, 17 (1972).
[59] M. C. Wani, H. L. Taylor, M. E. Wall, A. T. McPhail and K. D. Onan, *J. Amer. Chem. Soc.,* **97**, 5955 (1975).
[60] G. R. Pettit, J. J. Einck, C. L. Herald, R. H. Ode, R. B. Von Dreele, P. Brown, M. G. Brazhnikova and G. F. Gause, *J. Amer. Chem. Soc.,* **97**, 7387 (1975).
[61] R. B. Von Dreele and J. J. Einck, *Acta Crystallogr.,* **B33**, 3283 (1977).
[62] S. Neidle and G. Taylor, *Biochim. Biophys. Acta,* **479**, 450 (1977).
[63] J. C. Wang, *J. Mol. Biol.,* **89**, 783 (1974).
[64] H. M. Sobell, C. C. Tsai, S. C. Jain and S. G. Gilbert, *J. Mol. Biol.* **114**, 333 (1977).
[65] S. Neidle, A. Achari, G. L. Taylor, H. M. Berman, H. L. Carrell, J. P. Glusker and W. C. Stallings, *Nature,* **269**, 304 (1977).
[66] H. M. Berman, S. Neidle and R. K. Stodola, *Proc. Natl. Acad. Sci. U.S.A.,* **75**, 828 (1978).
[67] C. J. Alden and S. Arnott, *Nucleic Acids Research,* **4**, 3855 (1977).
[68] C. J. Alden and S. Arnott, *Nucleic Acids Research,* **2**, 1701 (1975).
[69] S. Neidle, *Cancer Treatment Reports,* **61**, 928 (1977).
[70] T. Skovsgaard, *Biochem. Pharmacology,* **26**, 215 (1977).
[71] N. R. Bachur, *in* 'Cancer Chemotherapy' (A. C. Sartorelli, ed.) *Amer. Chem. Soc. Symp. Ser.,* **30**, 58 (1976).
[72] A. Di Marco, personal communication.
[73] L. Lenaz, A. Necco, T. Dasdia and A. Di Marco, *Cancer Chemotherapy Reports,* **58**, 769 (1974).
[74] L. Lenaz and J. A. Page, *Cancer Treatment Reviews,* **3**, 111 (1976).
[75] P. M. Wilkinson, M. Israel, W. J. Pegg and E. Frie, *Abstracts of American Association for Cancer Research,* 188 (1977).
[76] A. Krishan, M. Israel, E. K Modest and E. Frie, *Cancer Research,* **36**, 2114 (1976).
[77] J. M. Varga, N. Asato, S. Lande and A. B. Lerner, *Nature,* 267, **56**, (1977).

[78] J. W. Lown, S.-K. Sim, K. C. Majundar and R.-Y. Chang, *Biochem. Biophys. Res. Comm.*, **76**, 705 (1977).
[79] C. E. Myers, W. P. McGuire, R. H. Liss, I. Ifrim, K. Grotzinger and R. C. Young, *Science,* **197**, 165 (1977).
[80] L. J. Anghileri, *Arnzeim. Forsch.*, **27**, 1177 (1977).
[81] C. Na and S. N. Timasheff, *Arch. Biochem. Biopjys.*, **182**, 147 (1977).
[82] K. Folkers, M. Liu, T. Watanabe and T. H. Porter, *Biochem. Biophys. Res. Comm.*, **77**, 1536 (1977).

# Index

## F



## G



## H



## I



## J



## K



## L



## M



## N

## W



## Z